INHERITED SUSCEPTIBILITY TO CANCER

Many cancers, both common and rare, are known to have a hereditary predisposition, and recent advances in genetics have clarified the risks, and in some cases the mechanisms, of cancer developing in an individual. This important contribution to the literature of cancer genetics covers all the key issues, reviewing both the technology behind genetic risk assessment and the ethical dilemmas it poses. It is divided into two parts. The first deals with ethical, legal and social issues, and also includes chapters on counselling, screening, and gene and mutation identification. The second systematically outlines current knowledge of the inheritance patterns of the many different cancer types, both from a site-by-site perspective and for special groups.

With a final chapter highlighting late-breaking developments, this up-to-date and authoritative volume will be of essential interest to oncologists, physicians and surgeons in other specialties, and to health professionals in the areas of primary care, counselling, and cancer risk assessment.

WILLIAM D. FOULKES is Assistant Professor in the Departments of Medicine and Human Genetics, McGill University, Montreal. He trained in cancer genetics in England and Canada, and studied the molecular genetics of ovarian cancer at the ICRF in London.

SHIRLEY V. HODGSON is Senior Lecturer in Clinical Genetics in the Department of Medical and Molecular Genetics, Guy's Hospital, UMDS, London. She is Director of Cancer Family Clinics at Guy's Hospital, and is the author, with Eamonn Maher, of *A Practical Guide to Human Cancer Genetics* (Cambridge University Press, 2nd edition, 1998).

INHERITED SUSCEPTIBILITY TO CANCER

Clinical, Predictive and Ethical Perspectives

Edited by

WILLIAM D. FOULKES
AND SHIRLEY V. HODGSON

Foreword by Francis S. Collins

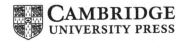
CAMBRIDGE
UNIVERSITY PRESS

CAMBRIDGE UNIVERSITY PRESS
Cambridge, New York, Melbourne, Madrid, Cape Town, Singapore, São Paulo, Delhi

Cambridge University Press
The Edinburgh Building, Cambridge CB2 8RU, UK

Published in the United States of America by Cambridge University Press, New York

www.cambridge.org
Information on this title: www.cambridge.org/9780521104746

First published 1998
This digitally printed version 2009

A catalogue record for this publication is available from the British Library

Library of Congress Cataloguing in Publication data

Inherited susceptibility to cancer : clinical, predictive, and ethical
    perspectives / edited by William D. Foulkes and S.V. Hodgson.
       p. cm.—(Cancer, clinical science in practice)
    ISBN 0-521-56340-2 (Hardback)
    1. Cancer—Genetic aspects. 2. Cancer—Risk factors. 3. Health risk assessment—Moral
and ethical aspects. I. Foulkes, William D. (William David), 1960– . II. Hodgson, S. V.
III. Series.
    [DNLM: 1. Neoplasms—genetics. 2. Disease susceptibility—genetics. 3. Mutation—
genetics. 4. Genetic Counseling. 5. Ethics, Medical. QZ 204 I55 1998]
RC268.4.I54   1998
616.99'4042—dc21
DNLM/DLC
for Library of Congress   97–35998   CIP

ISBN 978-0-521-56340-6 hardback
ISBN 978-0-521-10474-6 paperback

Contents

Contributors

Karin Au
Glaxo Wellcome Inc. Molecular Cell Biology, Five Moore Drive, PO Box 13398, Research Triangle Park, North Carolina 27709, USA

Howard Cuckle
Reproductive Epidemiology, Centre for Reproduction, Growth and Development, Research School of Medicine, 26 Clarendon Road, Leeds LS2 9NZ, UK

Gareth Evans
Region Genetics Service, Department of Medical Genetics, St Mary's Hospital, Hathersage Road, Manchester M13 0JH, UK

Gene Feder
Department of General Practice and Primary Care, St. Bartholomew's and the Royal London School of Medicine and Dentistry, Basic Medical Sciences, Mile End Road, London E1 4NS, UK

Harriet Feilotter
Departments of Paediatrics and Pathology, Queen's University, Kingston, Ontario K7L 3N6, Canada

Tamar Flanders
Department of Medicine, McGill University, Montreal General Hospital, Montreal, Quebec H3G 1A4, Canada

William Foulkes
Departments of Medicine and Human Genetics, McGill University, Montreal General Hospital, Montreal, Quebec H3G 1A4, Canada

and

Cancer Prevention Research Unit, Sir M.B. Davis-Jewish General Hospital, Montreal, Quebec H3T 1E2, Canada

Beatrice Godard
*Hotel Dieu Hospital Research Centre, University of Montreal, 3850
Urbain Street, Montreal, Quebec H2W 1T8, Canada*

David Goudie
*Human Genetics Laboratory, Department of Pathology, Ninewells
Hospital and Medical School, Dundee DD2 9SY, UK*

Nicholas Hayward
*Human Genetics Laboratory, Queensland Institute for Medical Research,
300 Herston Road, Queensland 4006, Australia*

Shirley Hodgson
*Department of Medical and Molecular Genetics, 8th Floor
Guy's Tower, St Thomas Street, London SE1 9RT, UK*

David Hogg
*Department of Medical Biophysics, University of Toronto, Medical
Sciences Building, 1 King's College Circle, Toronto
Ontario M5S 1A8, Canada*

Louise Hosking
*Glaxo Wellcome Medicines Research Centre, UK Genetics, Gunnels Wood
Road, Stevenage SG1 2NY, UK*

Bonnie King
*Department of Therapeutic Radiology, Yale University School of
Medicine, 333 Cedar Street, New Haven, Connecticut 06510, USA*

Bartha Maria Knoppers
*Centre de Recherche en Droit Public, University of Montreal, Pavilion
Maximilien Caron, Montreal, Quebec H3C 3J7, Canada*

Eamonn Maher
*Department of Paediatrics and Child Health, University of Birmingham,
Birmingham Women's Hospital, Edgbaston, Birmingham B15 2TG, UK*

Michael Modell
*Department of Primary Care, University College London Medical School,
Whittington Hospital, Highgate Hill, London N19 5NF, UK*

Lois Mulligan
*Department of Paediatrics and Pathology, Queen's University, Kingston,
Ontario K7L 3N6, Canada*

Steven Narod
*Department of Medicine, Women's College Hospital, 790 Bay Street, 7th
Floor, Toronto, Ontario M5G 1N8, Canada*

Dorothy Nelkin
Department of Sociology, New York University, 269 Mercer Street, 4th Floor, New York, New York 10003, USA

June Peters
Department of Human Genetics, University of Pittsburgh, Graduate School of Public Health, Crabtree A300, 130 DeSoto Street, Pittsburgh, Pennsylvania 15261, USA

Kathy Pritchard-Jones
Department of Paediatric Oncology, Institute of Cancer Research, Royal Marsden Hospital, Downs Road, Sutton, Surrey SM2 5PT, UK

Guy Rouleau
Centre for Research in Neuroscience and Department of Neurology, McGill University, Montreal General Hospital Research Institute, Montreal, Quebec H3G 1A4, Canada

Martin Ruttledge
Department of Medicine, Trinity College, University of Dublin, Dublin 2, Ireland

Philippe Sanséau
Glaxo Wellcome Medicines Research Centre, Genome Informatics Unit, Gunnels Wood Road, Stevenage SG1 2NY, UK

Stimson Schantz
Department of Surgery, Memorial Sloan-Kettering Cancer Center, 1275 York Avenue, New York, New York 10021, USA

Nicholas Schork
Departments of Epidemiology & Biostatistics and Genetics, Case Western Reserve University, 2109 Adelbert Road BRB 722, Cleveland, Ohio 44106-4955, USA

Pamela St. Jean
Department of Epidemiology & Biostatistics, Case Western Reserve University, 2109 Adelbert Road BRB 722 Cleveland, Ohio 44106-4955, USA

A. Malcom Taylor
CRC Institute for Cancer Studies, The University of Birmingham Medical School, Edgbaston, Birmingham B15 2T, UK

Zoltan Trizna
UTMB Department of Dermatology, 301 University Blvd., Route 0783, Galveston, Texas 77555–0783, USA

Preface

Cancer is a common disease in developed countries, and is becoming commoner in other parts of the world as mortality from competing causes, such as infection, decreases. The familial origins of susceptibility to cancer were first recognized as early as the nineteenth century. Advancing from anecdotal observations of extended pedigrees, with numerous cases of cancer, to the demonstration that a history of cancer is associated in many cases with increased risks of cancer to the relatives of cases, took many years. The development of statistical methods that allowed simultaneous analysis of numerous potential risk factors was an important step. Modelling of data using segregation analysis was another advance that clearly demonstrated the role of mendelian inheritance in human cancer. However, the real advance came when recombinant DNA technology allowed the generation of unlimited copies of fragments of human DNA. Minor variations in DNA between individuals could then be used to locate, at least approximately, the positions of genes which, when mutated, cause familial diseases.

This book is one of the first on inherited cancer that is not immediately out of date as it arrives on the shelves. This is because of the very success of the enterprise as most highly-penetrant cancer susceptibility genes have now been identified. The advances in our understanding of the herediatry basis of human cancer have been truly enormous, but these advances have not translated easily from the laboratory to the clinic, and there are some who see genetic testing for adult-onset disorders, such as cancer susceptibility as a dangerous new development. In this book we have combined descriptions of what is known about the inherited susceptibility to cancer with serious arguments as to the advisability of using this information at the present time. We hope that proponents of widespread genetic testing, and those who oppose such developments, will find the book an example of how, by presenting thesis and antithesis together, a new synthesis may occur.

This is not a text book for a cancer genetics course. We have had to select areas that seemed both relevant and interesting, but we believe that most of the important developments are discussed. As mentioned above, there are few highly-penetrant cancer susceptibility genes still to be identified, but finding genes is not an end in itself. Some of the dissatisfaction with genetic testing has arisen because prevention and treatment has lagged behind diagnosis. Perhaps this is an inevitable gap, but one we all hope will close sooner rather than later. Along with closing this gap, the next phase of research in inherited cancer susceptibility will probably focus on two areas, the much more difficult identification of common, low-penetrance cancer genes, and marriage of epidemiology and molecular genetics. In the concluding chapter, we attempt to keep the book as up-to-date as is possible by summarizing recent developments that were published after individual chapters were completed.

We would like to thank our teachers, colleagues, students and especially, our patients, for educating us. This book is dedicated to them.

William D. Foulkes and Shirley V. Hodgson
Montreal and London

Foreword

As a medical genetics fellow in 1983, I was asked to counsel a young woman whose mother and two sisters had all been diagnosed with pre-menopausal breast cancer. In one sister the disease had occurred bilaterally. Searching the literature turned up very little – just a few empirical studies, one of which suggested my patient's risk might be as high as 50%. While it occurred to me that this sounded a lot like a mendelian disorder, no compelling evidence existed then that highly penetrant autosomal gene mutations could play a role in common solid tumours.

How far we have come in those 15 years! From an era when familial cancer syndromes were considered to be relatively uncommon and generally recognizable by unique phenotypic features, we are now witnessing a paradigm shift where mendelian subsets of nearly all common cancers (breast, ovary, colon, prostate, etc.) are being rapidly defined at the molecular level. Spurred on by the tools and technologies arising from the Human Genome project, it is now also highly likely that weaker cancer susceptibility, resistance and modifier genes will emerge in significant numbers over the next few years.

This book thus arrives at a timely moment. Though the rapid pace of the field might discourage some from trying to generate an authoritative reference, Foulkes and Hodgson have assembled a group of visionary contributors who not only portray the present state of cancer genetics, but also provide helpful glimpses of the future for clinicians and researchers alike. A final chapter, written just as the book was going to press, assists this process by including major late-breaking developments that would otherwise have missed the publication deadline. Of particular note is that the editors have chosen to include in this book an in-depth analysis of the ethical, legal and social issues which arise as a consequence of the recent stunning advances in the molecular genetics of cancer. Placing these discussions side by side is highly appropriate. Until effective, non-toxic and accessible therapies are developed for individuals found to be at a high risk for cancer, the potential for discriminatory misuse of genetic information will remain. As the science of cancer genetics hurtles forward, we must put maximum energy into solving these vexing social and ethical problems.

Cancer genetics is thus the Starship Enterprise of the new genetic medicine. In all of medicine, it is likely to be the field where the molecular understanding of a common and often lethal disease advances most rapidly, where the use of widespread predictive testing to reduce future illness will get its first major application, where most health care providers will first come to grips with the need to incorporate genetics into their practice, where battles about genetic discrimination will be won or lost, and where the compelling paradigm of molecular medicine, that gene discovery will lead to better therapies, will first be put to a real test. It will be a fascinating ride. This book makes an excellent guide for the traveller.

Francis S. Collins, MD, PhD
Director,
National Human Genome Research Institute,
National Institutes of Health, USA

Part I

Ethical, legal and social issues, screening, counselling, gene and mutation detection

1

The inherited basis of cancer

SHIRLEY HODGSON and GARETH EVANS

Summary

This opening chapter serves as a summary of the topics discussed in this book and also, by way of an introductory section, adds a historical perspective. The authors outline some of the extraordinary leaps in knowledge concerning the molecular basis of both common and rare cancers, but note that it will take time for this to translate to clear clinical benefit. Predictive testing is of value for selected individuals, but its widespread, uncontrolled use has many ethical and solid-economic implications.

Introduction

Occasional families displaying a markedly increased incidence of cancers of a specific type have been described over many decades, for example, the Warthin family with autosomal dominant transmission of colon and uterine cancer (probably a family with hereditary non-polyposis colorectal cancer – see later), Broca's wife's family, in which many women – including, eventually, his wife – died of breast cancer, and indeed Napoleon's family displayed a high incidence of gastric cancer. It was, however, not until more recently that the possibility of a genetic predisposition to cancer being heritable was entertained with any seriousness – one of the first such reports being in 1948 when Penrose, McKenzie and Kean suggested that a tendency to breast cancer could have a hereditary basis. Indeed, when Henry Lynch and his son Patrick, in the 1960s, began to promote the idea of screening for colorectal cancer and to offer colonoscopies (from the 1970s) to first degree relatives of individuals who had developed colorectal cancer, and who had a strong family history of the condition, they were encouraged to give up the idea and concentrate on doing proper medicine! Thus, even then the suggestion that there might be an increased risk of specific cancers in individuals with a strong family history of cancer was considered to be somewhat heretical.

Recently, however, there has been a rapid acceptance not only of the existence of some rare families in which there appears to be a highly penetrant autosomal dominantly inherited susceptibility to specific cancers but also of the concept of 'familial clustering' of certain common cancers, with an increased risk of a cancer in close relatives of any affected individual. The degree of risk depends upon parameters such as the age at onset and number of primary tumours in the index case, and the number of close relatives they have who have developed the same cancer. A younger age at onset than average may thus indicate an increased chance that there is an underlying genetic predisposition. The data suggest that an hereditary predisposition to cancer may be of multifactorial aetiology, due in a small proportion of cases to the inheritance of genes predisposing strongly to specific cancers, and probably in a larger proportion of cases due to smaller inherited variations in susceptibility and interaction with environmental influences. Genes in which germline mutations can confer a high degree of susceptibility to certain cancers (up to 80–90% lifetime risk) have now been identified, and include the *BRCA1* and *BRCA2* genes (breast cancer), the *hMSH2*, *hMLH1*, and *APC* genes (bowel cancer), and the *TP53* gene (soft tissue sarcomas and leukaemias, childhood, and other cancers and in particular early onset breast cancer), but inherited pathogenic mutations in these genes have a low frequency in the population as a whole. It is likely that a much larger proportion of less pronounced familial clustering of cancer is due to mutations in other genes that confer lower but none the less significant risks for these malignancies. Interaction between such inherited variations and environmental factors may be important and complex.

There are also well-known rare syndromes, many with very characteristic phenotypes that can predispose to certain cancers. These syndromic forms of cancer predisposition have been the subject of detailed clinical and molecular studies. Screening programmes for individuals and families with familial adenomatous polyposis (FAP), von Hippel–Lindau disease (VHL), the neurofibromatoses and multiple endocrine neoplasias (MEN) have been developed. Many of these conditions are suitable for genetic registers with at-risk individuals being called up for screening as well as genetic testing at the appropriate age. Diagnosis and screening for these single gene disorders is now well established. FAP screening registers have been established for decades. Lockhart-Mummery described the autosomal dominant inheritance of this condition in 1925 (Lockhart-Mummery, 1934).

It is currently becoming possible to identify germline mutations in the first category of genes in certain (rare) families and to offer predictive genetic testing to unaffected members of those families for such mutations. This can differentiate between individuals with a very high risk of developing specific cancer from those who are probably at average risk. These high-risk individuals can then be offered screening for early cancer or premalignant lesions – or prophylactic surgery – and those individuals found not to have inherited the mutation can be released from surveillance. This would offer relief from anxiety for low-risk individuals, release from 'uncertainty' in high-risk individuals with the potential benefit of increased cancer surveillance, and the financial benefit to society of surveillance being targeted at individuals actually at high risk of developing cancer. The ability accurately to assess individual risks will enable them to make informed choices about their options. There has been considerable media interest about the possibility of offering tests for such mutations, perhaps even in the general population, but the recognition that these mutations are rare has not perhaps been kept in perspective. It is likely that the majority of cases of cancer occur because an individual has been exposed to certain carcinogenic environmental agents and that inherited genetic factors may have rendered them more susceptible to the effects of these agents. Genes conferring a small cancer susceptibility will be much more difficult to identify and counselling of individuals found to have such a susceptibility will be difficult. The reality of genetic testing for cancer susceptibility has, not surprisingly, led to a vigorous ethical debate about its uses. Such issues as whether to test children, or whether anyone should be tested in the absence of established surveillance programmes for the detection of cancer or premalignant lesions that are of proven benefit, are under intense scrutiny by the media. Implications for health and life insurance are of particular concern, and there is a growth industry in research into the psychological aspects of testing and the possible effects of testing and uptake of surveillance programmes.

Lessons from cancer predisposing syndromes

Much is being learned from the study of the syndromic forms of cancer predisposition mentioned above, and several important characteristics of familial cancer have been identified by examining families in which they occur. Thus, when FAP was described in the 1920s, the autosomal dominant pattern of inheritance, the appearance of premalignant lesions (multiple adenomatous polyps in the large bowel) and the early age at onset, and possible multiple incidence of colon cancer in affected individuals, was noted. Many individuals affected with these syndromes have characteristic phenotypic abnormalities other than the neoplasias, such as sebaceous cysts and osteomas in FAP, and melanin skin pigmentation in Peutz–Jeghers syndrome, suggesting that developmental genes may be involved in their aetiology. Much was learned from the paradigm of inherited retinoblastoma in the 1970s, when Knudson observed that unilateral retinoblastoma tended to be of considerably later onset (and non-familial) than cases of bilateral/multiple retinoblastoma, which characteristically occurred in young children and often in a familial setting. This led Knudson and others to postulate that children with multiple tumours have inherited a germline mutation in one of two alleles at a single locus, and that it required a second at the other allele in a retinal cell to initiate the tumour (Knudson 1971). In unilateral tumours both alleles had to be inactivated by acquired mutations, this fitted the mathematical model he developed to explain the difference in age at onset of the two types of tumour, and led to the development of the idea of germline mutations in tumour suppressor genes being the cause of some inherited causes of cancer predisposition. Subsequent work has defined the nature of the genes involved in several different cancer syndromes, and in most instances these function as tumour suppressors, notably the retinoblastoma gene, which can suppress the tumorigenicity of retinoblastoma cells (Huang et al., 1988). 'Loss of heterozygosity' – indicating loss of function of the remaining normal allele – can be demonstrated in the tumours, as would be expected under this model (Cavenee et al., 1983), indicating an autosomal recessive action at the cellular level. The main exceptions to this general rule are multiple endocrine neoplasia, where the inherited mutation is in the *RET* oncogene, and possibly the Li–Fraumeni syndrome, where the *TP53* gene product can act as a tumour suppressor, but in which mutations can confer oncogenic properties or a dominant-negative action.

Oncogenes are a family of genes which act in a dominant fashion to maintain or induce cell transformation. They are derived by mutation from normal cellular genes (proto-oncogenes) which have a role in controlling cell growth and proliferation. This change in function may be achieved by overproduction, gene amplification, point mutation or translocation resulting in activation of the proto-oncogene or by the development of fusion proteins. The functions of proto-oncogenes include protein phosphorylation, G-protein interaction and transcription regulation. Many of these actions regulate gene expression and cell-cycle dynamics. G-proteins (guanine nucleotide binding proteins) are also involved in signal transduction by exchanging GDP for GTP, stimulating other systems with the activated GTP:G complex; G-proteins have an intrinsic GTPase activity which terminate the signal. Certain oncogenes (e.g. *RAS*) resemble G proteins but maintain the protein in the GTP-bound activated state. Other oncogenes are derived from transcription factors and may interact with the products of tumour suppressor genes. Mutated proto-oncogenes are frequently detected in cancers (but rarely in the germline, outside MEN2), and each tumour type has a characteristic spectrum of oncogene alterations.

The role of tumour suppressor genes

Tumour suppressor genes were first identified by work in vitro showing that when normal cells were fused with malignant cells, their malignant behaviour was suppressed (Harris 1969), and loss of certain chromosomes from the hybrid resulted in the resumption of the malignant behaviour. The specific chromosomal region involved in different tumour types varied with the specific tissue. The retinoblastoma gene on chromosome 13 has been isolated and its gene product found to suppress tumorigenicity when introduced into retinoblastoma cells, to bind DNA tumour virus oncoproteins and interact with nuclear oncoproteins, to regulate transcription of *C-FOS* and *C-MYC* and proto-oncogenes and restrict cellular growth. The *TP53* tumour suppressor gene has a number of important functions including the suppression of cultured cell tumorigenicity and control of cell-cycle and apoptosis. Damage to DNA results in *TP53*-mediated cell-cycle arrest in GI to allow for DNA repair. *TP53* can induce apoptosis if DNA damage is too great, thus preventing mutations being passed to daughter cells. When mutated, *TP53* can act as an oncogene and also, by a dominant negative effect, reduce the activity of the normal gene. The Wilms' tumour gene possesses a zinc-finger motif and its product binds DNA. Many tumour suppressor genes are involved in the regulation of normal growth and development. Others may participate in cell–cell interactions in the cytoskeleton (e.g. the *APC* gene product – the FAP gene). Loss of heterozygosity of specific chromosomal regions may be detected which are characteristic for a particular tumour type, and study of these regions has led to the isolation of tumour suppressor genes involved in the development of specific cancers, and also to their identification in hereditary cancers (e.g. FAP and VHL disease). It appears that in many cases the tumour suppressor genes in which mutations occur somatically in sporadic cancers are the same as those which are involved in inherited cancer predisposition syndromes, suggesting that similar pathways of carcinogenesis are involved in the development of cancer in both instances. Fearon and Vogelstein's model for colorectal carcinogenesis postulates a series of mutations being necessary for the stepwise development of cancer (Fearon and Vogelstein, 1990). Each mutation is critical for the development of a clone of cells with a different behaviour and selective growth advantage, thus providing a seed-bed in which other mutations may occur, promoting the growth of a further clone of cells with more neoplastic potential but in which further mutations may be necessary for a fully carcinogenic phenotype to emerge. Subsequent mutations may determine metastatic and other characteristics of a tumour. Inherited mutations may be involved in changes early on in this sequence as in mutations in the *APC* gene (Powell et al., 1992) found in germline mutations in individuals with familial adenomatous polyposis and also in sporadic adenomas. Mutations in *K-RAS*, hypomethylation, loss or mutation of *DCC*, and *TP53* loss or mutations are changes which are seen sequentially in colon cancers, both sporadic and in individuals with FAP (although this is likely to be an over-simplification). This suggests that in some inherited cancer syndromes the development of premalignant lesions, such as colonic adenomas, provides the cell-pool with potential for cancers to develop within these lesions.

Activation and inactivation of tumour repressor genes and oncogenes may also occur as a result of genomic imprinting which may be dependant on the parent of origin. This may be exemplified by Beckwith–Wiedemann syndrome (BWS), characterized by prenatal overgrowth and an increased incidence of embryonal tumours – 20% of BWS patients have paternal uniparental disomy of the paternal chromosome 11p15; insulin growth factor 2 (IGF2) maps within this region and is imprinted, with monoallelic expression from the paternal allele and may act as a tumour growth promoter. *H19*, also on 11p15, appears to be expressed on the maternal allele, and may act as a tumour repressor. Both effects would result in tumour growth promotion in individuals endowed with two paternal contributions for this chromosomal region, by a combination of mechanisms. Preferential parental loss of heterozygosity may be seen in certain childhood cancers (Wilms' tumour and sporadic retinoblastoma) which may indicate parental imprinting effects in tumour repressor genes (Feinberg 1993).

Hereditary nonpolyposis colorectal cancer (HNPCC) is somewhat different, in that the inherited defect is in genes that repair DNA damage by replication errors. These replication errors can be detected in tumour DNA relative to genomic DNA and, as in HNPCC, tumours showing this characteristic tend to be proximally sited in the colon. In this syndrome there may be few colonic adenomas present and possibly no increased potential for these to develop, and *TP53* mutations may be less common in colorectal cancers in affected individuals (Kim et al., 1994), suggesting that the pathway to colorectal carcinogenesis may differ in this condition. Normal colonic epithelium in HNPCC patients does not demonstrate the microsatellite instability indicative of this type of repair defect and only about 50% of adenomas in affected individuals show this phenotype. It may thus be postulated that mutations causing a premalignant lesion (the adenoma) to develop are no more common in HNPCC than in normal individuals, but once those develop, cancer may evolve more rapidly because of an increased susceptibility to mutations within any premalignant lesion which arises. A high rate of mutation in the type II, the *TGFβ* receptor gene has, indeed, been demonstrated in colon cancer cell lines with microsatellite instability and this is not found in cells without this phenotype (Markowitz et al., 1995).

In each of the above situations (FAP and HNPCC), the phenotypic (neoplastic) abnormality is thought only to arise when there has been loss of, or mutation in, the wild-type allele, and there is good evidence to support this in tumours from individuals with FAP. A rather different situation is found in MEN type 2 (MEN2), where the germline defect is an activating mutation in the *RET* oncogene, but interestingly, mutations elsewhere in the gene (inactivating the *RET* gene product) cause Hirschsprung disease to develop, with failure of the enteric autonomic ganglion cells of the colon. In MEN2B there is hyperplasia of the autonomic ganglion cells, suggesting a role for the RET gene product in normal development. The *RET* gene is a tyrosine kinase receptor, and specific different mutations in the gene cause MEN2A, MEN2B or Hirschsprung disease.

Transfection of *RET* constructs with a MEN2A mutation into 3T3 cells causes transformation of these cells, and sporadic phaechromocytomas and medullary thyroid tumours may harbour MEN2B mutations. However, inactivation of the wild-type *RET* allele is not seen in MEN2 related tumours (as would have been expected if the inherited mutation was in a tumour suppressor gene), supporting the view that the familial susceptibility is indeed due to inappropriate activation of the germline *RET* gene.

Evidence that developmental genes may also function as tumour repressors comes from the recent identification of a gene in which mutations are found in Gorlin ('naevoid basal cell carcinoma') syndrome. This gene, *PTC*, has strong homology to the *patched* drosophila gene, a developmental gene expressed in the pharyngeal arches, neural tube, and posterior ectoderm of the limb buds. The gene product interacts with proteins involved in cell–cell interaction and cell signalling. It is postulated that homozygous loss of function of this gene product may cause both the developmental abnormalities found in Gorlin syndrome and the propensity to develop basal cell cancers in this condition (Hahn et al., 1996).

In the murine model, heterozygotes for mutations in the Wilms' tumour gene have congenital anomalies of the urogenital system, which may indicate that mutations in tumour suppressor genes do not only act in an autosomal recessive mode at the cellular level, as found in carcinogenesis (Pelletier et al., 1991). Other murine models provide more support for a role for tumour suppressors in development. For instance, homozygous inactivation of *RB-1* is lethal to mice, resulting in multiple developmental defects due to migration abnormalities in the brain. Homozygous Wilms' tumour gene (*WT1*) deficiency in mice results in renal agenesis and cardiac and diaphragmatic defects; also NF 'knockout' mice have cardiac defects and hyperplasia of the sympathetic ganglia, and some *TP53* deficient mice have exencephaly (reviewed by Hahn et al., 1996). It is interesting that in mice homozygous for *BRCA1* mutations, there is embryonic lethality with poor mesoderm formation and abnormal extra-embryonic tissue formation (Hakem et al., 1996).

Inherited cancer syndromes may thus be due to germline mutations in genes involved in various stages of the common carcinogenic pathways. Knowledge of the sequence of events should help to understand the pathogenesis of cancer and in the management and screening for these inherited conditions. A characteristic of mutations in inherited cancer syndromes, and indeed in sporadic cancers, is the notable tissue specificity of the effect of mutations involved in tumourigenesis. This is particularly seen with germline *RB-1* mutations leading to the development of retinoblastoma and osteosarcoma, *APC* mutations causing colorectal cancer and polyposis, and breast and ovarian cancers particularly occurring with *BRCA1* mutations. However, a wider spectrum of tumour susceptibility is seen in the Li–Fraumeni syndrome with inherited *TP53* mutations. Genomic imprinting may be important in the pathogenesis of some tumours, particularly embryonal tumours such as Wilms', rhabdomyosarcoma and osteosarcoma, where paternal alleles are preferentially retained in the tumour, possibly having been inactivated by genomic imprinting (Reik et al., 1990), and in inherited glomus tumours in which an autosomal dominant susceptibility to such tumours is only expressed in individuals who have the paternally inherited mutation – those inheriting it from their mother remaining clinically unaffected.

Recessive conditions causing cancer predisposition

Apart from the dominantly inherited conditions where the inherited defect is usually in a tumour suppressor gene, there are rare autosomal recessive or X-linked conditions which predispose to specific cancers by virtue of a defect in repair of DNA damage, or due to lowered immune surveillance mechanisms. Thus in ataxia-telangiectasia (A-T), homozygotes demonstrate progressive cerebellar ataxia, chromosomal instability, immunodeficiency and profound radiosensitivity, with a greatly increased susceptibility to the development of lymphomas and leukaemias. The gene for this condition, which was recently cloned, encodes a protein similar to a yeast protein kinase (Savitsky et al., 1995) It is interesting to note that A-T heterozygotes may be at increased risk of developing breast cancer (Swift et al., 1991).

Xeroderma pigmentosa is another autosomal recessive condition characterized by an increased tendency to develop skin cancers, and by a DNA repair defect specifically for DNA abnormalities induced by UV light. Affected individuals develop sun-sensitivity and multiple skin cancers due to an inability to perform excision repair of UV-C damage or (in variant types) related DNA repair mechanisms. There are several complementation groups, as a result of mutations in different genes, participating in the same pathway of DNA repair. Some of these genes encode helicases involved in repairing regions of UV damaged DNA. Excision repair of this type of DNA damage involves several interacting proteins (Li et al.,1993; Tanaka et al., 1990).

Fanconi anaemia is another autosomal recessive condition in which affected individuals are predisposed to cancer (e.g. leukaemia), demonstrate developmental anomalies, abnormal skin pigmentation, and bone-marrow failure. The basic defect appears to be a deficiency in repair of DNA cross-links (Gibson et al., 1993). Certain inherited conditions causing immune defects predispose to leukaemias and lymphomas.

It may be that even in conditions where there is clearly a strong inherited predisposition to certain cancers, the development of such cancers is dependent upon secondary factors, which include mutations at the same and other loci, environmental factors, and chance. The importance of the latter may be more pronounced in the more common situation of 'milder' inherited variations (i.e. inherited variations with less severe phenotypic effects) of susceptibility to cancer, which is likely to include inherited metabolic differences in handling carcinogens.

It is known that a large proportion of sporadic cancers are induced by environmental factors, notably tobacco smoke. Many chemicals only become carcinogenic after activation by metabolic enzymes – in particular phase I cytochrome-P450 (CYP) oxidative enzymes and phase II conjugating enzymes. Some polymorphisms in these enzymes have been associated with susceptibility to certain cancers, for example, defective glutathione S-transferase and N-acetyl transferase with susceptibility to lung and bladder cancer, but the 'jury is still out' with regard to assessing the importance of such variations (Raunio et al., 1995).

Public health implications and risk estimation

The current public perception of increased cancer risk in the presence of a family history of cancer is becoming heightened, resulting in increased requests for assessment of the risk for an individual of developing cancer based on family history. This assessment may be undertaken in a familial cancer genetic clinic, and will depend on a careful examination of many factors. Familial clustering of cancer may not necessarily indicate a highly penetrant autosomal dominant inherited susceptibility to cancer, particularly since these are rare, probably accounting for less than 5% of even breast, bowel and ovarian cancers. However, it could indicate shared environmental influences, chance effects, or the presence of less strongly predisposing genetic variations. Assessment of individual risk is often empiric, therefore, unless clear evidence of a cancer predisposing syndrome such as FAP or Gorlin syndrome is detected on clinical examination of the consultand or their affected relatives, use of mendelian genetics may not be appropriate.

Risk estimation

A careful family history is taken, noting the extent of such a history on the maternal and paternal side separately and confirming diagnoses where possible. Age at onset and multiplicity of cancer in relatives is important, since the chance that there is an hereditary predisposition present in an individual developing early onset – or metachronous or synchronous cancers – is significantly higher than where a single cancer develops at a later age. A personal history (particularly regarding cancer and related problems) and, where relevant, a clinical examination to exclude known cancer predisposing genodermatoses, is also required. The relative risk to an individual who has a first degree relative affected with a cancer is increased with many common cancers by a factor of 2 to 3 (e.g. colon cancer, breast cancer). This risk, however, is very much increased with earlier age at onset in the affected relative, and if there are several affected close relatives. Genetic models using segregation analysis suggest that this is probably due to the presence in the population of a small proportion of individuals who have a strong predisposition to the cancer. Thus in the case of breast cancer such a genetic susceptibility (due to mutation in one or more similar genes) may be present with a frequency of 0.0033 in the population, conferring a risk of 16% by age 40 years, 38% by age 50 years and 67% by age 70 years, accounting for 26% of cases of breast cancer diagnosed before 40 years, 15% by age 50 years and 8% by age 70 years (Figure 1.1; Claus et al., 1991) . None the less, the identification of *BRCA1* and *BRCA2*, with higher penetrance, probably means that these epidemiological estimates are an average of *BRCA1/2* and other less fully penetrant dominant genes. Families where *BRCA1/2* genes are segregating are likely to show many affecteds with an autosomal dominant pedigree (as most such susceptibility appears to segregate in this manner) whereas families with a less strong inherited or environmental susceptibility will not usually have such a strong family history of the cancer. In families demonstrating a clear autosomal dominant pattern of cancer susceptibility, genetic risk counselling is as for a dominantly inherited condition with incomplete penetrance. However, it is important to appreciate that an apparently unaffected male may transmit a breast cancer susceptibility

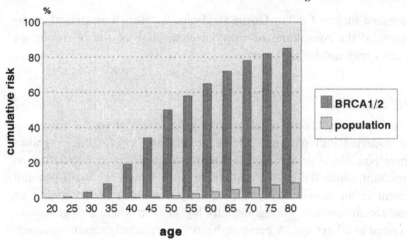

Figure 1.1. Cumulative breast cancer risk associated with mutations in *BRCA1/2*.

gene to his children, and age-related gene penetrance must be taken into account when calculating risks. Thus an unaffected woman aged 30 years at 50:50 risk of inheriting a *BRCA1* mutation would still have about a 40 to 45% chance of developing breast cancer over a lifetime, whilst the same woman at 50 years of age would have lived through most of her inherited risk of developing breast cancer, and would have less than a 20% chance of becoming affected.

In the more common situation where there is a less clear-cut family history, risk estimation is empiric and may be based on tables constructed using the cumulative risk of cancer at specific ages based on the age at onset of various combinations of affected first and second degree relatives – as in the CASH data set for breast cancer derived by Claus et al. (1994). An alternative method is to use empiric risk estimates for breast cancer modified by other risk factors including age at menarche and age at first live birth (Gail et al., 1989). It may be that presenting risk estimates as an estimate of risk over the next *n*-years is more comprehensible than a lifetime risk, since if an individual has a substantial risk of inheriting a gene that strongly predisposes to a cancer, their relative risk (for their age) of developing this cancer is much greater at a younger than at an older age. How important it is to specify this risk as accurately as possible is unclear. Studies are currently being undertaken to estimate the psychological impact of such information. It is very important that the receipt of a high risk estimate does not reduce an individual's willingness to undergo cancer surveillance!

The purpose of risk assessment could be seen to be twofold. In some cases it will be possible to reassure an individual who is over-estimating his or her risk of developing cancer that this risk is not so pronounced. In other cases a significantly increased risk of developing certain cancers may be determined, and in these cases it may be appropriate to offer a surveillance programme for the detection of cancer or premalignant lesions. In many situations the value of such screening has not yet been demonstrated conclusively by long-term trials, although regular endoscopies from the early teens have been shown to detect colonic adenomas in FAP before colon cancer usually occurs. In these cases prophylactic colectomy can be offered, which has been demonstrated to reduce the morbidity and mortality from colorectal cancer very substantially in this condition. In HNPCC, evidence is accumulating that regular colonoscopies from the mid-20s appear to detect adenomas and reduce mortality from colon cancers, although the optimal screening protocol has to be established. In this condition the lesion being detected is usually premalignant, with a good chance of benefit from its removal. Subtotal colectomy may be appropriate where multiple adenomas develop in an affected individual. However, in the case of ovarian and breast cancer, the value of surveillance programmes has not yet been established, and the lesion screened for in the case of breast cancer is malignant, not pre-malignant, thus reducing the chances of complete cure from its removal. Prophylactic oophorectomy and mastectomy can be considered in very high-risk cases, but this surgery cannot totally remove the risk of cancer (for instance, peritoneal ovarian cancer has been described after preventive oophorectomy) and is not without its own morbidity and mortality – not the least of a psychological nature. It could therefore be argued that such preventive measures are at least contentious and need careful long-term evaluation in many centres.

Impact of presymptomatic testing

In families where there is clear evidence for an inherited cancer susceptibility, it may be possible to identify the germline mutation responsible for this if blood (or tissue) can be obtained from an affected individual in the family, with fully informed consent for such testing. This generally requires an approach by the consultand who wishes to know whether they carry the mutation, and can in some families pose problems of confidentiality and conflict of interests. It is generally agreed that predictive testing in an unaffected individual for a defined cancer predisposing mutation should only be performed within the framework of careful genetic counselling, with several structured interviews allowing full consideration of the possible emotional, insurance and employment impact of the result, and the implications for the family. Such a counselling framework is being developed collaboratively, based on experience gained from predictive testing in Huntington disease. The implications of testing, however, are somewhat different from Huntington disease. The most obvious difference being that there are often preventive measures that can be taken in cancer. There are also the relatively unexplored implications of testing an individual who already has developed cancer, since the unexpected information that they could hand on a cancer predisposition to some of their children, combined with the additional appreciation that they themselves could develop further cancers, could be devastating. The demand for testing of this type is likely to be substantial; the age at which to offer predictive testing is an important issue – the consensus of opinion is that it is better not to test individuals under the age of adult consent for this type of genetic disorder. However, if, as in FAP, surveillance programmes should be instigated before adulthood it seems appropriate to test children; conversely, in the Li–Fraumeni syndrome, where tumours can develop in childhood, but screening for this condition is extremely difficult and of unproven benefit in affected individuals, one could argue that predictive testing at any age is inappropriate.

In conditions such as HNPCC where surveillance protocols appear to be of value in reducing morbidity and mortality from colorectal cancer, there have been those who advocate screening for germline HNPCC mutations in the general population rather than targeting individuals who are likely to be affected because of a family history of colorectal cancer and young age at onset. For many reasons this would seem to be inappropriate. The process of detecting mutations is laborious and incomplete (because there are multiple genes and mutations to be screened), so that only a proportion of mutations would be detected, and the pathogenic significance of a novel mutation might not be clear-cut. Genetic counselling for individuals in whom a germline mutation was detected would therefore be complex and demanding, and pre-test counselling likely to be inadequate. Cost-benefit analyses suggest that unless there is some form of selection for testing, based on family history, this type of population screening is not currently practical.

The identification of new genes has a number of implications. Recent attempts to patent gene sequences – ensuring obvious financial advantages for those holding the patents – have caused much debate. Should parts of the human genome be patentable? And if significant financial benefit can be attained by the study of DNA obtained from individuals who donated samples in good faith for research, do they have a claim on such benefits? Since this would be likely to cause significant administrative problems, consent forms for samples donated for research should perhaps have a disclaimer regarding such benefits.

As testing for genetic conditions predisposing to cancer becomes more widespread, issues such as confidentiality and who should have access to the results of predictive tests need to be faced. Currently there is much debate about whether insurance companies should have routine access to such test results. It might be argued that genetic tests, basically, are not any different from any other predictor of health, such as serum cholesterol or blood-pressure estimations, but it is likely that genetic tests are more open to misinterpretation and misuse than other tests. However, because of their potential implications for the whole family and the increased likelihood that confidentiality would be breached – with increasing numbers of parties being aware of the results – strict controls should be maintained on access to such data. Currently an individual with a first-degree relative affected with Huntington disease is penalized by life-insurers, whether or not he or she has had a predictive test. An individual who tests positive for an HNPCC germline mutation and who undertakes a successful surveillance programme may have a lower chance of dying of colorectal cancer than an individual who is at average risk of developing this cancer – but this is unlikely to be perceived by the average insurance company.

The way in which genetic information is used has many complicated implications not only for the individual but for their families, and the importance of keeping a sense of proportion when debating these issues cannot be over-estimated. There is much potential benefit to be gained from offering cancer surveillance to individuals at increased genetic risk, but the dangers of stigmatization and inappropriate use of such genetic information must not be ignored.

References

Cavenee, W.K., Dryja, T.P., Phillips, R.A. et al. 1983. Expression of recessive alleles by chromosomal mechanisms in Retinoblastoma. *Nature* **305**: 779–84.

Claus, E.B., Risch, N. and Thompson, W.D. 1991. Genetic analysis of breast cancer in the cancer and steroid Lannone study. *American Journal of Human Genetics* **48**: 232–41.

Claus, E.B., Risch, N., Thompson, W.D. 1994. Autosomal dominant inheritance of early-onset breast cancer. *Cancer* **73**: 643–51.

Fearon, E.R., Vogelstein, B. 1990. A genetic model for colorectal tumorigenesis. *Cell* **61**: 759–69.

Feinberg, A.P. 1993 Genomic imprinting and gene activation in cancer. *Nature Genetics* **4**: 110–13.

Gail, M.H., Brinton, L.A., Byar, D.P. et al. 1989. Projecting individualized probabilities of developing breast cancer for white females who are being examined annually. *Journal of the National Cancer Institute* **81**: 1879–86.

Gibson, R.A.,Buchwald, M., Roberts, R.G. and Mathew, C.G. 1993. Characterisation of the exon structure of the Fanconi Anaemia Group C gene by vectorette PCR. *Human Molecular Genetics* **2**: 35–8.

Hahn, H., Wicking, C., Zaphiropoulous, P.G. et al. 1996. Mutations of the human homology of drosophila patched in the nevoid basal cell carcinoma syndrome. *Cell* **85**: 841–51

Hakem, R., Luis de la Paupa, J., Sirard, C. et al. 1996. The tumour suppressor gene BRCA1 is required for embryonic cellular proliferation in the mouse. *Cell* **85**: 1009–23.

Harris, H., Miller, O.J., Klein, G., Worst, P. and Tachibaum, T. 1969. Suppresion of malignacy by cell fusion. *Nature* **223**: 363–8.

Huang, H.S.,Yeo, J., Shaw, Y. et al. 1988 Suppression of the neoplastic phenotype by replacement of the Rb gene in human cancer cells. *Science* **242**: 1563–6.

Kim, H., Jen, J., Vogelstein, B., Hamilton, S.R. 1994. Clinical and pathological characterisation of sporadic colorectal carcinomas with DNA replication errors in microsatellite sequences. *American Journal of Pathology* **145**: 148–56.

Knudson, A.G. 1971 Mutation and Cancer: Statistical study of retinoblastoma. *Proceedings of the National Academy of Science* (USA) **68**: 820–3.

Li, L., Balex, E.S., Peterson, C.A. and Legerski, R.J. 1993. Characterisation of the molecular defects in Xeroderma Pigmentosum Group C 1993. *Nature Genetics* **5**: 413–17.

Markowitz, S., Wang, J., Myeroff, L. et al. 1995. Inactivation of the type II TGF-B receptor in colon cancer cells with microsatellite instability. *Science* **268**: 1336–8.

Pelletier, J., Bruening, W., Li, F.P. et al. 1991. WT1 mutations contribute to abnormal genital system development and hereditary Wilms' tumour. *Nature* **353**: 431–4.

Lockhart-Mummery, J.P. 1934. The causation and treatment of multiple adenomatosis of the colon. *Annals of Surgery* **99**: 178–84.

Powell, S.M., Zilz, N., Beazer-Barclay, Y. et al. 1992. APC mutations occur early during colorectal tumorigenesis. *Nature* **359**: 235–7.

Raunio, H., Husgafvel-Pursiainen, K., Anttila, S. et al. 1995. Diagnosis of polymorphisms in carcinogen-activating and inactivating enzymes and cancer susceptibility: a review. *Gene* **159**: 113–25.

Reik, W., Romer, I., Barton, S.C., Surani, M.A., Howlett, S.K. and Klose, J. 1993. Adult phenotype in the mouse can be affected by epigenetic events in the early embryo. *Development* **119**(3): 933–42.

Savitsky, K., Bar-Sira, A., Gilad, S. et al. 1995. A single ataxia-telangiectasia gene with a product similar to P1-3 kinase. *Science* **268**: 1749–53.

Swift, A., Morrell, D., Massey, R.B. et al. 1991. Incidence of cancer in 161 families affected by ataxia telangiectasia. *New England Journal of Medicine* **316**: 1289–94.

Tanaka, K., Naoyuki, M., Satakata, I. et al. 1990 Analysis of a human DNA excision repair gene involved in group a xeroderma pigmentosum and containing a zinc finger domain. *Nature* **348**: 73–6.

2

Screening for cancer in those at high risk as a result of genetic susceptibility

HOWARD CUCKLE

Summary

This chapter begins with an examination of the general principles of screening, the expected benefits and rationale, the potential costs and how these all may change as the levels set for cut-off values for test positivity are altered. These themes are developed in the context of screening for cancer, examining the possible disadvantages of detecting a tumour earlier and thus increasing 'lead-time', particularly when the biology of tumour progression may not be well understood. Genetic-risk screening and testing is then considered and a distinction is made between testing for rare, high penetrant alleles of predisposing genes and genetic testing for commoner cancers, where most cases are not attributable to these genes. In this situation, the likely costs and benefits in will probably vary in different population groups.

Introduction

Screening is a systematic attempt to identify from among apparently healthy individuals those at high enough risk of a specific disease to warrant further investigation. The aim of the consequent investigation is to make a definite diagnosis and the diagnostic procedure used would be too expensive or hazardous to offer without prior selection. It attracts both enthusiasts and vociferous detractors. The enthusiasts generally emphasize the public health benefits – inroads that can be rapidly made into the incidence and mortality of disease – whereas the detractors are usually either concerned that the benefits might be illusory or that they must be paid for by unacceptable physical and psychological morbidity.

A balanced view is called for and this is best achieved by making explicit the benefits and costs, both human and financial, for the proposed screening program. In normal medical practice there is also frequently a conflict between the therapeutic and the iatrogenic but the action taken is influenced by the need to respond to a patient's demand for alleviation of symptoms. However, screening is not generally patient led, it is pro-active, and so there is a greater obligation to ensure that there is proof of greater good than harm before embarking on it.

It is fruitless to try to justify screening in general; each screening programme needs to be considered separately. Some will be found wanting and can be readily discarded. Others will show a clear-cut benefit and provided that sufficient funding were available could become routine practice. In many cases, however, the balance may be more finely poised and there is likely to be an element of value judgement. The purpose of this chapter is to demonstrate the general principles of screening and its evaluation with special reference to those at high genetic risk of cancer. It will first be necessary to introduce a few technical terms.

Screening terms

In its simplest form screening involves a single test and a disease. The *test* could be a biochemical assay, an imaging procedure or indeed any form of selection such as a questionnaire. It may be of its nature dichotomous, i.e. there are just two values with no 'grey' areas. The value associated with the disease would be labelled 'positive' and the other 'negative'. More often the test takes on a range of values and there is a general directional association between disease and increased or decreased level. Usually the *disease* relates to the health state of the individual being offered the test but in antenatal screening the mother is tested and the disease refers to the fetus. In diseases subject to preclinical progression and regression, like cancer, the individual being tested may be clinically healthy but his or her future presentation with clinical symptoms is being referred to. The terms 'affected' and 'unaffected' are used to include all these possibilities.

Ideally, the disease is well-defined in that each individual is affected or not and there is a 'gold standard' of diagnosis which is independent of the screening test itself. But that is not always the case. With a dichotomous test and a well-defined disease there are just four possibilities, namely positive and affected, negative and unaffected, positive and unaffected, and negative and affected. The former two are called 'true' positives and negatives respectively and the latter are 'false' positives and negatives. The discriminatory power of the test – its ability to distinguish affecteds from unaffecteds – is summarized by the 'detection rate' or the percentage of affecteds with positive test results and the 'false positive rate' or the percentage of unaffecteds with positive results. The detection rate is also known as the 'true-positive rate' or 'sensitivity', by analogy with a biochemical test whose sensitivity is the smallest amount it can detect. Some sources quote the 'true-negative rate' or 'specificity' instead of the false-positive rate, its obverse, but it is a misleading term. Thus, a marked improvement in a test that halves the false-positive rate from 2% to 1% may be unimpressive if expressed as an increase in specificity from 98% to 99%.

A multi-valued test can be dichotomized by choosing a 'cut-off level' to define positivity. In general the choice of cut-off is arbitrary – there will be no natural divide between affecteds and unaffecteds. Any change to a more extreme cut-off will lead to a reduction in the false-positive rate at the cost of a lower detection rate. Conversely, in order to increase detection more false-positives will be generated. One way of visualizing the discriminatory power of a given test is to draw the overlapping frequency distributions in affecteds and unaffecteds (directly as percentage histograms or by statistical modelling). Another method of displaying this is the 'receiver–operator curve' or ROC which is a plot of sensitivity against specificity for a range of possible cut-offs, again either directly or by modelling.

In practice the choice of cut-off is determined by two factors – the workload generated by carrying out diagnostic procedures in those with positive results and the risk of being affected given that the result is positive (i.e. the 'positive predictive value'). The latter is often referred to as though it were an index of the test performance *per se* but it is not. The predictive value is a function of the detection and false-positive rates but it also depends on the chance of having the disease prior to the test being done. A test with a low positive predictive value when applied to a population where the disease is rare will be expected to have a higher value when applied to high risk population. The only way in which this may not happen is if the distribution of test results is dependant on the prior risk. This will tend to occur when a test is applied to a group with positive results from another screening test and the two are measuring correlated factors.

The classic examples in which screening has been fully evaluated relate to antenatal screening for common serious congenital abnormalities that are largely well-defined disease states. These are neural tube defect, Down syndrome, haemaglobinopathy and cystic fibrosis which can be diagnosed in utero by invasive and hazardous procedures such as amniocentesis, chorionic villus biopsy and fetal blood sampling. At the end of pregnancy, or shortly thereafter, it will be possible to determine whether or not the fetus was in fact affected. Therefore the detection rate, false-positive rate and predictive value can be readily calculated. Assessing the value of screening for progressive diseases such as cancer is not so simple.

Cancer screening

The aim of screening for cancer is either to advance the diagnosis to a stage when the tumour is more readily treatable or to detect precancerous lesions whose treatment will be truly preventive. The central question in such screening is whether early or pre-cancer diagnosis can improve prognosis. Most sites of cancer show a marked gradient in average survival times according to the stage of clinical diagnosis. It would therefore appear to be obvious, even logically inevitable, that any screening test which leads to early diagnosis must improve prognosis. There is also a strong clinical impression in individual cases that this is so. But it is not necessarily the case because much, if not all, of the relationship between survival times and clinical stage can be due to bias.

For example, suppose a tumour started to grow in a 45-year-old woman, which was discovered by chance at an early stage when she was 50, but she refused treatment, symptoms presented at 55 and she died at 60. The survival time from incidental diagnosis was five years greater than had the tumour only been discovered symptomatically, but this, however, cannot be attributable to treatment. Therefore this 'lead time' bias can of itself account for survival time differences. Now suppose that there are a series of women with tumours of the same site, starting at age 45, but growing at different rates. Those with the more indolent tumours will spend a longer period at an early stage so that there will be more opportunities for early incidental diagnosis. It follows that intrinsically good prognosis is over-represented in individuals presenting with early diagnosis. This is known as 'length' bias.

Any study of screening for cancer must seek to avoid these powerful biases as well as the 'healthy screenee' effect whereby the group refusing an offer of screening tend to be deniers of symptoms and refusers of treatment with a shorter life expectancy than accepters. A direct but unethical study design would be to carry out a randomized trial of immediate versus deferred treatment in those presenting at an early stage and comparing not survival times but mortality rates. However, much the same results can be obtained by carrying out a randomized trial of screening itself. A new screening test is a limited resource and of unproven efficacy so that it is ethical to allocate it at random. In fact you could argue that it is unethical to do otherwise.

Cancers are not well-defined so the concepts of detection rate, false-positive rate and positive predictive value are of limited value. Affecteds in this context are cases that would have surfaced clinically in the absence of screening, but there is no reliable way of determining which they are. Some of the screen-detected cases may never have surfaced and represent over-diagnosis, whilst some of those missed at screening may surface clinically in the year following the test, others may not do so for many years and some of the late diagnosed cases may not have been present at the time of screening. With pre-cancerous lesions the problem is compounded by disease regression and by the possibility that some tumours will arise spontaneously without a pre-cancerous stage.

There are very few sites of cancer for which screening has been shown to be of enough benefit to establish national population-based programmes. In the UK this has only been done for cancers of the cervix and breast. Whilst the Pap smear was never subjected to the rigours of a randomized clinical trial there is sufficient proof of its ability to reduce cervical cancer mortality from other sources. Thus geographical comparisons and time trends indicate that well organized cervical cancer screening programs can yield 80% or higher reductions in mortality. Initially, cervical screening was poorly organized in the UK and had limited impact. However, this was eventually resolved by introducing a systematic scheme to call women for testing at a given age and to recall them at a fixed interval. Mammography has been examined in seven randomized trials and all of them showed a reduction in breast cancer mortality among those invited to be screened. The Swedish Two Counties Trial, which probably best reflects what might be achieved in routine practice with modern equipment, observed a 30% mortality reduction after only eight years. These results together with the non-randomized studies prompted the UK government to establish a national breast screening program (NHS-BSP). Women are called for the first mammogram at age 50 and recalled every three years until age 64.

Genetic risk screening

The purpose of genetic screening for a specific cancer is to identify those who are at high risk of developing the disease so that the harmful consequences can be reduced. The consequent action to be taken might include a regimen of cancer screening, primary prevention through a change to a healthier lifestyle and prenatal (or possibly in the future pre-conceptual) diagnosis to avoid passing the deleterious gene to their children. Not all activity aimed at identifying high risk individuals is screening. Only when it is undertaken in a pro-active and systematic way would the process be screening. Assessing risk among those who present themselves because of anxiety is not screening.

From the screening point of view there are two distinct types of genetic susceptibility to cancer. Firstly, there are rare types of cancer caused in the majority of cases by a germline mutation (e.g. retinoblastoma). Secondly, there are common cancers in which a germline mutation is only responsible for a minority of those affected (e.g. breast cancer).

The former situation is relatively straightforward and risk assessment does not differ substantially from other genetic disorders. First degree relatives of the individual presenting with the condition are likely to be referred to the clinical genetic services and have their risk assessed. The extent of risk will depend on factors such as the recessive or dominant nature of the inheritance, the new mutation rate and the degree of penetrance. As with other genetic conditions more distant relatives could also be drawn into the risk assessment process either to aid the verification of risk in closer relatives, or for their own sake. Once there is a simple way to determine the presence of one or more defective genes this process can be made more formal by systematically reaching out to more and more distant relatives. This is known as 'active cascade screening'.

With the more common cancers the problem has so far been to distinguish the inherited and sporadic cases. In the future when the principal genetic defects are known for a particular site of cancer, the genetically caused cases will be identifiable. It will then be possible to consider either active cascade screening or even more general population screening if the cancer was very common and a large minority of cases were hereditary. However, at present genetic tests are not generally available for common cancers and the identification of those likely to have inherited cancer is based on epidemiological considerations. With a germline mutation, genetically susceptible individuals will: (1) to some extent cluster in families; (2) tend to have multifocal lesions; (3) have a younger age of onset than those with sporadic disease; and (4) if there is a mutation in a tumour suppressor gene, affected families may have an excess of more than one type of cancer. Many family doctors are now aware of these risk factors and will refer close relatives of cancer patients to a specialist. However, unless the family doctor is given firm guidelines on who to refer and to whom, the system can become overloaded with too many referrals of relatively low risk patients (see Chapter 6). The problem is compounded by the increasing awareness by the lay public of genetic risks.

Screening for cancer among those at high genetic risk

Two obvious questions need to be asked about cancer screening among high risk individuals. Firstly, is it valid to assume that screening programmes shown to be of benefit in the general population will be efficacious when applied to the genetically susceptible? Secondly, is it justifiable to offer unproven screening procedures to high risk individuals? I will illustrate these questions in relation to breast cancer.

Screening results would be incomparable in hereditary and sporadic breast cancers if there were differences in: tumour or breast physiology affecting sensitivity, the natural history of preclinical disease, case-fatality or the harmful effects of mammography. There is no a priori reason to expect physiological or natural history differences for hereditary breast cancer although the possibility cannot be excluded. There is a suggestion of different case-fatality rates – four out of five studies examining this found longer survival in those with a family history compared to the general population (Langlands et al., 1976; Lynch et al., 1981; Albano et al., 1982; Anderson and Badzioch, 1986; Ruder et al., 1988). However, none of them controlled for age and only one allowed for the important confounding factor of clinical stage. Even the latter did not control carefully enough to avoid the lead-time bias that might be expected in anxious women. Therefore there is no strong reason to believe that there are case-fatality differences for breast cancer.

Of more concern are possible iatrogenic effects of mammography that might outweigh its benefits. For example, women who are homozygous for the ataxia-telangiectasia (A-T) gene are probably at high risk of breast cancer (in addition to lymphomas and leukaemia), and in vitro studies of their cells show dramatic radiosensitivity. Whilst few homozygotes live long enough to get breast cancer, heterozygotes do, and thus first degree relatives of patients with A-T may be at increased risk of breast cancer, particularly if they have been exposed to medical radiation. The evidence for this rests on epidemiological studies, and laboratory findings showing that cells of obligate heterozygotes demonstrate similar radiosensitivity to that found in A-T patients (Swift et al., 1987; Swift et al., 1991). Excluding known or suspected A-T carriers from screening will not completely avoid the problem. It is not known whether high risk women who are not A-T carriers are also radiosensitive. In the absence of hard evidence it would be difficult to exclude such women from the NHS-BSP, especially when they may have more to gain from it than most. A randomized trial of screening in high risk women would answer the question directly but it might be impractical.

The case of high risk women who are ineligible for the NHS-BSP because they are under 50 raises different issues. The programme begins at age 50 for reasons of cost efficiency (relatively few cancers occur in younger women) and because there is lack of evidence for a mortality reduction at earlier ages. There are a priori reasons to expect mammography to have relatively low sensitivity in premenopausal women due to breast density and this is borne out by studies of breast cancer incidence following negative mammography. Consequently the effect of screening on mortality is likely to be lower than in older women unless it is carried out much more frequently.

Information on mortality in young screened women is available from 11 published studies of which six were randomized trials (Verbeek et al., 1984; Palli et al., 1986; Andersson et al., 1988; Morrison et al., 1988; Shapiro et al., 1988; Tabar et al., 1989; Roberts et al., 1990; Frisell et al., 1991; Miller et al., 1992; Nyström et al., 1993; UK Trial of Early Detection of Breast Cancer Group, 1993). None of them included sufficient numbers of deaths to estimate reliably the effect on mortality and only three carried out annual mammography. Moreover, even in the only randomized trial with a mortality reduction approaching statistical significance some of the effect is attributable to the cancer being detected by screening when the women were over 50. Taken together, the published studies do not argue strongly either in favour or against a mortality reduction. A clearer conclusion will eventually emerge with longer follow-up of existing studies and from new trials including the large ongoing UKCCCR (UK Coordinating Committee for Cancer Research) Under-50s Trial of 195,000 women. Even if a mortality reduction is eventually established which is too small to warrant a change in NHS-BSP policy, it may be sufficient to encourage screening in young high risk women. The

28   *H. Cuckle*

reason would be that in absolute terms (i.e. in deaths prevented per 10,000 screens) the benefit may be as great as it is for older women without a genetic risk.

What then is to be done about young women with a high genetic risk of breast cancer? Currently many are being screened using regimens which vary: (1) the minimum age for the initial screen; (2) whether the youngest women have a baseline mammogram some years before starting routine screening; and (3) the screening interval. Some would argue that this is unjustifiable whilst others would say that the clinical benefit of providing the reassurance of negative mammographic findings to an anxious patient is sufficient justification. Naturally, if there is no evidence for a mortality benefit of screening, a negative result should not be taken to imply a reduced risk of dying from the disease. Indeed the complacency engendered by false reassurance might cause increased mortality if it leads to symptoms not being acted on readily. None the less women who are anxious because of their genetic risk may be seeking reassurance, not about eventually dying from cancer, but about having it now or in the near future, and that may be achievable.

Conclusion

Screening is a complex and potentially dangerous medical activity that should not be undertaken lightly. However, proper evaluation in advance is an ideal which may be difficult to achieve in the face of public demand, clinical freedom and the need to allay anxiety. The area of genetic susceptibility to cancer is a clear example of this. Recent advances in molecular biology are likely to lead to an increase in genetic screening using either the active cascade approach or in the general population. This, together with the current methods of identifying those at high genetic risk, will in turn generate more cancer screening. Whilst this process may be inevitable those involved should practise restraint and ensure that any new screening takes place within a well designed study.

References

Albano, W.A., Recabaren, J.A., Lynch, H.T. et al.,. 1982. Natural history of hereditary cancer of the breast and colon. *Cancer* **50**: 360–3.
Anderson, D.E., and Badzioch, M.D. 1986. Survival in familial breast cancer patients. *Cancer* **58**: 360–5.
Andersson, I., Aspegren, K., Janzon, L., Landberg, T., Lindholm, K., Linell, F., Ljungberg, O., Ranstam, J. and Sigfusson, B. 1988. Mammographic

screening and mortality from breast cancer: the Malmo mammographic screening trial. *British Medical Journal* **297**: 943–94.

Frisell, J., Eklund, G., Hellström, L., Lidbrink, E., Rutqvist, L.E. and Somell, A. 1991. Randomized study of mammography screening – preliminary report on mortality in the Stockholm trial. *Breast Cancer Research and Treatment* **18**: 49–56.

Langlands, A.O., Kerr, G.R. and Bloomer, S.M. 1976. Familial breast cancer. *Clinical Oncology* **2**: 41–5.

Lynch, H.T., Albano, W.A., Recabaren, J.A. et al. 1981. Survival in hereditary breast and colon cancer. *JAMA* **246**: 1197.

Miller, A.B., Baines, C.J., To, T. and Wall, C. 1992. Canadian National Breast Screening Study: 1. Breast cancer detection and death rates among women aged 40 to 49 years. *Canadian Medical Association Journal* **147**: 1459–88.

Morrison, A.S., Brisson, J. and Khalid, N. 1988. Breast cancer incidence and mortality in the Breast Cancer Detection Demonstration Project. *Journal of the National Cancer Institute* **80**: 1540–7.

Nyström, L., Rutqvist, L.E., Wall, S. et al. 1993. Breast cancer screening with mammography: overview of Swedish randomized trials. *Lancet* **341**: 973–78.

Palli, D., Rosselli Del Turco, M.R., Buiatti, E., Carli, S., Ciatto, S., Toscani, L. and Maltoni, G. 1986. A case-control study of the efficacy of a non-randomized breast cancer screening program in Florence (Italy). *International Journal of Cancer* **38**: 501–4.

Roberts, M.M., Alexander, F.E., Anderson, T.J. et al. 1990. Edinburgh trial of screening for breast cancer: mortality at seven years. *Lancet* **335**: 241–6.

Ruder, A.M., Moodie, P.F., Nelson, N.A. and Won Choi, N. 1988. Does family history of breast cancer improve survival among patients with breast cancer? *American Journal of Obstetries and Gynecology* **158**: 963–8.

Shapiro, S., Venet, W., Strax, P. and Venet, L. 1988. Periodic screening for breast cancer. In: *The Health Insurance Plan Project and its Sequelae, 1963–86.* Baltimore & London: Johns Hopkins University Press.

Swift, M,. Morrell, D., Massey, R.B. and Chase, C.L. 1991. Incidence of cancer in 161 families affected by ataxia-telangiectasia. *New England Journal of Medicine* **325**: 1831–6.

Swift, M., Reitnauer, P.J., Morrell, D. and Chase, CL. 1987. Breast and other cancers in families with ataxia-telangiectasia. *New England Journal of Medicine* **316**: 1289–94.

Tabar, L., Fagerberg, G., Duffy, S.W. and Day, N.E. 1989. The Swedish two county trial of mammographic screening for breast cancer: recent results and calculation of benefit. *Journal of Epidemiology Community Health* **43**:107–14.

UK Trial of Early Detection of Breast Cancer Group. 1993. Breast cancer mortality after 10 years in the UK trial of early detection of breast cancer. *The Breast* **2**: 13–20.

Verbeek, A.L.M., Hendricks, J.H.C.L., Holland, R., Mravunac, M., Sturmans, F. and Day, NE. 1984. Reduction of breast cancer mortality through mass screening with modern mammography. First results of the Nijmegen project, 1975–1981. *Lancet* **1**: 1222–6.

3
Ethical and legal perspectives on inherited cancer susceptibility

BARTHA MARIA KNOPPERS and BEATRICE
GODARD

Summary

There is a complicated interplay of public perceptions, expectations and demands upon professionals in relation to genetic testing for cancer susceptibility and the medical services offered. The ethical and legal aspects of these relationships are explored in this chapter, with particular reference to the issues of consent and confidentiality, employment and insurance, and testing of minors and incompetent adults. The chapter concludes with consideration of issues surrounding ownership and patenting of genetic information, and a proposal for principles to serve as a basis for shared responsibility for patient participation in the development of guidelines for such genetic testing.

Introduction

Much media debate tends to encourage taking sides for and against familial testing and population screening for genetic factors in common multifactorial diseases such as cancer. Positions are presented in phobic and polemic language. Typical, are allegations of 'slippery slope', 'playing God', 'biotechnological imperialism' or of 'scientific breakthrough' and 'gene for cancer found'.

New discoveries of the role of genetic factors in multifactorial diseases do not translate into treatments or cures but rather into information and in some cases, prevention. What we have then are scientific facts expressed in risk factors. Such at-risk information is often couched in incomprehensible probabilities and percentages using the language of susceptibility, predictivity, presymptomatic, expressivity, penetrance, late-onset, carrier status, and the like.

Furthermore, problems may arise in testing for late-onset diseases where the detection of the defect is possible before the clinical symptomatology has occurred.[1] The results of such testing do not provide an unequivocal answer; they only give probabilistic information on whether an increased risk exists. Also, there may be variable clinical expression in persons with an identical molecular defect, regarding the age of onset or the severity of the disease. A variety of modifying genes may alter clinical expression of a given molecular defect. Moreover, the mutations will differ between populations, and testing for many mutations that may be involved is usually not feasible.

This new phenomenon of susceptibility testing is important since little is known of the psycho-social impact of such genetic information. A recent study of breast cancer testing showed that normal results from genetic tests did not reassure women who had long believed that they were at risk for breast cancer because many of their relatives had died of the disease. Most of the women who were told that they did not have the disease gene still wanted frequent mammography and were thinking seriously about having their breast(s) removed as a form of prophylactic surgery (Vines 1994). Even in the case of Huntington disease, a monogenic disorder for which the gene has been identified, the uptake has been quite low and the behavioural responses unexpected (Anonymous 1994b).

Furthermore notions of 'normalcy' and 'disability' have long been culturally defined. Perception of being at risk as equivalent to being ill or disabled can only exacerbate discrimination and lead to the broader harm of geneticisation (Wolf 1995). Moreover, where present or future conditions can be discovered in the embryo, fetus or newborn, who decides what course of action to take?[2] Current guidelines governing research and clinical practice may not suffice in the ensuing ethical, legal, social, and personal dilemmas.

1 According to Annas (1992), important factors in determining whether a test should be offered include: (1) the frequency and severity of the disease; (2) the availability of a therapy of documented efficacy; (3) the extent to which detection by testing improves the outcome; (4) the validity and safety of the genetic tests; (5) the adequacy of resources to assure effective genetic testing and follow-up; (6) the costs in relation to the benefits; and (7) the acceptance of the genetic testing programme by the community, including both consumers and practicing physicians.

2 This chapter will not discuss embryo, prenatal or newborn testing. It is interesting to note, however, that in the case of prenatal diagnosis, the Royal Commission on New Reproductive Technologies (1993), recommended that physicians provide information concerning predisposition to serious late onset conditions as well as the availability of
continued on next page

There is no doubt that consumer pressure and expectations of profes-sionals will influence liability. Are there professional norms to guide researchers, physicians, and counsellors, or, will they simply assume responsibility, if not liability (see section 'Liability')? Furthermore, it may well be that ethical guidelines, where they exist, can do little to stem already accepted access to medical records. If treated as medical information so as not to distinguish genetic information as being 'differ-ent', neither confidentiality nor access rules are clearly defined in the public or private sectors (see section 'Privacy and confidentiality').

Selection and recruitment issues also come to mind since early infor-mation, detection and prevention may be the only 'cure'. Children and adolescents are particularly vulnerable groups not only because of vary-ing degrees of capacity to comprehend and consent but because of par-ental authority in the former and peer group pressure in the latter. While such vulnerability need not exclude them altogether, different evaluation and inclusion mechanisms could be necessary (see section 'Vulnerable populations').

Also present in the current debate is the possibility of socio-economic discrimination in terms of equitable access to employment and insurance (see section 'Employment and insurance'), to say nothing of the resulting stigmatization of genetic 'at-risk' families and individuals. It is at this point that the role of third parties such as employers, insurers and researchers as 'corporate citizens' becomes an issue. There may be both legitimate and illegitimate uses of genetic material and information. Screening employees to detect those at risk in certain work conditions or asking health questions on insurance questionnaires, or using DNA in research after obtaining consent and approval by ethics committees at first glance seems legitimate. But who verifies that the insurance indus-try's actuarial tables are scientifically valid and have included in the probabilistic value of this new at-risk information?

Closer to home for most researchers and for the participants them-selves is the question of the status of human genetic material as currently

continued from previous page
abortion but decided against recommending the same for susceptibility testing. The Royal Commission on New Reproductive Technologies (1993) recommended that: 'Prenatal diag-nosis not be offered for genes that increase susceptibility to disease' (p. 881). 'Prenatal susceptibility testing is even less appropriate than adult testing, because the benefits are even fewer and the potential harms greater. Like prenatal testing for late-onset single-gene disorders, prenatal susceptibility testing puts children in a very vulnerable position if they are shown to be at greater risk' (p. 880).

sampled and banked. Is DNA, as found in all cells, to be treated as any other sample? To whom does it belong? What can be patented and when? (See section 'Ownership and patents'.)

Finally, even if clear legal and ethical parameters would be adopted after public debate, the very principles of autonomy, privacy, justice, and equity could well be undermined by systemic failures and frailties (Knoppers and Chadwick, 1994). Informatic and technological capabilities of access and possibly of abuse, surpass even the imagined protection of genetic material and information. Moreover, equitable access is threatened by private clinics that operate in the failure of governments both to integrate the new genetics into the health care infrastructure and to determine priorities and future directions. Current international, national, or state statutes and professional codes have yet to be officially and openly debated and interpreted in order to determine their adequacy in face of this challenge.[3] The controversies surrounding inherited cancer susceptibility studies encompass all these issues. An attempt at their solution may serve as a prototype for other multifactorial conditions.

Liability

Beginning then with the issue of medical liability and genetic testing, a recent study of professional norms in the practice of human genetics, stated that 'medical malpractice law is expensive, time consuming and is arguably not an effective mechanism for quality assurance' (Knoppers et al., 1996). As we move from the monogenic to the multifactorial arena of human genetics, with the concomitant increase in knowledge and in communication skills that this will require, genetic malpractice may well become an issue since there are few formal standards of requisite education or competence through which to protect the public. Genetic susceptibility being only one factor amongst environmental, socio-economic, cultural and familial factors, the very nature and art of counselling and communication or even the opportunity to express the desire not to know, will require a fundamental restructuring of the physician–patient relationship. Medical advice becomes an important issue when a condition can be prevented or treated (Motulsky, 1994). Non-directive advice, which is strongly advocated in reproductive counselling, may be inappropriate, since at-risk, probabilistic information must be explained and the relevant medical recommendations of how to avoid and prevent the

3 There is little statutory law on genetic testing (Knoppers and Chadwick, 1994).

disease under study must be given. Often, as in predictive diagnosis of cancer, no clear therapeutic intervention other than more frequent monitoring may be available. It is difficult to provide recommendations that apply equally to predictive diagnosis of all late-onset diseases, since every condition raises somewhat different scientific, medical and psychosocial issues (Motulsky, 1994).

Physicians are not obliged to perform genetic testing on demand when it is not indicated. As with any genetic test, the physician should explain the test, its purpose, what could be learned and what action could be taken on the basis of this knowledge, as well as the possible alternatives and the consequences of not undergoing the test. The basic concept is that people have a right not to be touched without their consent because of their interests in bodily integrity and self-determination. The patient is the one who must experience the test and live with its consequences. There is no obligation on the part of the patient to accept any medical test or medical treatment.

It should be emphasized that if the physician believes genetic testing is indicated for a particular patient and recommends it, and the patient refuses, the physician has an obligation to make sure that the refusal is an informed one, that the patient knows why genetic testing is being offered, what can be learned from it and what could happen if the test is not performed. The refusal should be explored and the reasons documented in the patient's chart. A Californian case held that a family physician, whose patient had refused a Pap smear on two occasions and later died of cervical cancer, had a legal obligation to obtain an informed refusal from her before accepting her refusal at face value (Annas, 1992).

In addition to the issue of competence then, liability will be increasingly centred on failure to communicate actual or potential 'at-risk' information rather than on classical malpractice during an intervention or diagnostic technique. This duty to communicate is not only complicated by the at-risk nature of susceptibility information but also by the fact that the duty implies providing choices and in that the duty may continue over time.

As concerns choices, different levels of participation should be presented so that a person can decide to participate fully or to know fully, partially or not at all. This means that choices must be offered – i.e. to be contacted, to participate, to provide DNA, to be informed of results, to allow different forms of research with that DNA, to allow family access to that DNA, and finally, for the DNA to be banked or not (Knoppers and Laberge, 1995).

The continual refinement of genetic knowledge and testing, also expands the duty to follow up. To this duty now may be added a new duty, that of 'look-back' – also a variant of the duty to recall as developed in cases of defective products or of HIV infected blood. In a recent Canadian case, the Court held that the family physician was in breach of his duty to disclose when the head of the hospital blood bank advised him that his patient's transfusion years earlier had been with a potentially HIV-contaminated blood component. The patient died of HIV-related pneumonia without knowing his status and in that same year, the widow learned that she was HIV positive (Pittman, 1994). As tests become more refined to the point where there are significant changes in the diagnostic interpretation of patients already tested or, where new tests become available that could be performed on banked samples for which originally no tests were available, does the duty to look-back 'activate'? What will be its limits?

Privacy and confidentiality

Genetic information is personal but also necessarily familial (and as we shall see later, socio-economic, as concerns insurers and employers). The first time that the familial nature is likely to arise is long before a test is even available, that is, during linkage studies.

In linkage studies, each family member who may be potentially 'of interest' must first consent to be contacted by the researcher. It is the patient or family informant who should contact other informants in the family so as to complete the family medical history. It is here that the emergence of the 'right not to know' raises specific problems with regard to consent. Surely, the exercise of that right must be based on some knowledge. Yet, when does 'some knowledge' become subtle coercion? How far should family members or professionals push a person toward confronting the possibility of an 'incurable' disease when the person is ambivalent or resists that knowledge, even if early detection and treatment increase long-term survival?

Another issue is that of family members possessing genetic information but who refuse to communicate such information. Is the duty to warn, if it exists, that of the physician or the family? Is it a legal or only a moral duty? As early as 1983, the US Presidential Commission recommended that, in the situation where the patient/research participant refuses to inform other family members of their at-risk status, the following four conditions should be met before refusal is overridden (President's Commission, 1983):

(1) All efforts to persuade the individual to disclose information voluntarily have failed.
(2) There is a high probability of harm to the relatives (including future children) if the information is not disclosed, and there is evidence that the information would be used to prevent harm.
(3) The harm averted would be serious.
(4) Only genetic information directly relevant to the relative's own medical status would be revealed.

More recently, the moral nature of this obligation has been underscored (Baumiller et al., 1996; ASHG, 1998). It is interesting to note however that the Quebec Code of Ethics includes the possibility for notification by the physician in spite of the obligation of confidentiality 'if there should be a just and imperative motive related to the health of the patient or the welfare of others' (Article 3.04, Code of Ethics, 1981). European texts have similar provisions (Knoppers, 1995) and the recent opinion of the French National Ethics Committee acknowledges that there may be a duty to rescue (Comité Consultatif, 1996).

Even in the absence of a legal duty, a physician may have the privilege to warn family members that could serve as a defence (Dickens and Park, 1996). Moreover, since genetic information about a patient has potential to benefit that entire patient's family, the physician may question why that patient should have a right to prevent disclosure of the information (Knoppers, 1996). Or, the physician may see the patient's genetic profile as 'family property' and if the information is treated as such, that physician may be in conflict between duties to the family and to the patient (Gevers, 1988). To date, no court has held that there is a legal duty on physicians to warn relatives of patients that they may be at risk of a genetic disorder (Dickens and Park, 1996). The patient with a genetic susceptibility is not putting relatives at risk by carrying the gene (in comparison with the disclosure of HIV infection where it is the patient who harms others by his or her actions) (Dickens and Park, 1996). One circumstance in which a breach of confidentiality could be considered is when health care providers screening for genetic conditions inform their patients in advance of that eventuality. This would permit patients to refuse testing or to seek medical advice and services elsewhere (Macklin 1992).

Generally, in spite of legislative and regulatory mechanisms as well as professional obligations, the confidentiality of a patient's medical record is never absolute. Statutes may create duties to disclose confidential medical information based upon the rationale that the public good or interest, specifically avoiding doing harm to others, sometimes justifies breaching patient's privacy (Knoppers, 1996). For example, a physician may be obliged to report, for purposes of public safety or public health, medical conditions that impair capacity, contagious diseases or psychiatric illness.

Vulnerable populations

Certain participants in genetic testing, such as incompetent adults, adolescents, and children do not have the legal capacity to consent. While the duties of competence, of due care in testing and informing and of follow-up remain, genetic testing with vulnerable populations raise specific issues due to the need to protect and to include such populations. Usually, studies or programmes using responsible adults who are adequately informed and who freely give consent create no special problems with regards to the issue of consent. It is more difficult when persons are not capable of giving consent for themselves, as is often the case with incompetent adults but this population would not in all likelihood be involved in susceptibility testing.

The genetic testing and treatment of children, however, has expanded to include testing for susceptibility, testing for the benefit of others, for research purposes, or including them in protocols for somatic cell therapy (Malkin and Knoppers, 1996; Skene and Charlesworth, 1996). The role of physicians with regard to genetic testing of children remains ambiguous as do the rights of children to be tested or not (Wertz et al., 1995). Few arguments for testing can be made in the absence of direct and immediate medical benefits to the children. Thus, testing for susceptibility raises more complex issues, and has not been accepted (Council of Europe 1990, 1996; Nuffield Council on Bioethics 1993; Sharpe 1994; ASHG/ACMG 1995). It is interesting to note that in Canada, the National Council of Bioethics and Human Research recommended in 1993 that any decisions made by the parent, with a physician, for a child concerning DNA banking, be subject to review and ratification when the child becomes capable.

Adolescents participate in the medical decision-making process to the extent that they are capable (Wertz et al., 1994). DNA testing is already offered to adolescents in the context of familial adenomatous polyposis-coli or familial hypercholesterolemia, or from ethnic groups at risk for thalassemia or Tay-Sachs (Scriver and Fujiwara, 1992). Currently, carrier testing for cystic fibrosis is problematic. The information conveyed is of a probabilistic nature in cases where no mutation can be detected and cannot definitively identify or exclude the person. In these cases, education and counselling become essential.

Following the example of the report of the Working Party of the British Clinical Genetics Society (1994) on the genetic testing of children, the American Society of Human Genetics and the American College of Medical Genetics (ASHG/ACMG, 1995) established important points to consider before testing children and adolescents for disease susceptibilities and carrier status in regard to: (1) the impact of potential benefits and harms on decisions about testing; (2) the family's involvement in decision-making; and (3) considerations for future research. On the first aspect, medical benefit to the child should be the primary justification for genetic testing in children and adolescents, as well as substantial psychosocial benefits to the competent adolescent. If the medical or psychosocial benefits of a genetic test will not accrue until adulthood, as in the case of carrier status or adult-onset diseases, genetic testing generally should be deferred. Also, if the balance of benefits and harms is uncertain, the provider should respect the decision of competent adolescents and their families. Testing should be discouraged when the provider determines that potential harms of genetic testing in children and adolescents outweigh the potential benefits. Regarding the family's involvement in decision-making, the provider should obtain the permission of the parents and, as appropriate, the assent of the child or consent of the adolescent. The provider is obligated to advocate on behalf of the child when he or she considers a genetic test to be – or not – in the best interest of the child. In the same way, a request by a competent adolescent for the results of a genetic test should be given priority over parents' requests to conceal information. Finally, among considerations for future research, as genetic testing for children and adolescents becomes increasingly feasible, research should focus on the effectiveness of proposed preventive and therapeutic interventions and on the psychosocial impact of tests (ASHG/ACMG, 1995).

The American Society of Human Genetics and the American College of Medical Genetics also recommend that providers who receive requests for genetic testing in children and adolescents should weigh the interests of children and adolescents and those of their parents and families. The provider and the family both should consider the medical, psycho-social, and reproductive issues that bear on providing the best care and on promoting the well-being of children and adolescents. Finally, because children and adolescents are part of a network of family relationships, as they grow through successive stages of cognitive and moral development, parents and professionals should be attentive to the child's and adolescent's increasing interest and ability to participate in decisions about their own welfare.

Employment and insurance

Employment and insurance are two of the most tangible ways in which genetic information may be used (Rothstein and Knoppers, 1996). Out of fear of not obtaining employment or insurance, many individuals who are at risk of genetic disorders may forego genetic testing. As we have seen above in regard to privacy and confidentiality of genetic information, the disclosure of genetic information to employers or insurers is not foreclosed, especially considering the fact that in order to obtain insurance or employment, access to medical records is usually requested.

Workplace testing for harmful, environmental agents has long been ongoing. Today, genetic testing can be used to predict which asymptomatic workers are likely to develop late-onset disorders or multifactorial disorders. While employers have the right to select the employees qualified for the position, the problem with genetic disorders is that individuals can be identified before the onset of symptoms.[4] Pre-employment genetic testing should only be undertaken when it is scientifically shown to be directly job-related.

Genetic testing is being introduced into the insurance underwriting process (Masood, 1996). In 1991, a report of the American Council of Life Insurance and the Health Insurance Association of America concluded that as genetic testing becomes more available, genetic information should be as relevant and accessible as any other medical

---

4 In Europe, many jurisdictions have adopted prospective policy positions regarding genetic testing. The European Parliament (1990) has declared that selection on the basis of genetic predisposition must never be an alternative to cleaning up the workplace, that employees should have the right to refuse genetic testing without consequences, and there should be no storage of genetic data on workers. As for the Council of Europe (1996), it recommended that all predictive testing of genetic disease be specifically restricted to that which is performed for health purposes or for scientific research linked to health purposes only. The House of Commons Select Committee on Science and Technology in Great Britain supported these recommendations while the French National Ethics Committee asked for a specific legislative prohibition (Rothstein and Knoppers, 1996).

information. In the USA, a NIH-DOE task force on genetic information and insurance recommended that until participation in a programme of basic health services is universal, alternative means of reducing the risk of genetic discrimination should be developed (Rothstein and Knoppers, 1996). Insurers should consider a moratorium on the use of genetic tests in underwriting and should undertake educational efforts within the industry to improve the understanding of genetic information. In Canada, where health care is universally available, a study paper for the Law Reform Commission of Canada as well as the Science Council of Canada made the same recommendation – that some form of basic life insurance be universally available at the same premium, with additional insurance optional and contingent upon genetic information provided by the applicant (Knoppers, 1991; Science Council of Canada, 1992).

In Europe, the World Medical Association adopted a position against any testing by insurers and against asking specific questions about the results of genetic tests (Last World Medical Assembly, 1992). The UNESCO Declaration and the proposed European Convention on Bioethics recommend that genetic data be protected from third parties except where the law provides otherwise or where justified by general interest (Council of Europe 1996; UNESCO 1996).

Ownership and patents

The failure of the November 1996 European Directive on the legal protection of biotechnology, inventions, and more specifically, on patents on living forms, had as much to do with the real world of competition in the gene hunt, as it did with public misunderstanding of DNA banking and the function of patent law (Council of Europe, 1996). Several notorious events contributed to this controversy. The first was the famous 1988 American case of Mr Moore whose 'interesting' and rare form of leukaemia led to the development of a cell line and profits for the researchers and institution involved but not for Mr Moore who was quite unaware of these mercantile developments. When he sued for a share of the profits on the basis of the fact that his body was his property, he failed. The Court reasoned that the implications for research, for organ donation and indeed for the biotechnology industry itself were enormous. The Court did say, however, that liability could be based on a failure to obtain an informed consent and to reveal commercial interests (Moore v. Regents, 1988). The second occurred in 1991 when a NIH researcher, C. Venter, applied for a patent on partial DNA sequences of unknown function.

While the American Patent Office rejected the claim since it did not meet the traditional requirements of patentability, it threw a chill on traditional, international collaboration and exchange between scientists. Such speculation on the actual or future worth of DNA as well as an increasing mistrust by the very human 'sources' of DNA of the hidden biotech-university or government sponsored research alliance has spawned a new debate on the ownership of DNA.

Also, there is the proprietary approach to the samples themselves, typified by the Genetic Privacy Act where sample 'sources' own their DNA. At the level of databases, this approach is paralleled by the proprietary rights attached to the sequence data held by commercial entities such as Human Genome Science (HGS). Scientists can access such data if they agree to give HGS first refusal on any commercial development they find (Anonymous, 1995).

In contrast to the HGS proprietary approach, Genethon in France and more recently, Merck, have advocated open access to sequence data (Anonymous, 1994a). This approach has its parallel in the concept of DNA as being a part of the person which is given to a DNA bank subject to certain conditions based on personal values and beliefs (Knoppers et al., 1996).

Myriad Genetics has filed a patent on the *BRCA1* gene. This patent claims the rights to the gene and to all possible mutations that can give rise to the disease. The company intends to develop a diagnostic test based on the gene – 'a high-quality and inexpensive test' (Brown and Kleiner, 1994). Some collaborators are opposed to this commercializing of DNA and consider it is too early to develop a test, because *BRCA1* is a complicated gene and many mutations in the gene trigger disease (Brown and Kleiner, 1994). Other collaborators in the *BRCA1* research disagree with the patenting approach because they 'wish to offer families under their care, a prediction service based on the techniques they have developed with their own research, and thus refuse to pay a license to a company to do it' (Anonymous, 1994a). Partly in reaction to the way that the *BRCA1* patent is being handled, research teams have decided to form a consortium to share family data and primers between themselves (Anonymous, 1994a).

In December 1995, the race to unearth the second hereditary breast and ovarian cancer gene, *BRCA2*, was concluded (Wooster et al., 1995). Scientists at Myriad Genetics, who had isolated *BRCA1* in 1994, rushed to submit a patent application for *BRCA2* coinciding with the publication of Wooster et al. (1995). Two rival patent applications have been submitted in the UK and USA. Each group feels it has a case – the European group was the first to publish evidence that *BRCA2* has been cloned. The Myriad team points to having been the first to compile the full-length sequence of the gene. There is the possibility that the two teams will reach some form of cross-licensing agreement.

There is no doubt that the whole area of intellectual property and human genome research in general, as well as that of patents in particular require further study (Knoppers et al., 1996). The position of the research community and that of legislation as well as the international debate reflects the value placed on rewarding scientific discoveries and the individual and collective contributions to those discoveries (Beardsley, 1996).

Conclusion

Susceptibility testing for inherited cancers not only raises the usual array of ethical and legal issues inherent to all genetic testing – liability, privacy and confidentiality, vulnerable populations, employment and insurance, and ownership and patenting – but also serves to highlight the increased uncertainty as to their resolution because of the probabilistic nature of the information it provides. While classical legal principles will provide some guidance, much more discussion of the issues is needed. If such cancer testing is a forerunner, the frameworks put in place will require input from the patients and families, not just the scientific or legal experts. Traditional ethical principles too, while certainly applicable, should be revisited.

It goes without saying that genetic testing and counselling should embrace the four ethical principles of autonomy, beneficence, non-maleficence, and justice. But to these standard principles could be added those particular to communication within relationships. In the context of human genetics, we have recommended three new ethical principles: (1) the principle of reciprocity or exchange of knowledge and provision of choices – this principle recognizes an inequality between the knowledge held by individuals and that held by practitioners of medical genetics. Justice requires that such knowledge and thus power, be redistributed in a way that is beneficial to the individual; (2) the principle of mutuality or civic responsibility – genetic disease implicates not only the individual but also the family and future generations. This fact imposes a duty on the individual to help family members in the communication of genetic information and understanding of genetic disease; and (3) the principle of solidarity – the State in return for the free and willing participation of its citizens in research and testing should put in place legal and other regulatory mechanisms to protect them from untoward socio-economic discrimination. These three principles may constitute a solid basis for shared responsibility and for patient participation with a view to establishing genetic justice based on genetic responsibility (Knoppers, 1991).

The message emerging is 'that much more work needs to be done, both at the research and development level and in terms of basic research, before genetic testing for susceptibility to common diseases is accepted as a valid service' (Harper, 1995). Certainly, the same can be said for ethical and legal issues.

References

ASHG/ACMG. 1995. Report. Points to consider: ethical, legal, and psychosocial implications of genetic testing in children and adolescents. *American Journal of Human Genetics* **57**: 1233–41.

ASHG/Social Issues Committe. 1998. Professional disclosure of familial genetic information. *American Journal of Human Genetics* **63**. (In press.)

American Council of Life Insurance and the Health Insurance Association of America. 1991. *Report of the ACLI-HIAA Task Force on Genetic Testing.* Washington DC: US Government Printing Office.

Annas, G.J. 1992. Breast cancer screening in older women: law and patient rights. *The Journal of Gerontolgy* **47** (Special Issue): 121–5.

Anonymous. 1994a. NIH files counter-patent in breast cancer gene dispute. *Nature* **372**: 118.

Anonymous. 1994b. Genetic testing set for takeoff. *Science* **265**: 464–6.

Anonymous. 1995. A survey of biotechnology and genetics. *The Economist* (25 February): 2–18.

Baumiller, R. C. et al. 1996. Code of ethical principles for genetics professionals. *American Journal of Medical Genetics* **65**: 177–83.

Beardsley, T. 1996. Vital data. *Scientific American* (March): 100–5.

Brown, P., and Kleiner, K. 1994. Patent row splits breast cancer researchers. *New Scientist* (24 September): 4.

Code of Ethics of Physicians. R.R.Q. 1981. c. M-9. r. 4.

Comité Consultatif National d'Éthique pour les Sciences de la Vie et de la Santé (France). 1996. Génétique et médecine: de la prédiction à la prévention. *Médecine/sciences* **12**: 125–9.

Council of Europe. 1990. Recommendation No. R(90)13 of the Committee of Ministers to Member States on prenatal genetic screening. prenatal genetic diagnosis and associated genetic counselling. *International Digest of Health Legislation* **41**(4): 615.

Council of Europe. 1995. *Convention for the Protection of Human Rights and Dignity of the Human Being with regard to the Application of Biology and Medicine: Bioethics Convention.* Strasbourg: Directorate of Legal Affairs.

Dickens, B. and Park, N. 1996. Legal and ethical issues in genetic prediction and genetic counselling for breast, ovarian and colon cancer susceptibility. In *Proceedings of Critical Choices Symposium*, Princess Margaret Hospital, Toronto.

European Parliament. 1990. *Resolution on the Ethical and Legal Problems of Genetic Engineering in Ethical and Legal Problems of Genetic Engineering and Human Artificial Insemination. Committee on Legal Affairs and Citizen's Rights.* Luxembourg: Office for Official Publications of the European Communities.

Gevers, J.K.M. 1988. Genetic testing: the legal position of relatives of test subjects. *Medicine and Law* 7: 161–3.

Harper, P. 1995. Genetic testing, common diseases, and health service provision. *The Lancet* 346(23/30): 1646.

Knoppers, B.M. 1991. *Human Dignity and Genetic Heritage: Study Paper*, pp. 69–72. Ottawa: Law Reform Commission of Canada.

Knoppers, B.M. 1995. Professional norms: towards a Canadian consensus. *Health Law Journal* 3: 1–18.

Knoppers, B.M. (Project Director). 1996. *Genetic Testing.* Toronto: The Ontario Law Reform Commission.

Knoppers, B.M., Caulfield, T. and Kinsella, D. (Eds.). 1996. *Legal Rights and Human Genetic Material.* Toronto: Edmond Montgomery.

Knoppers, B.M. and Chadwick, R. 1994. The Human Genome Project: under an international ethical microscope. *Science* 265: 2033–4.

Knoppers, B.M. and Laberge, C. 1995. Research and stored tissues persons as sources. samples as persons? *JAMA* 274(2): 1806–7.

Last World Medical Assembly (44th). 1992. Declaration on the Human Genome Project. Marbella Spain. *International Digest of Health Legislation* 44(2): 150.

Loi N. 1994. 94-548 du 1er juillet 1994 relative au don et à l'utilisation des éléments et produits du corps humain à l'assistance médicale à la procréation et au diagnostic prénatal. *Journal de Officiel République Française* pp. 11060–8.

Macklin, R. 1992. Privacy control of genetic information. In *Gene Mapping: Using Law and Ethics as Guides*, ed. G.P. Annas and S. Elias. pp. 159–70. New York: Oxford University Press.

Macklin, R. and Knoppers, B. M. 1996. Genetic predisposition to cancer – issues to consider. *Cancer Biology* 7: 49–53.

Masood, E. 1996. Whose right to genetic knowledge? *Nature* 379: 389-92.

Moore *v.* Regents of the University of California. 249 Cal. Rptr. 494 (Cal. App. 2 Dist. 1988); 252 Cal. Rptr. 816 (Sup. Ct. 1988).

Motulsky, A.G. 1994. Predictive genetic diagnosis. *American Journal of Human Genetics* 55: 603–5.

National Council of Bioethics and Human Research (Sub-Committee). 1993. *Report of the Working Group on Research with Children with Genetic Disorders*, Communiqué 33(4): 1-33.

Nuffield Council on Bioethics. 1993. *Genetic Screening: Ethical Issues*, pp. 89–90. London: Nuffield Council on Bioethics.

Pittman Estate *v.* Bain. 1994. 112 D.L.R. (4th), pp. 257–482. Ontario Genetics Division.

President's Commission for the Study of Ethical Problems in Medicine and Biomedical and Behavioral Research. 1983. *Screening and Counseling for Genetic Conditions.* Washington DC: The Commission.

Rothstein, M.A. and Knoppers, B.M. 1996. Legal Aspects of Genetics. Work. and Insurance in North America and Europe. *European Journal of Health Law* 3: 143–61.

Royal Commission on New Reproductive Technologies. 1993. *Proceed with Care*, vols. 1 and 2. Ottawa: Minister of Government Services Canada.

Science Council of Canada. 1992. *Genetics in Health Care. Report 42.* Ottawa: Minister of Supply and Services Canada.

Scriver, C. and Fujiwara, T.M. 1992. Invited editorial: cystic fibrosis genotypes and views on screening are both heterogeneous and population related. *American Journal of Human Genetics* **51**: 943–50.

Sharpe, N. 1994. Psychological aspects of genetic counselling: a legal perspective. *American Journal of Human Genetics* **50**: 234–5.

Skene, L. and Charlesworth, M. 1996. The new genetics: legal and ethical implications for medicine. *Medical Journal of America* **165**: 301–3.

UNESCO. 1996. *Revised Outline of a Declaration on the Protection of the Human Genome.* Paris: International Bioethics Committee.

Vines, G. 1994. Gene tests: the parents' dilemma. *New Scientist* (12 November): 40–4.

Wertz, D., Fanos, J.H. and Reilly. P.R. 1995. Genetic testing for children and adolescents: who decides? *JAMA* **272**(11): 875–81.

Wolf, S.M. 1995. Beyond 'Genetic discrimination': toward the broader harm of geneticism. *Journal of Law Medicine and Ethics* **23**: 345–53.

Wooster, R. et al. 1995. Identification of the breast cancer gene BRCA2. *Nature* **378**: 789-91.

Working Party of the British Clinical Genetics Society. 1994. The genetic testing of children. *Journal of Medical Genetics* **31**: 785-7.

4

Cancer genetics and public expectations

DOROTHY NELKIN

Summary

The public understanding of genetic issues is influenced by the prevailing popular culture and media coverage. This may lead to unrealistic expectations as to what the geneticist can provide, with a gulf of communication between the public and the professional. The impact of genetic testing on insurance premiums and social stigmatization depends on this public perception of the meaning of the results of such tests, and the moral and social judgements made depend inextricably upon the cultural and social attitudes. This chapter discusses and develops these issues, using examples of the way words such as 'gene' are used in the popular media.

Introduction

In September 1995, geneticists from the National Institutes of Health held a press conference to announce their discovery that a particular mutation (185delAG) of the *BRCA1* gene, associated with hereditary susceptibility to breast and ovarian cancer, occurred with unusual frequency among Ashkenazi Jewish women. The scientists, who were about to publish a paper describing their research results in *Nature Genetics* (Struewing et al., 1995), worried that millions of alarmed Jewish women might rush to their doctors demanding a genetic test. They therefore convened Jewish community leaders to discuss the research and its limitations, to caution against alarm, and to announce their plans for the follow-up research necessary to establish the significance of the initial findings. They also negotiated with biotechnology firms to delay the marketing of genetic tests.

Some sense of the significance of the association was revealed through a population survey of Ashkenazi Jewish women, selected without regard to their family history of cancer. This survey found that approximately 1% carry the 185delAG mutation, suggesting that the alteration is present not only in high risk families but in the broader population as well (Struewing et al., 1995). But, in the light of continued biological uncertainties and the ethical, social, and legal implications of widespread testing, Francis Collins, Director of the National Center for Human Genome Research, again warned in January 1996 against the marketing and clinical application of tests (Collins, 1996). Predictably, however, companies were already developing tests and, barely six months after the early agreement to delay, several companies began to market the test for the *BRCA1* variant and later introduced full sequence commercial testing of the *BRCA2* gene as well.

The goal of genetic testing is to detect susceptible individuals – those who are currently asymptomatic, but predisposed to a genetic condition. Given the very large numbers of women potentially at risk for breast cancer, commercial laboratories are eager to market genetic tests. Developing a test can be technically straightforward, involving the identification of a single alteration on a gene located in a known position. However, in many cases there is great heterogeneity of mutations necessitating complex mutation detection methods and difficulties in the interpretation of results. There are also biological and social uncertainties about the meaning of 'susceptibility'. The relation between a DNA sequence of a gene and the corresponding phenotype is not simple (Hubbard and Lewontin, 1996). Moreover, testing is socially problematic, for tests have only statistical, not absolute validity, and no satisfactory therapeutic options are available. A woman confronted with an abnormal test result would not know what it means in terms of her actual risk, nor would she have any certain way to protect herself against the disease. Discovering her future risk of cancer could expose this woman and her family, also implicated by the genetic information, to insurance or employment discrimination (Billings et al., 1992)

Thus, a healthy woman diagnosed as genetically predisposed to breast cancer would face a series of difficult practical choices as she seeks to integrate the information from a test – should she undergo a prophylactic mastectomy even though that is not a certain solution? How can she control access to genetic information so as to avoid discrimination and stigmatization? Should other family members, who may also be at risk, be informed? Should her children, potentially at risk, be tested? What are the implications for her future family planning?

The social and ethical dilemmas of presymptomatic testing have been much discussed in the context of Huntington disease and other relatively rare mendelian disorders (Holtzman, 1989; Nelkin and Tancredi, 1994; Wexler, 1992). As scientific attention turns to more common and complex conditions such as cancer, these problems will be greatly amplified (Marteau and Richards, 1996). Yet, given the pace of discovery, there are too few trained genetic counsellors available to help people under-stand genetic information, its implications, and make informed choices about how to respond. Responses will rest in part on public understand-ing of genetic research, on people's expectations, and on their beliefs about the meaning of genetic information.

One approach to the public understanding of science is through the messages and images conveyed through the news media and other vehi-cles of mass culture. The gene has a ubiquitous presence in popular culture. Reports about genetic research and stories about its clinical and social implications appear repeatedly in media reports, magazine articles, television programmes, talk shows, advertisements, and childcare books (Nelkin and Lindee, 1995). These media messages matter. They help create the unarticulated assumptions and fundamental beliefs under-lying personal decisions, social policies, and institutional practices. And they influence the demand for genetic tests and the way people respond to genetic information. In her study of women in genetic counselling clinics, for example, anthropologist Rayna Rapp found that their responses were directly influenced by the world of medicalized melodramas – *Dallas, St. Elsewhere*, and the *Jerry Lewis Telethon* (Rapp, 1988).

This chapter explores the representation of genetics in popular culture, describing repeated stories, metaphors, and images that convey the clin-ical and social implications of genetic research. The frequent media reports of new discoveries encourage optimistic expectations about the predictive power of genetic testing and the possibility of genetic therapy. Science seems to resolve the uncertainties of dread disease and provide an effective means of therapeutic control. But, countering the technological optimism of media reports are repeated warnings about the risks of genetic discrimination and the moral dilemmas involved in 'tampering' with genes. I will describe these themes as they appear in media reports and popular culture narratives, suggesting their importance in shaping the public meaning of genetic information.

The powers of prediction

The announcement of the cloning of the *BRCA1* gene and the discovery of the gene alteration prevalent among Ashkenazi women attracted vast media attention that often overstated its implications (Goldgar and Reilly, 1995). These stories played to receptive readers, primed by popular expectations about the meaning of genetic predisposition and the predictive power of genetic tests.

The gene in popular culture is an agent of destiny, an oracle, a blueprint, a medical crystal ball. Journalists convey this sense of determinism, 'Our fate is in our genes' (Jaroff, 1989, p. 62). The message appears in visual images – a cartoon portrays 'Ms Tena, reader advisor' standing in front of her shop. Next door is her competitor, 'Madame Rosa, geneticist'. Both women are in the business of predicting fate (Downes, 1987).

Journalists describe geneticists as sleuths deciphering the genetic text, pioneers working on the genetic frontier, hunters 'stalking the killer' (Nelkin, 1995). Every new discovery of a marker or a gene becomes a 'breakthrough' that will 'unlock the key to human ailments', and reveal the 'secret of life'. Deterministic language pervades mass media messages about the meaning of the genes.

Presenting personal stories, the media encourage hopes and expectations about the value of genetic testing. In one often repeated tale, a woman from a 'cancer family' is about to have a double mastectomy when, just days before her operation, a genetic test reveals that she does not, in fact, carry the mutant gene. Another story is about a family with a history of colon cancer. They have all submitted to painful annual colonoscopies in order to detect early signs of the disease, but now, because of genetic testing, they know who is susceptible and who will be spared.

Parental advice books and magazines are an important source of public information, and they too convey the promise of genetic prediction. Readers of *Child* magazine find out that tests can provide an 'early peek at genetic endowments' (LaForge, 1991). Women's magazines advise parents to discover their children's predispositions, to decipher the 'script' imposed by the genes (Shute, 1988). A medical journalist suggests that parents make a genogram with all the information they can find about their relatives. A gene data bank, Vivigen Genetic Repository, advertises its services to parents – 'Here's a healthy gift that really counts: DNA for your loved ones for future genetic analysis' (Chavez, 1991). The idea is to store genetic data so that children will benefit from the eventual availability of diagnosis and cure. Seldom do such media accounts dwell on the multiple, complex, and poorly understood causes of cancer, and the statistical meaning of being 'predisposed'.

The popular view of genetic predisposition differs in significant ways from scientific understanding. For scientists, the concept of genetic predisposition signals that an individual may suffer a future disease. A predisposition to cancer is less a prediction than a statistical risk calculation, and many variables may influence its future expression. In popular media reports, this statistically driven concept becomes reduced to cause – there are persons or families 'at risk'. And possible future states are often defined as equivalent to current status. We read about cancer genes, alcohol genes, criminal genes, or obesity genes as if a predisposition will be expressed regardless of the influence of dietary, social or environmental factors. We are, the media tell us, victims of a molecule, captives of heredity, fated by our genes. But media stories also offer hope that genetic information will enhance our ability to control disease in this 'long awaited era of genetic therapy'.

Therapeutic controls

Reports on the genetics of cancer are reaching a vulnerable public that is eager for solutions to devastating diseases and hopeful about genetics as the medicine of the future. Futuristic scenarios and hyperbolic headlines encourage optimistic expectations. 'Genetic research leaves doctors hopeful for cures', 'New hope for victims of disease', 'The long awaited era of genetic therapy has at last arrived'. The popular science magazine, *Discover*, describes 'The Ultimate Medicine . . . Genetic surgeons can now go into your cell to fix those genes with an unlikely scalpel: a virus' (Montgomery, 1990, pp. 60–8). Interviewed for the *Discover* article, molecular biologist Richard Mulligan declared, 'We can use gene transfer to make a cell do whatever we want. We can play God on that cell'.

US News and World Report tells its readers that gene therapy, 'the medicine of the future', is a potent weapon against cancer. 'No disease has given up more of its secrets to genetic sleuths than cancer.' Genetics, promised the writer, will allow doctors to identify diseases and 'do something about them' (Silberner 1991, p. 64). Another journalist covered genetics as 'the medical story of the century, [which] will dramatically cure cancer, heart disease, aging, and much more' (Rosenfeld, 1992).

Such reports often just reiterate the enthusiastic promises of scientists. In 1993, *Science* celebrated the discovery of a tumor suppressor gene as

'The molecule of the year', encouraging reports about the possibilities of preventing and curing 'a terrible killer in the not too distant future' (Koshland, 1993, p. 1953). A clinical investigator wrote, 'It seems the long awaited era of genetic healing has at last arrived' (Culver, 1993). Dr. W. French Anderson informed a *Time* Reporter that 'Physicians will simply treat patients by injecting a snippet of DNA and send them home cured' (Dewitt, 1994). The isolation of a colon cancer gene in 1993 prompted a scientist to tell a *New York Times* reporter that, 'The great thing about the diagnostic implications of this work is that deaths are entirely preventable' (Angier, 1993).

Such reports turn tentative experimental findings into magic bullets. They are encouraged by scientists and the press offices of their institutions as they seek the publicity that they hope will create a positive public image of science and help to attract research funds. A press release from Scripps Research Institute in January 1995, for example, promised a cure for cancer through a small injection of a protein that would cut off the blood supply from tumors and cause them to shrink, while leaving normal tissue intact. The press release was about a laboratory observation, there had been no experimental trials to test the relevance of the observation to human pathology (Altman, 1995).

In our entrepreneurial culture, commercial interests contribute to media hype. Biotechnology companies believe that media coverage will help create a market for their products. In the light of the huge potential market for cancer therapies, every advance in this area becomes a business event. *Forbes*, featuring a gene therapy company in San Diego that specializes in cancer, announced 'the birth of a mega-market'. Corporate advertisements promise 'a great leap forward in the treatment of disease'. An advertisement for a pharmaceutical product reads: 'Bad Genetics?' Use Opti-genetics – 'The first genetic optimizer'. A pharmaceutical company advertisment, appearing soon after the discovery of the *BRCA1* breast cancer gene, admits that 'finding a cure for breast cancer will not be easy'. But, it reads, 'Our researchers are working to find a breakthrough . . . new treatments and ultimately the cure for breast cancer'.

Such messages repeatedly suggest the immanence of therapeutic benefits from genetic research. They reflect the pressures from aggressive sources of information, eager to promote the latest techniques, as well as a sense of what consumers, hoping for panaceas, want to hear. But there is a counterside to promotional hyperbole, for exaggerated promises that dovetail with people's hopes and expectations open the way to cynicism should promises falter or fail. In the case of cancer research, a growing realization of the practical difficulties of extending laboratory studies of gene therapies to clinical applications is puncturing inflated expectations, and this is increasingly reflected in media reports. Describing the research on the unusual frequency of the 185delAG mutation among Ashkenazi Jews, for example, a journalist questioned whether it 'makes sense to screen healthy people for the defect, given that there is now no good therapy to offer those in whom it is found' (Kolata, 1995).

The distance between diagnostic understanding and the availability of therapeutic solutions is an old story. The development of diagnostic techniques has always outpaced the ability of medical practitioners to provide appropriate treatment (Nelkin and Tancredi, 1994). Until the twentieth century, clinicians had focused most of their attention on the art of diagnosis, because few treatments were available for the many existing diseases. Lacking therapeutic options, they emphasized the importance of describing their patients as accurately and scientifically as possible. The process of discovery became an objective in itself and the value of a test rested less on therapeutic implications than on its contribution to the refinement of medical evaluation.

Today, with access to more and more knowledge about bodily processes, the public expects results. But understanding genetic diseases does not necessarily lead to benefits beyond the ability to predict. Indeed, the growing access to genetic information has left us in a state of what Robert Proctor has called 'enlightened impotence' (Proctor, 1995, p. 247). And the value of enlightenment is increasingly tempered by awareness that predictive information about genetic status may expose an individual to stigmatization and discrimination.

Genetic discrimination

News about genetic tests often include stories about families who have lost their insurance or employment on the basis of a genetic predictions. In the contemporary political economy, preoccupied with cost-containment and efficient planning, predictive information becomes an institutional resource, a way to avoid costly decisions and to reduce future risks. Discrimination on the basis of their genetic predisposition is a growing problem, and this is part of the story of genetics conveyed in the press. Describing discoveries of new markers or the development of new tests, journalists warn of the problems in maintaining confidentiality of test results. We read that genetic tests for breast cancer offer a 'Faustian bargain . . . Patients who carry mutations can lose their insurance'

(Rubin, 1994, p. 61). Given the risks of discrimination, asks another journalist, 'Do you really want to peek into this crystal ball?' (Monson, 1995, p. 64).

Such warnings are influencing personal decisions. Some people who know from their family history that they are vulnerable to a disease are choosing not to be tested even when tests are available. And when they are tested, they worry about the abuse of genetic information. Personal accounts reveal the concerns of people whose 'lives are lived in the shadow of genetic disease' (Marteau and Richards, 1996). Two sisters who had been diagnosed as having the alteration in the *BRCA1* gene that increased their susceptibility to breast and possibly colon cancer decided to keep their genetic status secret. Insisting on anonymity, they spoke as 'Jackie' and 'Emma' at a workshop on insurance discrimination – to protect their family from discrimination, they said they were often forced to lie (National Action Plan, 1995). Their worries are well founded. A 1993 survey of insurance companies from 32 states found that 44% believed that a family history of breast cancer would be an acceptable reason to deny a woman insurance coverage (NIH/DOE, 1993). And a 1995 survey of people with a known genetic condition in their family found that 22% had been refused health insurance because of their genetic status (Lapham, 1995).

Beyond such warnings about the practical implications of genetic prediction, the media express a set of moral reservations that mainly revolve around two issues: the practice of genetic manipulation and the eugenic implications of genetic prediction; and the patenting of genes.

Moral reservations

Genetic manipulation and eugenic implications

The gene has assumed an iconic importance in American culture where DNA is often treated as an essential entity, the 'secret of life', the way to define the essence of personhood and identity. Scientists have encouraged essentialist images by calling the genome the 'Bible', the 'Holy Grail', or the 'Book of Man', and conveying the idea that this molecular structure is more than a biological entity – 'DNA is what makes us human', said James Watson, the first director of the Human Genome Project. In this context, any research that suggests genetic manipulation is taboo.

Body parts – for example, the pineal gland, the heart, the blood, the brain – have all at various times in human history, represented the essential human self. Today the genes are seen as the essence of humanity. DNA, in many media stories, appears as sacred territory, a taboo arena that should never be manipulated. These concerns are most explicit in religious publications that question the right to 'tamper' with genes, to 'play God'. To manipulate genes is to move them to the profane realm of engineering and technology. This, it is feared, will compromise their sacred status.

While such views are often dismissed as a marginal response from groups with religious agendas, concerns about genetic manipulation extend well beyond such groups. In his 1995 Morgenthau Memorial lecture on 'The New Dimensions of Human Rights', Zbigniew Brzezinski defined what he believes to be one of the most critical problems of human rights today – 'the rapidly growing potential for the actual alteration of human individuality and for the inequitable social exploitation of that potential'. This 'momentous challenge' posed by science threatens 'dehumanization and destruction' (Brzezinski, 1995).

The 'peril' in 'uncontrolled tampering' is also a common theme in popular magazine reports. 'Lurking behind every genetic dream come true is a possible *Brave New World* nightmare', writes a *Time* reporter (Dewitt, 1989). 'To unlock the secrets hidden in the chromosomes is to open up the question of who should play God with man's genes'. An accompanying image portrayed scientists balancing on a tightrope of coiled DNA. A writer in *US News and World Report* worries about 'tinkering with destiny' (Rubin, 1994). And an illustration for a *New York Times* article on gene therapy features a drawing, imitative of the famous Edvard Munch painting 'The Scream' in which a figure stands horrified, mouth ajar, eyes wide open, its hair a mass of coiled DNA (Goldenburg, 1990).

Moral reservations about advances in genetic understanding include the ever-present fear of its eugenic implications. Anti-abortionists often cite a comment they attribute to geneticist Sir Francis Crick, 'No newborn infant should be declared human until it has passed certain tests regarding its genetic endowment . . . If it fails these tests, it forfeits the right to live' (Chamberland, 1986, p. 20). This remark is an extreme expression of an increasingly urgent set of questions – 'Is it right to bring a damaged child into the world?' Do carriers of genetic diseases have a duty to prevent their perpetuation?

Questions of family planning present dramatic dilemmas for those who discover they are predisposed to a genetic disease, and they have also become a plot in fictional dramas that reach throusands of television viewers. In 1991, an episode of the TV series *Northern Exposure* featured a man who was reluctant to marry because of a history of violence in his family. Would he perpetuate his potentially destructive genes? His situation was described in the TV episode as a 'Genetic Chernobyl'. A *Star Trek* programme revolved around a society that had 'controlled procreation to create people without flaws'. And a talk show program debated the decision of anchorwoman Bree Walker Lampley to have a baby. Lampley, who has a genetic condition called ectrodactyly, was questioned on the air about her 'genetic responsibility'. Such popular narratives are suggesting an expansion of parental responsibility, implying that those who plan to bear a child should consider not only the emotional cost of a disability but also the economic and social burden of a less than perfect offspring on the state.

Media discussions of germline therapy that would alter the reproductive lineage explicitly raise the threat of eugenic implications. Those who welcome germline engineering view it as a humane technology of great benefit to people with severe genetic conditions who want to bear children. But some perceive such techniques as interfering with 'God's Will'. And others see a slippery slope towards the use of the technology to enhance desired physical or behavioural traits. Critics regard genetic engineering in the context of the commercialization of genetics – the interest of biotechnology firms in expanding the applications of new techniques.

Commercialization and gene patenting

The ties between the science of genetics and its commercial applications – the conflicts of interest when 'profits and ethics collide' – have invited public cynicism. The media repeatedly call attention to the non-medical interests – the investments, the quest for profits, the intense competition for priority – that are driving research and the development of clinical applications such as genetic tests. Troubled journalists report debates over patenting genes and question the very fact that genes – that 'life itself' – can be patented and owned. They describe the 'genetic gold rush', driven by an expanding biotechnology industry where profits may prevail over people. The legal aspects of the patenting issue in genome research is discussed in Chapter 3.

The media express several concerns about commercialization in this field of science, its influence on the direction of research, its implications for our view of the body, and its meaning for the integrity of science.

Some worry that patenting possibilities are skewing the direction of
research. A newsletter published by a cancer prevention group, asks
why so much more 'hoopla' is focused on the race to pin down the breast
cancer gene than on a method of reducing potentially harmful substances
in the environment (Arditte and Schreiber, 1994). Cancer prevention
groups argue that the genes are only one part of a complex picture,
and that we cannot afford to ignore the role of environmental pollutants
if we are to understand and control the growing cancer rates. The nearly
exclusive focus on cancer genetics, they believe, is diverting attention
away from more critical questions.

Religious forces have organized against biotechnology research for
quite different reasons – the implications of manipulating the body and
commodifying life. Since the 1980 US Supreme Court decision authoriz-
ing the patenting of new life forms, religious leaders have demanded
government review of developments in genetic engineering. 'New life
forms may have dramatic potential for improving human life' said the
National Council of Churches in 1980, but 'the cure may be worse than
the original problem.' In June 1983, fifty religious leaders signed a resolution opposed to 'efforts to engineer specific genetic traits into the germline of the human species.' And in 1995, eighty religious leaders resolved
to oppose patenting of genes as a form of 'commodification of life'. While
their statement focused on patenting and took no formal stand on genetic
manipulation, the implications were obvious, for without the right to
patent, there would be less incentive for industries to assume the high
costs of developing new diagnostic tools or therapeutic products.

The corporate ties of geneticists, their shares in biotechnology firms,
have inevitably attracted media skeptics who are disillusioned by the
changes in the culture of science. Science writers have long admired –
even adulated – the norms of science and the ideals of scientific objectivity (Nelkin, 1995). That scientists should have commercial interests vio-
lates their image of science as pure and unsullied by profits (Lyon and
Gorner, 1995). Their critiques of corporate-driven science reflect a
broader public ambivalence about science – whether it is to be supported
as an abstract pursuit of objective truth or as a useful and marketable
endeavour. Journalists these days are describing scientists not only as
sleuths and pioneers, but as 'greedy entrepreneurs', 'gene merchants',
or 'molecular millionaires', driven by economic interests that threaten
their objectivity and override concerns about abuse. Cartoon images of
geneticists include corporate graphs and dollar signs. They portray
geneticists in less than flattering terms as naive, squabbling over patent

rights, and unaware of the social implications of their work. This image of the modern scientist, tainted by a relentless drive for commercial profit, also appears in some of the most popular films about science such as *The Fugitive* and *Jurassic Park*.

Conclusion

In this chapter, I have described some of the themes and images that pervade reports and representations of the gene in popular culture. The messages are complex – they project a mix of futuristic fantasies and moral reservations, of inflated optimism and cautious cynicism. They reflect the perpetual hope of finding technological solutions to dread disease, but also the pervasive scepticism that is a part of the broader public image of science in the 1990s. These media messages are shaping the public understanding of genetics. They influence the decisions of individuals about whether or not to be tested and their choices of how to deal with the predictive information from genetic tests. They set a framework for the public expectations that will affect clinical practices and institutional policies concerning the use of predictive information. And they will bear on the future of a powerful science that offers promising applications, but also possibilities for pernicious abuse.

Acknowledgements

This chapter was developed with support from the National Center for Human Genome Research of the NIH: Grant 1R01 HG0047-01. Some of the material appears in Dorothy Nelkin and Susan Lindee, *The DNA Mystique: The Gene as a Cultural Icon*, W.H. Freeman, 1995. I would like to thank Dr. William Foulkes for supplying some useful reprints.

References

Altman, L. 1995. Promises of miracles. *New York Times* (January 10):C3.
Angier, N. 1993. Scientists isolate gene that causes cancer of colon. *New York Times* (December 3): A1.
Arditte, R. and Schreiber, T. 1994. Breast cancer: organizing for protection. *Resist* 3: 1–8.
Billings, P., Kohn, M. A. and de Cuevas, M. 1992. Discrimination as a consequence of genetic testing, *American Journal of Human Genetics* 50: 475–575.
Brzezinski, Z. 1995. The new dimensions of human rights. Morgenthau Memorial Lecture, Carnegie Council on Ethics and International Affairs, New York

58

Chamberland, D. 1986. Genetic engineering: promise and threat. *Christianity Today* (7 February): 20.

Chavez, L. 1991. Brochure. Santa Fe: Vivigen Genetic Repository, New Mexico.

Collins, F. S. 1996. *BRCA1* – Lots of mutations, lots of dilemmas. *New England Journal of Medicine* 334: 186–88.

Culver, K.W. 1993. Splice of life: gene therapy comes of age. *The Sciences* 1: 18–24.

Dewitt, P.E. 1989. The perils of treading on heredity. *Time* (20 March): 70.

Dewitt, P.E. 1994. The genetic revolution. *Time* (17 January): 46–57.

Goldenburg, S. 1990. Drawing. *New York Times* (16 September): editorial.

Goldgar, D. and Reilly, P. 1995. A common *BRCA1* mutation in Ashkenazim. *Nature Genetics* 11: 113–14.

Holtzman, N. 1989. *Proceed With Caution*. Baltimore: Johns Hopkins Press.

Hubbard, R. and Lewontin, R.C. 1996. Pitfalls of genetic testing. *The New England Journal of Medicine* 334: 1192–1194

Jaroff, L. 1989. The gene hunt. *Time* (20 March): 62–7.

Kolata, G. 1995. Tests to assess risks for cancer raising questions. *New York Times* (27 March): A9.

Koshland, D. 1993. Molecule of the year. *Science* 262: 1953.

LaForge, A.E. 1991. Born brainy. *Child* (November): 88–90.

Lapham, E.V. and Weiss, J.O. 1995. Survey of the Alliance of Genetic Support Groups. Cited by K. Hudson et al. Genetic Discrimination and Health Insurance. *Science* 270: 391-3.

Lyon, J. and Gorner, P. 1995. *Altered Fates*. New York: Norton.

Marteau, T. and Richards, M. (eds). 1996. *The Troubled Helix*. Cambridge: Cambridge University Press.

Monson, N. 1995. Family Affairs. *Weight Watchers Magazine* (April): 32–7, 64.

Montgomery, G. 1990.The Ultimate Medicine. *Discover* (March): 60–8

National Action Plan on Breast Cancer. 1995. One family's experience. Workshop on Genetic Discrimination in Health Insurance, Sponsord by the National Action Plan and the ELSI working Group of the Human Genome Project, Bethesda, July 11,

NIH/DOE 1993. *Genetic Information and Health Insurance*. Washington DC: USGPO.

Nelkin, D. 1995. *Selling Science: How the Press Covers Science and Technology*, 2nd edn. New York: W. H. Freeman.

Nelkin, D. and Lindee, M.S. 1995. *The DNA Mystique: The Gene as a Cultural Icon*. New York: W. H. Freeman.

Nelkin, D. and Tancredi, L. 1994. *Dangerous Diagnostics: The Social Power of Biological Information*, 2nd edn. Chicago: University of Chicago Press, 1994.

Proctor, R. 1995. *Cancer Wars*. New York: Basic Books.

Rapp, R. 1988. Chromosomes and communication: the discourse of genetic counselling. *Medical Anthropology Quarterly* 2: 143–57.

Rosenfeld, A. 1992.The medical story of the century. *Longevity* (May): 42–53.

Rubin, R. 1994. Tinkering with destiny. *US News and World Report* (22 August): 56–61.

Shute, N. 1988. How healthy is your family tree?' *Hippocrates* (January/ February): 88–9.

Silberner, J. 1991. The age of genes. *US News and World Report* (4 November): 64–37.

Struewing, J.P., Abeliovich, D., Peretz, T. et al. 1995. The carrier frequency of the *BRCA1* 185delAG mutation is approximately 1 percent in Ashkenazi Jewish Individuals. *Nature Genetics* **11**: 198-200.
Wexler, N.1992. Clairvoyance and caution. In *The Code of Codes*, eds. D. Kevles and L. Hood, pp. 211–43. Cambridge: Harvard University Press,.

5
Genetic counselling
JUNE PETERS

Summary

This chapter focuses primarily on genetic counselling for susceptibility to the common familial cancers such as breast and colon, with occasional reference to other hereditary cancer syndromes. Genetic issues commonly encountered by health professionals who are seeing families with cancer clusters are discussed. The chapter first addresses the general field of genetic counselling and education, then turns to familial cancer risk counselling, and finally to genetic, medical, psychological, ethical, and social concerns in genetic susceptibility testing.

Introduction: what is genetic counselling?

The worldwide effort to map the human genome is already having major effects on medical care. A wide variety of health professionals will soon be dealing routinely with applications of numerous technological advances in cancer genetics. These developments will increasingly be applied to clinical use in cancer diagnosis, prevention, treatment, monitoring for recurrence, and susceptibility, and the role of the genetic counsellor in the provision of information relating to the risk of adult-onset diseases, such as cancer, is likely to become more important.

Genetic counselling definition

Genetic counselling during the twentieth century has evolved from several streams of input: eugenics, public health, academic study of human genetics, health psychology, and medicine (Kenen, 1984; Fine, 1993; Sorenson, 1993). Reed coined the modern term 'genetic counselling' and defined it as 'encompassing knowledge of human genetics, respect for the sensitivities, attitudes and reactions of the client, and the desire to teach the truth to the full extent that it is possible' (Reed, 1955).

In the 1970s an attempt was made by professional societies to make this definition more explicit. Since that time, genetic counselling has been defined as a communication process which deals with the human problems associated with the occurrence, or risk of occurrence of a genetic disorder in a family (Ad Hoc Committee of ASHG, 1975). Explicitly included in this definition are helping the individual or family to: (1) comprehend the medical facts; (2) appreciate the way that heredity contributes to the disorder, and to the risk of recurrence in specified relatives; (3) understand the alternatives for dealing with the risk of occurrence; (4) choose among alternative courses of action; and (5) make the best possible adjustment to the diagnosis of the disorder in an affected family member and/or to the risk of recurrence of that disorder.

Genetic counselling requires the following elements: (1) eliciting a complete individual and family social, reproductive, and health history; (2) assessing genetic risk; (3) consulting with the individual and family about available clinical evaluation and testing options including risks, benefits, limitations, interpretation and possible psychological and economic consequences of genetic testing and diagnosis; (4) assessing psychosocial needs and making psychosocial interventions; (5) facilitating medical and reproductive decision-making in a non-directive fashion; (6) anticipatory grief and crisis counselling; and (7) facilitating medical screening, testing, or management options as requested by the individual or family.

Genetic counselling is likely to evolve further with the pressures of providing counselling for new diagnostic genetic tests for an increasing and diversified client population (Kenen and Smith, 1995). Changes are probable in both genetic service delivery systems and the development of alternative models of the genetic counselling process itself.

Genetic issues in genetic counselling

Genetic counselling involves the collection and documentation of genetic information in the family history, the educational opportunity to disseminate genetic information, and the establishment of statistical risk for occurrence or recurrence of disease. These are covered below with respect to cancer.

Family history

A detailed family history is elicited from the consultand (the person coming for consultation) and recorded as a pedigree (Resta, 1994). In the US, a Pedigree Standardization Task Force (PSTF) established recommendations for universal standards in human pedigree nomenclature (Bennett et al., 1993, 1995). These data include information about births, deaths, miscarriages, and abortions in a minimum of three generations, plus mention of mental retardation, birth defects, genetic conditions, and other illnesses such as cancer and heart disease. The ratio and pattern of affected and unaffected individuals influences risk analysis.

Genetic education

An important part of the genetic counselling process is to explain in understandable terms the principles of medical genetics, patterns of inheritance, and probability. Specific mention is made of reproductive recurrence risks, availability of genetic diagnostic testing, and reproductive options including availability of prenatal diagnosis.

Risk assessment in genetic counselling

Transmission and interpretation of risk information is difficult due to: problems for the layperson in understanding the laws of probability; applying an average population risk to the individual whose personal risk may in fact be much higher or lower than the average; preconceived notions about whether or not one will be affected; and the tendency to simplify ambiguous risks into simple binary categories that resolve uncertainty about outcome (Lippmann-Hand and Fraser, 1979a,b,c; Kessler and Levine, 1987; Evans, 1993; Palmer and Saintfort, 1993; Richards et al., 1995). Risk assessment may be offered in a variety of ways, including proportions, percentages, qualitative estimates of low, moderate or high, and the chances of not getting the disease as well as chances of having it. Sometimes risk figures are compared to another more familiar point of reference such as having another disease or accident.

The content of the genetic couselling session is generally recorded in a lengthy letter both to the referring physician and to the family. In addition, appropriate written literature, such as brochures and fact sheets, may be offered. For expediency, the content of some of the education for now commonplace procedures (e.g., amniocentesis or CF carrier testing) may be standardized in a set of slides, video, or even by using an interactive computer programme.

Medical content of genetic counselling

The scope of genetic counselling includes discussion of disease diagnosis, including the criteria for and certainty of diagnosis, the natural history of the disease over the lifespan, and whether the disease is expected to alter the natural lifespan. Although the presenting problem may involve just one organ, genetic diseases often involve disruption of multiple biological systems. Medical testing may be ordered to confirm diagnoses or to find occult signs of the disease in affected individuals and their relatives. Prenatal diagnosis refers to the diagnosis of genetic disease before birth and is accomplished by ultrasound, chorionic villus sampling, amniocentesis, percutaneous umbilical blood sampling, or fetal biopsy. Effective prevention or curative treatments rarely have been available for genetic diseases, so most medical interventions for genetic conditions involve secondary or tertiary prevention and symptom treatment.

Psychosocial assessment in genetic counselling

General areas of assessment include current mental status, mood, and the person's behaviour and responses during the genetic counselling process. Psychosocial information should include cultural background, childhood traumas, losses, or abuse; relationships and sexual history, family cohesiveness and communication styles; coping strategies, competencies, and support resources; and general psychosocial history. In addition, it is important to discuss beliefs, attitudes, and experiences when the specific genetic condition is being considered.

Psychosocial interventions in genetic counselling

The more cognitive aspects of genetic counselling will not be successful unless the counsellor attends to the emotional aspects concurrently (Epstein, 1975; Kessler, 1980). The genetic counsellor may need to help the consultand adjust to the knowledge of a genetic condition in the family (Peters, 1995).

Counsellors should be familiar with indications for psychiatric referral when signs of mental illness or distress are noted (Schneider, 1994). Suicide has been reported in some persons with high risk for expressing genetic disorders and the genetic counsellor should be aware of this possibility (Peters, 1994c). Other indications for referral are: clinical levels of depression, guilt, or anxiety; unresolved grief; obsessive, intrusive thoughts; overzealous health vigilance; severe sleep or eating disturbance;

drug or alcohol addiction; somatization; or disruptions in sexual functioning or satisfaction.

Genetic counselling process

Genetic counselling is practised in a variety of settings – academic medical centres, private testing sites, inter-disciplinary specialty clinics, and in research settings. In the US and Canada, performance of the various tasks of genetic counselling are often shared by a team of individuals including PhD or MD geneticists, post-doctoral fellows, masters level genetic counsellors or genetic nurses, and sometimes a variety of other medical specialists are needed to care for persons with multiple manifestations of genetic disease. Frequently, entire families are seen conjointly.

Directive counselling and non-directive counselling are generally taken to mean the offering or withholding of direct advice, often about reproduction and abortion (Kessler, 1992). Non-directiveness generally implies an assumption that consultands can and should make their own decisions about certain aspects of their healthcare.

Although non-directiveness is endorsed in the UK, a number of investigators have observed that all genetic counselling involves some element of direction given to participants, be it overtly delivered as medical advice, or covertly conveyed by counsellor selection of which information is given (Kessler, 1992). Cross-cultural experiences show that receiving advice from an expert is preferable to individual autonomy for a number of consultands of certain ethnic and cultural groups (McGoldrick, 1982; Weil and Mittman, 1993; Geller et al., 1995).

Familial cancer risk counselling

This is a communication process between healthcare professionals and individuals concerning the occurrence, of cancer in their families (Peters, 1994a; Table 5.1). These families are often seeking more information about the hereditary basis of cancer in the family, genetic testing, and advice about medical surveillance. These needs can most often be met by multi-disciplinary teams consisting of individuals with expertise in oncology, surgery, genetics, and counselling psychology.

The scope of this counselling is wide (Figure 5.1; Kelly, 1991; Schneider, 1994; Peters and Stopfer, 1996, table 1) and its aim includes reducing mortality through prevention and early detection, enhancing quality of care, establishing a co-ordinated approach to ascertainment,

Table 5.1. *Suggested components of comprehensive familial cancer risk counselling*

- Full, three-generation pedigree taken and extended as necessary
- Primary diagnosis documentation on all affected relatives
- Background information on genetics, oncology, and testing
- Statistical genetic risk assessment and counselling
- Identification of genetic susceptibility syndromes
- Psychosocial assessment and interventions
- Genetic susceptibility testing as appropriate
- Pre-test informed consent
- Susceptibility test result notification
- Post-test counselling and follow-up
- DNA banking on affected relatives as needed
- Recommendations for medical surveillance
- Referral to prevention trials
- Participate in multidisciplinary management teams
- Establish/liaison with hereditary disease registries
- Referral for additional consultations as needed
- Advocacy for patient rights to healthcare
- Establish/sustain support groups

Source: Adapated from Peters (1994a), with permission.

screening, diagnosis, treatment, and follow-up care for cancer, and implementation of future genetic technology such as gene-based treatments.

Family history screening and indications for referral

Ascertainment may occur at the time of diagnosis of a cancer, when considering reproductive options during medical screening, or when considering genetic susceptibility testing (Petersen, 1996b). Each consultand should have a family history taken, particularly noting relatives diagnosed with cancer, their age at diagnosis, current age, bilaterality, and occurrence of multiple different cancers.

Documentation of diagnoses is necessary by review of the pathology reports of biopsies and surgical specimens (reviews of diagnoses on death certificates may be inaccurate) or with reference to disease registries.

Genetic education

Families with cancer need varying degrees of background information about biology, genetics, oncology, epidemiology, and probability in order to comprehend fully the risk information they will later be given (Kelly,

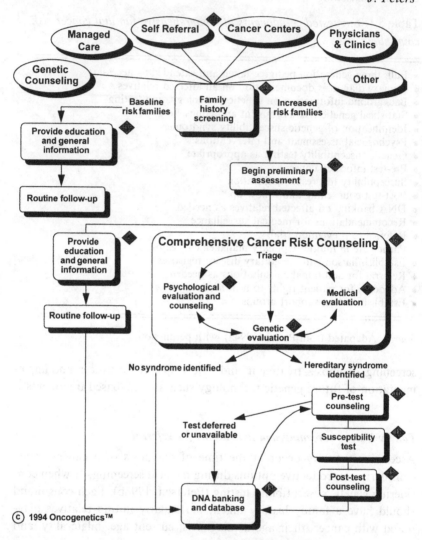

Figure 5.1   Cancer risk assessment and counselling protocol.

1991, 1992; Peters, 1994a,b, 1995; Schneider, 1994; Hoskins et al., 1995; Peters and Stopfer, 1996).

Popular sources of information that can be provided are books, brochures, newsletters, etc., written at the level of lay audiences (e.g., Kelly, 1991; Cooper, 1993), many of which are provided by specific hereditary cancer registries and support groups (e.g., in the US, The Von Hippel Lindau Family Alliance, and the *Hereditary Colon Cancer Newsletter*).

The National Cancer Institute of the US also provides written information, slide sets, telephone consultations, referral directories, and internet sites for supplemental cancer genetics information. In the US, these can be accessed by calling 1-800-4CANCER or through the NCI cancernet website at: www.cancernet.nci.nih.gov.

Familial cancer risk assessment

Cancer risk assessment refers to the process of quantifying the probability for an individual to develop cancer due to the presence of variables such as family history, environmental exposures, lifestyle, and chance, often in comparison to the general population 'baseline risk' of cancer.

Hoskins et al. (1995) present a guide for primary care clinicians for use in evaluating inherited breast cancer risk. Offit and Brown (1994) reviewed four different models for breast cancer risk assessment based on family history and other recognized risk factors. The most commonly used means of measuring risk are by estimating relative risk or cumulative risk. Individuals seem better to be able to understand and integrate cumulative risks over time in order to make concrete life decisions, for example, about career, family planning, and prophylactic surgery (Kelly, 1992). Methods for this analysis are detailed elsewhere (Anderson and Badzioch, 1985, 1989; Gail et al., 1989; Claus et al., 1994; Hoskins et al., 1995).

Diagnosing hereditary cancer syndromes

If the pedigree suggests a mendelian inheritance pattern of a cancer-predisposing condition and particularly when such a condition has been diagnosed in the family, risk assessment involves the discussion of two individual probabilistic events: (1) the chance that they will inherit the cancer susceptibility gene mutation; and (2) the manifestation of the disorder and the chance that people with this specific mutation will eventually develop cancer (penetrance). Reaching a correct diagnosis is crucial for genetic counselling. Hodgson and Maher (1993) have compiled a very useful text of known hereditary cancer syndromes, organized by site of origin and by syndrome.

When no specific syndrome can be identified, DNA banking from affected relatives within these families may be appropriate. The purpose would be for relatives at risk to have DNA available for testing when new gene discoveries are made. However, tissue storage itself has many ethical, legal, and social ramifications and should be undertaken only with fully informed consent.

Medical recommendations

Richards et al. (1995) have noted that for many consultands the central issue of genetic risk counselling is what to do about a risk they already perceive as high. Surveillance and prophylactic measures should therefore be discussed. Counsellors may also help the family to implement any recommendations made, and to address anxieties and explore obstacles to surveillance (Peters and Stopfer, 1996).

Medical treatment

Knowledge of genetic risk status may alter the appropriate treatment and the decision-making process for some individuals who learn that they are at high risk for development of subsequent tumours.

Psychosocial issues

Cancer risk counselling is conducted simultaneously on two different levels – the medical and the emotional (Royak-Schaler and Benderley, 1992). Lerman and colleagues (1995) have noted that efforts to counsel women about their breast cancer risks are not likely to be effective unless their breast cancer anxieties are also addressed.

Psychosocial assessment

The counsellor should explore the meaning of cancer to the individual and to the family and their theories of causation (Kenen, 1980; Kelly, 1992; Green et al., 1993; Richards et al., 1995; Grosfeld et al., 1996). Cancer may be perceived as a punishment, or risk status may be assumed to be based on physical or personality resemblance to an affected individual. Information offered by geneticists that is not in accordance with family explanations and expectations may be disregarded (Kenen, 1980; Grosfeld et al., 1996), so it is wise for counsellors to elicit underlying beliefs before undertaking genetic education.

Assessment should also include the emotional reactions to cancer and risk. Investigators in the Utah (USA) study of a large *BRCA1* family have observed that consultands with close relatives with cancer often expressed strong, long-term emotional effects of this legacy (Baty et al.,

1995) including, anxiety, anger, fear of developing cancer, fear of disfigurement and dying, grief, guilt, lack of control, negative body image, comparisons to affected relatives, altered sexual functioning and sense of isolation (Baker, 1991; Kelly, 1992; Wellisch et al., 1992; Lynch and Watson, 1992; Lynch and Lynch, 1993; Peters, 1995). Such anxiety and fear can have a major impact on daily activities, life decisions, and healthcare behaviour (Kash et al., 1992; Lerman et al., 1993), and may fluctuate with time. Genetic disorders also affect relationships, and adequate marital and family assessment, therefore, may be necessary.

There may also be differences in psychosocial issues depending on whether the family is newly ascertained or whether it has been known for years to have a hereditary cancer predisposition (Berk, 1996) and, on which cancers the relatives develop (Baker, 1991; Williams, 1991; Peters, ASHG lecture, 1994). In western culture, for example, breasts are symbolic of women's identity, nurturing, and sexuality, whereas the functions of the colon are often seen as dirty, shameful, and secret.

Psychosocial interventions

Grief counselling is often necessary and discussing the family history is an opportunity for relatives to remember and grieve their personal losses.

Many consultands enter the counselling process feeling fatalistic about getting and dying from cancer. Demonstrating a genetic model that gives a basis for believing that he or she has an equal chance of *not* getting cancer can be very therapeutic. Dispelling misconceptions can also serve to relieve emotional burdens. Individuals having trouble making decisions about genetic testing or about their healthcare may benefit from learning problem-solving or other decision-making skills (Lerman et al., 1996).

Kash et al. (1992), studying women at high risk who were attending a high risk surveillance programme, has shown that women at risk of breast cancer have psychological distress levels as great as women with actual cancer. A substantial subset of women who have an interest in breast cancer susceptibility testing have intrusive thoughts and other signs of anxiety and distress (Lerman et al., 1994b). Psychoeducational support group experience has been shown to improve surveillance adherence in this at-risk group, as has been demonstrated for women with cancer (Fawzy et al., 1990a,b; Spiegel, 1992).

Process of counselling

A key to advising consultands lies in knowing which proposed interventions have proven risks, benefits, and limitations, and which do not. A non-directive approach is particularly appropriate for reproductive decisions and in situations in which options have relatively equal risk:benefit ratios (e.g., choosing lumpectomy plus radiation versus mastectomy for certain breast cancers).

Schneider and Marnane (1995) conducted a survey of a subset of 50 genetic counsellors within the US who are currently conducting cancer risk counselling sessions. Whereas the majority believed that it was appropriate for counsellors to advise clients to follow widely accepted screening and lifestyle guidelines, many felt that it was inappropriate to advise regarding DNA testing options, prophylactic surgery, or disclose information to other family members at risk.

Organization of service

Peters (1994a, b, 1995) has adapted a comprehensive breast centre model (Lee et al., 1992a,b) to the development of genetic cancer risk counselling programmes (Figure 5.1). It is important for clinicians to consider how this might fit into various parts of their medical practice from referral through screening, triage, assessment, treatment and follow-up to optimize use of limited genetic counselling resources (Peshkin et al., 1995). Even some private laboratories have made testing available primarily within a genetic counselling infrastructure (e.g. OncorMed, Genetic Education and Testing Packets, 1996) or at the very least, profess a responsibility to prepare educational materials for physicians and their patients (Skolnick, 1996).

In contrast to this heterogeneity of approaches, co-ordinated national approaches are possible in smaller European countries. For example, in the Netherlands, genetic counselling is provided by clinical geneticists (with a genetic associate) at eight clinical genetics centres all linked to a university hospital. There is co-operation among the three main medical centres in Amsterdam in dealing with families in accordance with a single protocol known as the Amsterdam Protocol for Familial and Hereditary Tumours. This protocol specifies medical diagnosis and management recommendations as well as providing information for patients and family members (Fred Menko, 1995, pers. comm.).

Susceptibility testing – general concerns

Nature of genetic susceptibility tests

Cancer genetic susceptibility testing poses challenges due to genetic heterogeneity, profound personal and familial implications of results, and the possibilities of stigmatization, discrimination, misunderstanding and misuse of the information (Kenen, 1980; Durfy and Peters, 1993; Nelkin and Lindee, 1995; Biesecker, 1997; Peters and Biesecker, 1997). Genetic testing historically has been voluntary, available only for rare genetic conditions with a known monogenic basis, offered within the context of genetic counselling that supports autonomous decision-making, and with thorough informed consent about possible implications prior to test-taking. It is now being introduced for common diseases, in larger populations, and within mainstream medicine.

Laboratory selection

Laboratories performing research studies are often not the same as those providing clinical diagnoses for purposes of counselling. Not all laboratories perform all tests, and different laboratories may use non-overlapping methodologies, making comparisons difficult. The technical aspects of susceptibility testing are discussed in Chapter 8.

Selection of a laboratory that also offers tissue storage capabilities leaves open the possibility for testing at a later date.

Regulation of laboratory quality control

Assuring quality control for molecular testing is essential, and laboratories should adhere closely to general quality assurance programmes, be licensed, and participate in all applicable external proficiency testing programmes. In the US, clinical laboratories performing an examination of materials derived from the human body for the purpose of providing information for diagnosis, prevention, prognosis, or treatment of humans must obtain certification from the Health Care Finance Administration (HCFA) under the Clinical Laboratory Improvement Amendment (CLIA) of 1988 (Andrews et al., 1994).

Test interpretation, sensitivity, specificity, and genotype–phenotype correlations

It is appropriate to expect the laboratory to provide up-to-date information regarding test sensitivity and specificity (Boland, 1966; Menko et al., 1996). For example, interpretation of a particular genetic alteration may be influenced by whether it has ever been observed before in high risk families; whether the alteration causes a change in protein length, configuration, or function; how closely the family medical history of the current patient resembles those of the research families on which test interpretation is being based; family ethnic background; and the state of technology development being used by the laboratory selected. The laboratory report should take into account relevant genetic risk factors and be sufficiently clear and specific about limitations (Petersen and Brensinger, 1996).

Indications for cancer susceptibility testing

Genetic testing up to this point has been undertaken largely in the context of research studies where indications were selected based on research needs. There is a number of policy statements urging caution in this until more information is known about test characteristics and implications (Li et al., 1992; Evans et al., 1992, 1994; Lynch and Watson, 1992; Biesecker et al., 1993; King et al., 1993; ASHG, 1994; National Advisory Council for Human Genome Research, 1994; ASCO Sub-committee on Genetic Testing for Cancer Susceptibility, 1996).

Professional organizations are beginning to establish standardized indications for genetic testing for cancer susceptibility in an individual affected with cancer. For example, the American Society of Clinical Oncology (ASCO) has issued a statement that includes recommended indications for referral (ASCO Sub-committee on Genetic Testing for Cancer Susceptibility, 1996). These are: (1) the person has a strong family history of cancer or very early onset disease; (2) the test can be adequately interpreted; and (3) the results will influence the medical management of the patient or family member. Combinations of these criteria are then used to create three categories of indications for cancer predisposition testing.

Group 1 consists of tests for families with well-defined hereditary syndromes for which either a positive or negative result will change medical care, and for which genetic testing may be considered part of the standard management of affected families (see Table 5.2). Most practitioners now agree that genetic diagnostic and susceptibility testing under controlled circumstances is indicated for these diseases.

Group 2 includes tests for known cancer susceptibility genes, for which the medical benefit of the identification of a heterozygote carrier is presumed but not established. The potential clinical value and reliability of the test is based on research studies. Included in group 2 are hereditary

Table 5.2. *Selected hereditary cancer predisposition syndromes*

Syndrome	Gene
Hereditary breast and breast–ovarian	*BRCA1, BRCA2*
Li–Fraumeni syndrome (LFS)	*TP53*
Cowden syndrome	*PTEN*
Familial adenomatous polyposis (FAP)	*APC*
Hereditary non-polyposis colorectal cancer (HNPCC)	*MSH2, MLH1, PMS1, PMS2, MSH6*
Multiple endocrine neoplasia type 1 (MEN1)	*MEN1*
Multiple endocrine neoplasia (MEN2A,B)	*RET*
Neurofibromatosis 1 (NF1)	*NF1*
Neurofibromatosis 2 (NF2)	*NF2*
von Hippel–Lindau syndrome (VHL)	*VHL*
Basal cell venus syndrome (Gorlin syndrome)	*PTC*
Retinoblastoma	*RB1*
Wilms' tumour	*WT1, FWT1* (not identified)
Ataxia-telangiectasia (AT)	*ATM*
Peutz-Jeghers syndrome	Not identified

non-polyposis colorectal cancer (HNPCC), hereditary breast–ovarian cancer syndrome, and Li–Fraumeni syndrome. There is some controversy about whether, when, how and for whom testing should be offered in this group. A subset of members of the ASCO sub-committee differed from the majority report. In their view, genetic testing for beast cancer susceptibility should not be offered outside the context of hypothesis-driven research approved by institutional review boards.

Finally, group 3 is the most controversial. Included in this group are tests for individuals without a family history of cancer, conditions in which the significance of the detection of a germline mutation is not clear, and tests for hereditary syndromes for which the germline mutations have been identified in only a small subset of families.

Several commentaries to the ASCO Statement were published concurrently by representatives of the National Breast Cancer Coalition (Visco and the National Breast Cancer Coalition, 1996), Myriad Genetics Inc. (Skolnick, 1996), and the National Action Plan on Breast Cancer (Collins and NAPBC, 1996). The two statements from the consumer coalitions call for partnerships between patients, physicians, and researchers in attempts to recognize and address the many unanswered questions regarding the ramifications of susceptibility testing, and urge consumers to be wary of testing outside of research protocols.

Technical advances in the ability to detect mutations with improved levels of sensitivity, specificity and speed are evolving. These developments will undoubtedly alter indications for testing; however, the technical ability to perform tests for mutations should not be confused with a mandate to offer them (Collins and NAPBC, 1996).

Susceptibility test context

Genetic susceptibility testing should always occur within the context of a supportive professional relationship between counsellor/physician/nurse and the consultand (ASHG, 1994). This can be accomplished through a co-ordinated research investigation or a clinical programme.

With informed consent, individuals in the family who are affected with cancer are tested first to search for mutations in a particular gene known to cause a hereditary cancer syndrome. If a pathogenic mutation is found in one or two family members with cancer, the testing of their relatives will be informative.

Genetic counselling for susceptibility testing

Biesecker et al. (1993) set out the genetic counselling necessary for susceptibility testing for inherited breast cancer. This approach had a strong emphasis on the importance of pre-test counselling, the multi-disciplinary team approach, and the necessity of follow-up for family members tested. Grosfeld et al. (1996) has described genetic counselling for multiple endocrine neoplasia type 2 (MEN2), Lynch et al. (1996) and Menko et al. (1996) for HNPCC, and Petersen (1996b) for familial adenomatous polyposis (FAP).

Currently, testing is being offered mainly to self-referred persons within high risk families or from registries. As testing becomes more commonplace, the possibility of testing may be introduced to people who have never heard of susceptibility testing or who had never previously thought much about it. Presumably this group will need more basic pre-test education.

Schneider (1994) discusses genetic principles for genetic susceptibility testing, and observes that there are at least three distinct aspects of the testing process: (1) informed consent during pre-test counselling; (2) disclosure of results; and (3) follow-up counselling.

Informed consent

Informed consent refers to a communication process (usually both oral and written) between health care providers and consultands in which participants are provided with sufficient information to decide whether or not to be tested, and if so, when and how. The legal aspects of informed consent are discussed in Chapter 3, but here the focus is on the role of the genetic counsellor in ensuring that the rights and welfare of the individual are protected. Two worrisome sources of possible undue influence are professionals (including the counsellors themselves) and family members.

Informed consent and professional biases

Difficulties in achieving non-directiveness, and counsellor biases colouring the transmission of information from counsellor to consultand, may occur. Firstly, there is a pro-testing bias typical of medicine in which testing is generally viewed in a positive light. Aware of this bias, the genetic counsellor is challenged to present a balanced view of the risks, benefits, and limitations of genetic susceptibility testing in order to refrain from overtly or covertly swaying the consultand's decision regarding testing. For example, if a counsellor tells an individual, 'If you were my spouse, I would advise you to take the test', the consultand might agree to undergo a test just to please the counsellor, who is in a powerful role of trustee. In a more subtle scenario, the counsellor who believes that knowing genetic status is better than not knowing might bias the consultand towards testing in more subtle ways, such as overstating the potential for cancer prevention or therapy as one of the benefits of genetic testing, gently persuading the consultand to be tested. When clear-cut benefits of testing have yet to be demonstrated for some syndromes such as breast–ovarian cancer, it may be prudent to let individuals who are undecided wait to be tested until more data are available.

Informed consent and family biases

Another layer of potential interference with autonomous decision-making about genetic susceptibility testing could come from family and friends. Families have cultures, beliefs about health and illness, testing biases, spiritual and religious beliefs and dynamics of their own. The influence of loved ones can be a source of strength and camaraderie, but they may have an interest for themselves in persuading that relative to be tested.

When the family history is positive, members have already experienced multiple relatives developing cancer and thus, have had previous encounters with the medical system. These prior experiences may make relatives either wary of the medical profession, more motivated to use medical care, or in conflict about wanting the best of care. The counsellor needs to help the consultand sort through and become more aware of the effects of these family biases while also striving to protect the privacy of individuals. This can be delicate when the individual is being pushed toward testing by zealous relatives determined to stamp out cancer through genetic testing, or conversely, impeded from testing by relatives who do not wish to co-operate with family testing efforts. Some individuals do not consider a test decision to be solely for their own benefit (considering this selfish), and prefer to construe their decision to be tested altruistically, for example, for the sake of a spouse or the children.

Informed consent and culture

Another issue to be considered in the informed consent process regarding testing is the class and cultural characteristics of the person. Cross-cultural issues are increasingly important. For example, it was estimated in 1990 that one in four Americans was foreign-born or a member of a racial minority group (US Bureau of Census, 1990) and by the year 2010, one in three Americans who will be non-white or Hispanic (US Bureau of Census, 1992). Racial and ethnic minority groups have already achieved majority status in certain cities such as Los Angeles and San Francisco (US Bureau of Census, 1990). In addition to facing many barriers to general health care, members of these minority cultural groups may have very different needs and perceptions of the use of genetic testing (Weil and Mittman, 1993).

Geller et al. (1995) and colleagues held a series of consumer focus groups to explore ethnically and socially diverse participants of beliefs about the causes of cancer, what they would want to know about a genetic test for breast cancer, their attitudes about the advantages and disadvantages of having such a test, what they would do with the test results, and their expectations of their role in decision-making. In comparisons of women in different socio-economic strata (SES), marked differences were found in preferences for the content of the informed consent. Women in high SES groups wanted information on the validity and accuracy of the test, cost of testing, follow-up recommendations and implications of test results for other family members. Women in low SES groups wanted answers to practical questions regarding testing – for example, does testing involve drawing blood?; who will do the test?; when will the results be available?; does the test detect cancers? Overall, higher SES women preferred more autonomy than lower SES women. However, participants across SES groups believed that written materials would be a welcome addition to the informed consent process.

Working with a Navajo family with HNPCC that they have been following for about 12 years, Lynch et al. (1996) found other cross-cultural issues interacted with and altered the genetic counselling process. The use of some culturally familiar analogies such as those of agricultural and animal husbandry met with some success in explaining biological and genetic principles in ways that would not be upsetting or degrading to the traditional tribal beliefs. Investigators observed that the process would be enhanced further by incorporating a member of the native group into the genetic counselling process as an active participant.

Informed consent and declining testing

The 'right not to know' is one that should not be overlooked. From their work on the effects of carrier testing in childhood on adult siblings of cystic fibrosis patients, Fanos and Johnson (1995) concluded that remaining unaware of carrier status may serve a significant psychological function for some individuals at risk for genetic disorders. Research to determine whether the same may apply to hereditary cancers is not yet available.

The health psychology literature suggest that the benefits of prior awareness of risk may depend on individual coping styles. Among women seeking amniocentesis, those who coped by seeking information or 'monitoring' were significantly more likely to experience anxiety and depression than those who coped by 'blunting' information-avoidance (Miller, 1995). Lerman and colleagues (Lerman and Croyle, 1994; Lerman et al., 1994a,b) studying first degree relatives of women with cancer found results consistent with this. Those with more cancer worries and monitoring coping styles were significantly more likely to anticipate negative psychological consequences of *BRCA*1 testing.

Denial is commonly addressed in the genetic literature (Lubinsky, 1994). Some people may ignore or decline counselling because they do not think of themselves as having a risk for inherited cancer. Grosfeld et al. (1996) have pointed out that the decision to have a genetic test can be seen as a sign that the individual is facing the threat of genetic disease consciously. Consultands may engage in advance-and-retreat strategies of making and breaking appointments in repeated cycles that parallel their internal conflicts over accepting and rejecting new cancer risk information about themselves (author's pers. obs.). In light of this, it is important to consider the timing of offering genetic testing. Situations in which testing might be counterproductive are when a person is in denial about risk, is currently caring for an ill relative, or is immobilized by anxiety about cancer. All of these individuals need supportive counselling, with deferral of testing until a more receptive time.

Informed consent in cancer patients versus in relatives at risk for cancer

There are important differences between couselling relatives considering predictive testing and counselling persons with cancer who are considering testing to help establish the presence of a disease-conferring mutation in the family. Affected individuals will be getting information that elucidates the genetic basis for their cancer as well as information about risk for possible additional cancers. As Peshkin (1996) points out, the counsellor should be sensitive to the timing of an invitation for the affected individuals to participate. They may be currently undergoing treatment and concerned primarily about their recovery. Others may have had cancer years ago and want to keep all thought of cancer behind them. The prevention and early detection options for them may not be as much of a benefit as for the younger susceptible consultand.

Pre-test counselling for cancer susceptibility testing

The psycho-oncology literature suggests that genetic testing produces greater distress among persons who previously were unaware of the risk status (Croyle and Lerman, 1994). Therefore, it is essential that the foundational work for the risk notification session is laid during the pre-test counselling and informed consent process.

There is general agreement that samples should not be obtained without thorough pre-test counselling (Table 5.3; Schneider, 1994).

Testing motivations and expectations

The reasons for seeking cancer predictive testing are varied. Some people may value knowledge both for the sake of knowing and for the control over one's life that this knowledge implies. Others may hope to put uncertainty to rest. Some may wish to avoid expensive, risky, and uncomfortable medical surveillance programmes if they were to test negative. Many have altruistic reasons such as helping research or for the sake of

Table 5.3. *Issues in pre-test counselling*

- Motivation and expectations
- Review medical and genetic facts
- Possible results and implications
- Accuracy and limitations
- Risks and benefits
- Assess and support coping
- Privacy and confidentiality
- Programme specifics

protecting their children. Others may want to know their risk status when starting or continuing a family (Petersen and Boyd, 1995; Burt and Petersen, 1996). Sometimes patients and their families want more information to understand the biological basis of their cancer.

Surveys of the general population have demonstrated that the public is very interested in genetic susceptibility testing for cancer (Chaliki et al., 1995; Smith and Croyle, 1995). Over 90% of relatives of breast cancer patients and of ovarian cancer patients reported that they would want to be tested, once a test is available (Lerman et al., 1994b; Struewing et al., 1995). Women's interest in testing for any cancer susceptibility is usually greater than men's and there is greater interest among those with high self-perceived (rather than calculated) risk of cancer (Struewing et al., 1995; Lerman et al., 1994a).

Motivation for testing may be based on misconceptions about the nature of testing, for example, 'the test will give me a definitive answer about cancer'. It may also be based on assumptions about possible medical interventions. There is widespread belief in the general population that the medical community would not be offering cancer susceptibility testing if there were nothing that one could do about one's risk. These test expectations can be a source of later disappointment if the testing fails to meet the person's underlying needs and wishes.

For some genetic conditions, studies, however, find few people are presenting themselves for predictive testing. Schneider and her colleagues have shown that only 12 of 48 members of the first six extended kindred with Li–Fraumeni syndrome invited to be tested actually enrolled and completed an initial visit (Schneider and Marnane, 1995). The most common reasons for declining participating in the testing process were recent cancer diagnosis or death in a relative, fear of insurance problems, lack of options for prevention, inconvenience, 'not a good time in life', and not interested. The investigators conclude that the demand for testing will be difficult to predict given the complex issues faced.

Most participants in one research study on susceptibility testing felt strongly that they knew what the outcome would be and were seeking testing as confirmation of that intuition (Grosfeld et al., 1996). There is some evidence from Huntington disease testing that those persons who receive results congruent with prior expectations show better adjustment, whereas those who receive results that differ significantly from what they expected will have the most long-term adjustments to make (Huggins et al., 1992). The genetic counsellor, therefore, should ascertain at the outset whether the participant believes that the results will turn out positive or negative.

Medical and genetic facts

Many consultands have little prior knowledge of genes, chromosomes and the relation of these to cancer. Richards and colleagues observe 'the fact that lay people use technical terms such as gene or chromosome does not necessarily mean that they understand these terms in the same way as geneticists' (Richards et al., 1995, p.229). Grosfeld et al. (1996) found that much of what passes for genetic knowledge is often derived from personal or family experience with a particular disease. Patterns unique to a given family – for example, only first born offspring are affected – may be erroneously generalized to a principle. Others may correctly understand a principle, for example, 50% risk, but inappropriately apply it to count up the number of affected persons in their own sibship and decide about one's own risk based on whether that 50% ratio has been met or not.

The primary genetic facts about the common inherited cancers that are essential are: basic laws of inheritance; gene penetrance; variable phenotypic expression; and occurrence of non-genetic cases even within hereditary families (Richards et al., 1995).

Prior to testing, the persons considering testing should also understand the medical options available for prevention, early detection, and treatment. Being at increased risk for cancer, they should be following surveillance recommendations that differ from the general public. These recommendations may change as the result of genetic testing.

In the first year of a study of *BRCA1* counselling and presymptomatic testing in Utah, qualitative observations of subject responses to genetic counselling showed that subjects often lacked certain knowledge prior to counselling, for example, they did not know of the increased risk of gene positive males for cancer and the relative lack of increased risk for male breast cancer. Female subjects often did not know that they were at risk for both breast and ovarian cancer because their own nuclear family may have expressed only one or the other. Many were surprised to learn of the possibility of prophylactic mastectomy and oophorectomy (Baty et al., 1995).

Prophylactic surgery is a prevention option that is offered in many of the hereditary cancers, but the efficacy varies considerably form one condition to the next. For example, it is very effectively used in FAP (Petersen, 1996b) and MEN2. These conditions are also characterized by a very early onset of symptoms, almost 100% penetrance, and the ability to remove the organ at risk for cancer. The situation is much less clear-cut for hereditary colon (except FAP), breast, and ovarian cancer, because of heterogeneity, variable age at onset of cancer, reduced penetrance and a number of organs at risk for malignancy; also prophylactic surgery leaves tissue which remains at risk for malignant transformation.

Prophylactic mastectomy and oophorectomy are emotionally charged areas of prevention, with strong proponents and critics within both professional and lay groups (Lynch and Watson, 1992; King et al, 1993; Stefanek, 1995). There is lack of research regarding the decision-making process about using these procedures and only sporadic case reports about the effectiveness of the procedures. Because genetic risk is rarely the only factor that goes into making a decision about surgery, there is a strong need for multidisciplinary input, and thorough psychosocial counselling regarding use of prophylactic surgery to prevent cancer (Peters, 1994b). For recent ELSI (ethical, legal, and social issues) recommendations, see Chapter 20.

Susceptibility test implications

Participants should be prepared for results of genetic susceptibility testing that are negative, positive, or inconclusive (see Tables 5.4, 5.5a and 5.5b).

The implications differ depending on several factors:

(1) The test result.
(2) Whether or not the person being tested has already had cancer.
(3) Whether a cancer-causing mutation has already been identified in the family or this is the first person to be tested.

Table 5.4. *Possible implications of positive results of cancer susceptibility test*

Genetic	The mutation can be passed on to offspring Notify other relatives at risk
Medical	Explanation for cancers in self and/or relatives Increased lifetime risk of one or more cancers Specialised surveillance and prevention advised Risk to more than one organ system
Psychological	Psychological difficulties common during adjustment May alter self-perception
Social/economic	Family relationships can be strained or altered Insurance and employment discrimination Possible stigmatization

Source: Adapted from Schneider (1994), with permission.

Participants can have much greater confidence that negative results are truly negative when a mutation is already known to occur in a given family than when one must be discovered and demonstrated to be causative of cancer. The clinical significance of a particular mutation found in a high risk research population cannot necessarily be generalized to different populations without such high a priori risks (Schatzkin et al., 1995).

Accuracy/limitation of testing

The counsellor will need to be very clear with the family at the outset as to what types of genetic alterations will and will not be found, and the implications of each. When results are negative, there is a possibility that a mutation was missed or the results unclear. A test may be inconclusive if a missense alteration cannot be distinguished from a benign polymorphism. If a mutation is found, it does not mean that the person will definitely get cancer, which type, or when.

Risks of genetic susceptibility testing

The main risks of testing are psychological, social, and economic. These are summarized in Table 5.6. The psychological reactions often start at the time of informed consent, with high levels of anxiety, depression, sleep and other somatic complaints documented one week following

Table 5.5a. *Implications of negative result of susceptibility test when a* mutation is already known *to be in the family*

Genetic	This person does not have the mutation seen in affected relatives; does not exclude other genetic alterations Cancers in this person have other causes, which may be genetic, environmental, multifactorial, or chance This person cannot pass on this mutation
Medical	Cancer risks return to baseline unless other risk factors exist Medical surveillance resumes population recommendations
Psychological	May be relief or guilt at being spared May be disbelief in result after a lifetime at risk
Social/economic	May create gap between relatives with and without mutation Insurance risk status may improve

Source: Adapted from Schneider (1994), with permission.

Table 5.5b. *Implications of negative result of susceptibility test when the* cause of familial cancers is *unknown in the family*

Genetic	Cannot distinguish false negative from true negative The person could still be at risk for a different mutation Risk to offspring remains increased
Medical	Cancer remains elevated Continue high risk medical surveillance
Psychological	Uncertainty about genetic risk continues Unable to obtain closure May become disillusioned with testing after repeated negative results in the face of obvious increased risk
Social/economic	Family relationships may be affected Insurance and employment status remain vulnerable

Source: Adapted from Schneider (1994), with permission.

Table 5.6. *Potential risks associated with positive results of cancer susceptibility testing*

Genetic	May offer inaccurate risk information due to: • inappropriately applying cancer risks derived from one population to another; • failing to account for gene–gene and gene–environmental interactions; • unrecognized variations in penetrance and expressivity
Medical	Increased lifetime cancer risk estimates uncertain regarding: individual age of onset, type and number of tumours Problems obtaining adequate medical surveillance
Psychological	Altered sense of personal identity, self-esteem, mood, function
Social/economic	Couple and family relationships altered Confidentiality and privacy threatened Insurance and employment vulnerable Financial burden of extra surveillance

Source: Adapted from Schneider (1994), with permission.

pre-test counselling and remaining high for the interim months until test results are available (Grosfeld et al., 1996).

The risk of adverse social implications within the family are common (Biesecker et al., 1993). There is the risk of communication barriers going up between those who chose testing and those who declined testing, as well as between those who tested positive and those who tested negative. As a result, family relationships and dynamics could be altered. Grosfeld et al. (1996) found that asymptomatic carriers were often stigmatized within the family as already sick. As a result, the family became preoccupied with looking for symptoms or for re-evaluation of past events as symptomatic. Some individuals felt almost no relief when they learned that they were non-carriers, but rather, felt empty and isolated from family members who were carriers. Lynch and Watson (1992) noted that some of those who tested negative for *BRCA1* expressed disbelief and wished to continue with intensive surveillance and still consider prophylactic surgery.

Benefits of cancer susceptibility testing

Reduction of uncertainty for at risk individuals and increased compliance with screening recommendations are important benefits of testing programmes (Petersen, 1996a,b). Some families have reported increased supportiveness and better communications (Giambarresi and Kase, 1995, pers. comm.; Grosfeld et al., 1996). Risks for offspring may be clarified. Testing may provide an increased ability to plan for the future, such as choice of career, geographic location near a medical centre, or planning a family. For those whose test results are negative in a family with a known mutation, results can be reassuring and release them from surveillance programmes.

The benefits are summarized in Tables 5.7a and 5.7b.

Table 5.7a. *Potential benefits associated with cancer susceptibility testing when results are positive for a mutation*

Genetic	Have a better understanding of the biological basis of the cancer Provide accurate risk analysis for relatives
Medical	Alter cancer prevention and detection
Psychological	Resolution of uncertainty about risk status Explanation for cancer Improve motivation for healthcare Opportunity for active coping strategies
Social/economics	Increased supportiveness and communications Children can be started on healthy habits Motivation to plan for future

Source: Adapted from Schneider (1994), with permission.

Table 5.7b. *Potential benefits associated with cancer susceptibility testing when no mutation is found in person from family with known mutation*

Genetic	Person does not have the mutation causing cancer in a branch of the family Children cannot inherit mutation from parent who does not bear it
Medical	Cancer risk decreases to general population risk in absence of other risk factors Reduce unnecessary medical surveillance
Psychological	Feelings of relief and elation Enables chance to get on with life
Social/economic	Increased communication and support Financial savings from unnecessary medical visits and procedures

Source: Adapted from Schneider (1994), with permission.

Coping resources and strategies

It is important to discuss the anticipated impact of results upon the client and his or her family and to identify maladaptive coping styles before the decision to be tested is made. Adaptive coping approaches can then be encouraged.

Privacy and confidentiality

Because the dangers of discrimination are very real to families with hereditary cancer susceptibility, issues of privacy and confidentiality should be discussed. Confidentiality pertains to the treatment of information that an individual has disclosed in a relationship of trust and with the expectation that it will not be divulged without permission to others in ways that are inconsistent with the understanding of the original disclosure (see Chapter 3).

Test specifics

The genetic counsellor (or nurse) is often the one to discuss other more mundane matters regarding the testing programme, including fees, that testing requires a tissue specimen (usually blood), how the test will be done, when results will be available, at what points clients can change their minds or withdraw from the testing programme, and who to contact for questions and support.

Cancer susceptibility test notification

See Table 5.8. The way in which results are to be given should be negotiated between participant and counsellor prior to the risk notification visit. Results are usually given in person, preferably with a support person in attendance. Most counsellors agree that results should be given near the beginning of the session once it is established that the person still wishes to receive the results. The content of the session should again cover the genetic, medical, and psychosocial issues raised in the pre-test counselling (Biesecker et al., 1993). Discussions of children's risk for inheriting a mutation are appropriate at this time. The issue of testing children will be dependent largely on whether the disease is manifested in childhood and what medical benefits can be derived from testing.

Medical issues at this point switch from theoretical generalizations to being applied to the individual who has just learned that the cancer risk

Table 5.8. *Susceptibility test result notification*

- Consider family preferences regarding setting and format
- Disclose in person when possible
- Invite a supportive relative/friend
- Confirm that person still wants results
- Offer results in simple, direct way
- Allow for emotional reactions
- Encourage active coping, increased social support, stress management
- Personalize genetic and medical information
- Be prepared for issues arising during pre-test counselling to re-emerge
- Re-visit privacy, confidentiality, insurance issues
- Discuss short-term and long-term plans

---

has substantially increased or decreased based on the test results. It is important for those who have learned that they are likely to develop cancer to feel that they can be active in trying to lower their risks.

Dealing with the potentially strong psychological reactions to hearing the results of testing is one of the primary functions of this meeting (Biesecker et al., 1993; Lynch and Watson, 1992; Grosfeld et al., 1996). Some people might subsequently feel differently about themselves or lower their goals, or be too frightened to seek medical care.

It is often wise to provide written or tape-recorded information about the genetic and medical consequences of the test result, since participants may be too stunned at the time of the visit to absorb much information. Additional telephone contacts or referral to an appropriate support group are often helpful.

Follow-up

Because the emotional impact of receiving test results may vary widely from person to person and over time, a significant duration may be necessary to work through the implications of test results emotionally (Table 5.9).

No variables have yet been found to predict infallibly who will have long-term trouble in adjusting to results, which may be important whether the results are favourable or unfavourable. Studies are in process through the NIH-ELSI hereditary cancer consortium to assess this. One key predictor may be the extent to which the consultand equates a positive test result with cancer and death. Results of a prospective cohort

Table 5.9. *Susceptibility test counselling follow-up*

- Coming to terms with test result implications
- Positive, negative, and inconclusive results can all generate emotional reactions
- Short-term contact for acute reactions
- Offer at least one year long-term contact post-test
- Update personal and family histories
- Check understanding of test implications
- Review medical surveillance plans
- Enroll in prevention trials when available
- Consider reproductive implications
- Notify appropriate relatives of testing options
- Explore family relationships and communications

---

study of 279 adult men and women of families with *BRCA1*-linked hereditary breast–ovarian cancer showed that of the almost 200 persons who completed a baseline interview, genetic education, and counselling, 60% requested test results (Lerman et al., 1996). At one-month follow-up, non-carriers of *BRCA1* mutations showed statistically significant reductions in depressive symptoms and functional impairment compared with carriers and non-tested individuals. However, individuals identified as mutation carriers did not exhibit increases in depression and functional impairment. Among unaffected women with no prior prophylactic surgery, 17% of carriers intended to have mastectomies and 33% to have oophorectomies.

Grosfeld and colleagues (1996) counselling families undergoing MEN-2 testing found that 43% of participants expressed anxiety complaints, 34% depression, 37% had somatic complaints, and 49% had sleep disturbances two weeks after disclosure. Psychological distress remained for up to a year following disclosure, although the levels dropped significantly.

Petersen and colleagues have reported on testing of 47 adults and 36 minors at risk for FAP (Petersen and Boyd, 1995). There was some evidence that family relationships and identity was linked to gene status. The value of counselling included reduction of uncertainty and adjustment of misperceptions. Testing of minors presented additional counselling challenges; predictive genetic testing of 41 children at risk for FAP showed that at three-month follow-up, there were no significant changes in the levels of clinical depression or anxiety in the children or in their parents. However, mutation-positive children with affected mothers had significantly higher depression scores at follow-up, and regardless of test results, children with affected mothers had significantly increased anxiety scores after testing. In families with both mutation-positive and muta-tion-negative children, FAP-unaffected parents experienced significantly increased depressive symptoms at follow-up.

In grief counselling, counsellors generally caution consultands to avoid making any irrevocable life decisions within the first few months follow-ing a loss or crisis because the strong emotional response to the test result itself may be colouring decisions at this time. The same principle may be applied to susceptibility testing.

Individuals with negative results are often reluctant to return for fol-low-up, but experience with Huntington disease has shown that they had the comparable rates of psychological distress at one year post-testing as did those with positive results. These observations have been confirmed in MEN-2 (Grosfeld et al., 1996). Thus, the provider should make every effort to maintain contact with all tested individuals.

Conclusion

There are many technical, ethical, and counselling issues yet to be resolved about hereditary cancer susceptibility. Some of the ethical dilem-mas include establishing policy about testing of fetuses and minors for adult-onset risks; how to maintain the confidentiality of results without impinging on family or primary care patient relationships; how to handle desires for different levels and types of information with families; how to provide equitable access to information with geographically dispersed families and with different socio-economic groups (Biesecker, 1997).

Richards and colleagues (1995) have suggested areas of research that are needed: consultands' accuracy of perception of their own and their close relatives genetic risk; knowledge and understanding of inheritance of susceptibility genes; communication within families about genetic risk; family patterns in use of appropriate screening and risk reduction meth-ods; effects of genetic counselling and of genetic testing on levels of worry and anxiety; establishing the ideal levels of worry and anxiety to energize positive health behaviours; selective use or avoidance of genetic testing by various sub-sets of the population; and effective use of resources in pro-viding genetic services including counselling, education, and testing.

As knowledge about inherited susceptibility to cancer increases and additional susceptibility genes are identified, there will be an increased need for multidisciplinary teams to form in order to care for the medical,

genetic, and psychosocial needs of families with hereditary cancer syndromes. It is hoped that forming familial cancer risk counselling programmes now will offer not only a suitable context for susceptibility
testing, but could also serve as a framework for many of the technological
advances to follow in every aspect of cancer care, from surveillance to
diagnosis, treatment, and follow-up.

Acknowledgements

The author is deeply indebted to those who have shared the wisdom
gained from their genetic counselling experiences, both counsellors and
consultands. Special thanks to Henry Lynch, Barbara Bowles Biesecker
and Donald Hadley who allowed me to sit in on their genetic counselling
sessions. Specific input from the following colleagues was essential in the
development of the present chapter: Barbara Bowles Biesecker, Eileen
Dimond, Leo Giambaresi, Donald Hadley, and Regina Kenen.

References

Ad Hoc Committee of the American Society of Human Genetics (ASHG). 1975.
    Genetic counselling definition. *American Journal of Human Genetics* **27**: 240–
    2.
American Society of Clinical Oncology (ASCO) Sub-committee on Genetic
    Testing for Cancer Susceptibility. 1996. Statement of the American Society
    of Clinical Oncology: genetic testing for cancer susceptibility. *Journal of
    Clinical Oncology* **14**(5): 1730–6.
American Society of Human Genetics (ASHG). 1994. Statement of the ASHG on
    genetic testing for breast and ovarian cancer disposition. *American Journal of
    Human Genetics* **55**: 1–4.
Anderson, D.E. and Badzioch, M.D. 1985. Risk of familial breast cancer. *Cancer*
    56:383-7.
Anderson, D.E. and Badzioch, M.D. 1989. Combined effect of family history and
    reproductive factors on breast cancer risk. *Cancer* **63**: 349–53.
Andrews, L.B., Fullarton, J.E., Hotzman, N.A., Motulsky, A. (Eds.). 1994.
    Assessing Genetic Risks: Implications for Health and Social Policy, pp. 10, 27,
    51, 297. Institute of Medicine Report. Washington, DC: National Academy
    Press.
Baker, N.C. 1991. *Relative Risk: Living With a Family History of Breast Cancer.*
    New York: Penguin Books.
Baty, B., Botkin, J., Croyl, R. et al. 1995. BRCA1 counselling and
    presymptomatic testing: protocols and lessons from the first year. *Journal of
    Genetic Counselling* **4**: 318–19.
Bennett, R.L., Steinhaus, K.A., Uhrick, S.P. et al. 1993. The need for developing
    standardised family pedigree nomenclature. *Journal of Genetic Counselling* **2**:
    261–73.

Bennett, R.L., Steinhaus, K.A., Uhrick, S.P. et al. 1995. Recommendations for strandardised human pedigree nomenclature. *American Journal of Human Genetics* **56**: 745–52. (Reprinted in *Journal of Genetic Counselling* **4**: 167–79).

Berk, T. 1996. Review of article on genetic counselling for familial adenomatous polyposis. *Oncology* **10** (1): 97–8.

Biesecker, B.B. Boehnke, M., Calzone, K. et al. 1993. Genetic counselling for families with inherited susceptibility to breast and ovarian cancer. *JAMA* **269**(15): 1970–4.

Biesecker, B. B. 1997. Genetic testing for cancer predispostion. *Cancer Nursing* 20(4): 285–300.

Boland, C.R. 1996. Review of article on genetic counselling in HNPCC. *Oncology* **10**(1): 81–2.

Burt, R.W. and Petersen, G.M. 1996. Familial colorectal cancer: diagnosis and management. In *Prevention and Early Detection of Colorectal Cancer*, ed. G.P. Young, P. Rozen and B. Levin. London: Saunders.

Chaliki, H., Soader, S., Levenkron, J.C., Logan-Young, W., Hall, W.J. and Rowley, P.T. 1995. *American Journal of Public Health* **85**(8): 1133–5.

Claus, E.B., Risch, N. and Thompson, W.D. 1994. Autosomal dominant inheritance of early onset breast cancer. *Cancer* **73**: 643–51.

Codori, A.M., Petersen, G.M., Boyd, P.A., Brandt, J., Giardiello, F.M. 1996. Genetic testing for cancer in children: short-term psychological impart. *Archives of Pediatric and Adolescent Medicine* **150**: 1131–8.

Collins, F.S. and the National Action Plan on Breast Cancer (NAPBC). 1996. NAPBC commentary on the ASCO statement on genetic testing for cancer susceptibility. *Journal of Clinical Oncology* **14**(5): 1738–40.

Cooper, G.M. 1993. *The Cancer Book.* Boston: Jones and Bartlett.

Croyle, R. and Lerman, C. 1994. Psychological impact of genetic testing. In *Psychosocial Effects of Screening for Disease Prevention and Detection*, ed. R. Croyle. New York: Oxford University Press.

Durfy, S. and Peters, J. 1993. For the benefit of all: case study and commentary on breast cancer susceptibility. *Hastings Center Report* **25**(5): 28–30.

Epstein, C.J. 1975. Genetic counselling: present status and future prospects. In *Early Diagnosis and Prevention of Genetic Disease*, ed. L.N. Went, Vermeij-Keers and A.G. van der Linden, pp. 110–28. Leiden: Leiden University Press.

Evans, D.G.R., Burnell, L.D., Hopwood, P. and Howell, A. 1993. Perception of risk in women with a family history of breast cancer. *British Journal of Cancer* **67**: 612–14.

Evans, D.G.R., Fentiman, I.S., Mcpherson, K., Asbury, D., Ponder, B.A.J. and Howell, A. 1994. Familial breast cancer. *British Medical Journal* **308**: 183–7.

Evans, D.G.R., Ribiero, G., Warrell, D. and Donnai, D. 1992. Ovarian cancer family and prophylactic choices. *Journal of Medical Genetics* **29**: 416–18.

Fanos, J.H. and Johnson, J.P. 1995. Barriers to carrier testing for adult cystic fibrosis sibs: the importance of not knowing. *American Journal of Medical Genetics* **59**: 85-91.

Fawzy, F.I., Cousins, N., Fawzy, N.W., Kemeny, M.E., Elashoff, R. and Morton, D. 1990a. A structured psychiatric intervention for cancer patients. I. Changes over time and methods of coping and affective disturbance. *Archives of General Psychiatry* **47**: 720-5.

Fawzy, F.I., Cousins, N., Fawzy, N.W., Kemeny, M.E., Elashoff, R. and Morton, D. 1990b. A structured psychiatric intervention for cancer patients.

II. Changes over time in immunological measures. *Archives of General Psychiatry* **47**: 729-35.

Fine, B.A. 1993. The evolution of nondirectiveness in genetic counselling and implications of the Human Genome Project. In *Prescribing Our Future: Ethical Challenges in Genetic Counselling*, ed. D.M. Bartels, B.S. LeRoy and A.L. Caplan, pp. 101–18. New York: Aldine de Gruyter.

Gail, M.H., Brinton, L.A., Byar, D.P. et al. 1989. Projecting individualized probabilities of developing breast cancer for white females who are being examined annually. *Journal of the National Cancer Institute* **81**: 1879–86.

Geller, G., Bernhardt, B.A. and Holtzman, N.A. 1995. Involving consumers in the development of a model informed consent process for BRCA1 testing: what do they want to know? *Journal of Genetic Counselling* **4**(4): 322–3.

Green, J., Merton, F. and Stratham, H. 1993. Psychosocial issues raised by a familial ovarian cancer registry. *Journal of Medical Genetics* **300**: 101–5.

Grosfeld, F.J.M., Lips, C.J.M. and TenKroode, H.F.J. 1996. Psychosocial consequences of DNA analysis for MEN type 2. *Oncology* **10**(2): 141–6.

Hodgson, S.V. and Maher, E.R. 1993. *A Practical Guide to Human Cancer Genetics*. Cambridge: Cambridge University Press.

Hoskins, K.F., Stopfer, J.E., Calzone, K.A. et al. 1995. Assessment and counselling for familial breast cancer risk: a guide for clinicians. *Journal of the American Medical Association* **273**: 577–85.

Huggins, M., Bloch, M., Wigins, S. et al. 1992. Predictive testing for Huntington disease in Canada: adverse effects and unexpected results in those receiving a decreased risk. *American Journal of Medicine and Genetics* **42**: 508–15.

Kash, K.M., Holland, J.C., Halpern, M.S. and Miller, D. G. 1992. Psychological distress and surveillance behaviors of women with a family history of breast cancer. *Journal of the National Cancer Institute* **84**: 24–30.

Kelly, P. 1991. *Understanding Breast Cancer Risk*. Philadelphia: Temple University Press.

Kelly, P.T. 1992. Breast cancer risk analysis: a genetic epidemiology service for families. *Journal of Genetic Counselling* **1**(2): 155–68.

Kenen, R.H. 1980. Negotiations, superstitions, and the plight of individuals born with severe birth defects. *Society, Science and Medicine* **14A**: 279–86.

Kenen, R.H. 1984. Genetic counselling: the development of a new interdisciplinary occupational field. *Society, Science and Medicine* **18**(7): 541–9.

Kenen, R.H. and Smith, A.C.M. 1995. Genetic counselling for the next 25 years: models for the future. *Journal of Genetic Counselling* **4**(2): 115–24.

Kessler, S. 1980. The psychological paradigm shift in the genetic counselling. *Social Biology* **27**: 167–85.

Kessler, S. 1992. Directiveness. *Journal of Genetic Counselling* **1**(1): 9–17.

Kessler, S. and Levine, E.K. 1987. Psychological aspects of genetic counselling. IV. The subjective assessment of probability. *American Journal of Medical Genetics* **28**: 361–70.

King, M.C., Rowell, S. and Love, S.M. 1993. Inherited breast and ovarian cancer: what are the risks, what are the choices? *Journal of the American Medical Association* **269**: 1975–80.

Lee, C.Z., Coleman, C. and Link, J. 1992a. Developing comprehensive breast centers. Part 1: Introduction and overview. *The Journal of Oncology Management* **1**(1): 20–3.

Lee, C.Z., Coleman, C. and Link, J. 1992b. Developing comprehensive breast centers. Part 2: Critical success factors. *The Journal of Oncology Management* **1**(2): 20–6.

Lerman, C., Audrain, J. and Croyle, R.T. 1994a. DNA-testing for heritable breast cancer risks: lessons from traditional genetic counselling. *Annals of Behavioural Medicine* **16**(4): 327–33.

Lerman, C. and Croyle, R.T. 1994. Psychological issues in genetic testing for breast cancer susceptibility. *Archives of Internal Medicine* **154**: 609–15.

Lerman, C. and Croyle, R.T. 1996. Emotional and behavioral responses to genetic testing for susceptibility to cancer. *Oncology* **10**(2): 191–9.

Lerman, C., Daly, M., Sands, C. et al. 1993. Mammography adherence and psychological distress among women at risk for breast cancer. *Journal of the National Cancer Institute* **85**: 1074–80.

Lerman, C., Daly, M., Masny, A. and Balshem, A. 1994b. Attitudes about genetic testing for breast-ovarian cancer susceptibility. *Journal of Clinical Oncology* **12**(4): 843–50.

Lerman, C., Lustbader, E., Rimer, B. et al. 1995. Effects of individualized breast cancer risk counselling: a randomized trial. *Journal of the National Cancer Insitute* **87**: 286–92.

Lerman C., Narod, S., Schulman, K. et al. 1996. BRCA1 testing in families with hereditary breast-ovarian cancer: a prospective study of patient decision making and outcomes. *JAMA* **275**(24): 1885–92.

Li, F., Garber, J., Friend, S. et al. 1992. Recommendations on predictive testing for germline p53 mutations among cancer-prone individuals. *Journal of the National Cancer Insitute* **84**(15): 1156–60.

Lippman-Hand, A. and Fraser, F.C. 1979a. Genetic counselling: provision and reception of information. *American Journal of Medical Genetics* **3**: 113–27.

Lippman-Hand, A. and Fraser, F.C. 1979b. Genetic counselling: the post-counselling period. I. Parents' perceptions of uncertainty. *American Journal of Medical Genetics* **4**: 51–71.

Lippman-Hand, A. and Fraser, F.C. 1979c Genetic counselling: the post-counselling period. II. Making reproductive choices. *American Journal of Medical Genetics* **4**: 73–87.

Lubinsky, M.L. 1994. Bearing bad news: dealing with the mimics of denial. *Journal of Genetic Counselling* **3**(1): 5–12.

Lynch, H.T., Drouhard, T., Vasen, H.F.A. et al. 1996. Genetic counselling in a Navajo hereditary non-polyposis colorectal cancer kindred. *Cancer* **77**: 30–5.

Lynch, H. T., Lemon, S. J., Durham, C. et al. 1997. A descriptive study of BRCA1 testing and reactions to disclosure of test results. *Cancer* **79**: 2219–28.

Lynch, H.T. and Lynch, J.F. 1993. Familial predisposition and cancer management. *Contemperary Oncology* : 12–25.

Lynch, H.T. and Watson, P. 1992. Genetic counselling and hereditary breast-ovarian cancer. *Lancet* **339**: 1181.

McGoldrick, M., Pearce, J.K. and Giordano, J. (Eds.). 1982. *Ethnicity and Family Therapy*. New York: Guilford Press.

Menko, F.H., Wijnen, J.T., Meera Khan, P., Vasen, H.F.A. and Oosterwijk, M.H. 1996. Genetic counselling in hereditary nonpolyposis colorectal cancer. *Oncology* **10**(1): 71–6.

Miller, S. M. 1995. Monitoring vs blunting styles of coping with cancer influence the information patients want and need about their disease: implications for cancer screening and management. *Cancer* **76**: 167–77.

National Advisory Council for Human Genome Research. 1994. Statement of use of DNA testing for presymptomatic identification of cancer risk. *JAMA* **271**(10): 785.

Nelkin, D. and Lindee, S. 1995. *The DNA Mystique*. New York: W.H. Freeman & Co.

Offit, K. and Brown, K. 1994. Quantitating familial cancer risk: a resource for clinical oncologists. *Journal of Clinical Oncology* **12**(8): 1724–36.

Palmer, C.G.S. and Sainfort, F. 1993. Toward a new conceptualization and operationalization of risk perception within the genetic counseling domain. *Journal of Genetic Counselling* **2**(4): 275–94.

Peshkin, B., Benkendorf, J., Hughes, C. and Lerman, C. 1995. An education and counselling hierarchy for BRCA1 susceptibility testing and cancer prevention: optimizing resources and meeting the demand. *Journal of Genetic Counselling* **4**(4): 331–2.

Peshkin, B. 1996. Review of the role of genetic counsellor in familial cancer. *Oncology* **10**(2): 176–82.

Peters, J.A. 1994a. Familial cancer risk. Part 1: Impact on today's oncology practice. *Journal of Oncology Management* (Sept/Oct.): 20–30.

Peters, J.A. 1994b. Familial cancer risk. Part 2: Breast cancer risk counselling and genetic susceptibility testing. *Journal of Oncology Management* (Nov/Dec.): 18–26.

Peters, J.A. 1994c. Suicide prevention in the genetic counseling context. *Journal of Genetic Counseling* **3**(3): 199–213.

Peters, J.A. 1995. Breast cancer genetics: relevance to oncology practice. *Cancer Control* (May/June): 195–207.

Peters, J.A. and Biesecker, B.B. 1997. Genetic counseling and hereditary cancer. *Cancer Supplement* **83**(3): 576–86.

Peters, J.A. and Stopfer, J. 1996. The genetic counsellor's role in familial cancer. *Oncology* **10**(2): 159–66.

Petersen, G.M. 1996a. Genetic counselling and predictive testing for colorectal cancer. *International Journal of Cancer* **69**(1): 53–4.

Petersen, G.M. 1996b. Genetic counselling and predictive testing in familial adenomatous polyposis. *Seminars in Colon and Rectal Surgery* **6**(1): 55–60.

Petersen, G.M. and Boyd, P.A. 1995. Gene tests and counselling for colorectal cancer risk: lessons from familial polyposis. *Journal of the National Cancer Institute Monograph* **17**: 67–71.

Petersen, G.M. and Brensinger, J.D. 1996. Genetic testing and counselling in familial adenomatous polyposis. *Oncology* **10**(1): 89–94.

Reed, S. 1955. *Counselling in Medical Genetics*. Philadelphia: W.B. Saunders.

Resta, R.G. 1994. The crane's foot: the rise of the pedigree in human genetics. *Journal of Genetic Counselling* **2**: 235–60.

Richards, M.P.M., Hallowell, N., Green, J.M. et al. 1995. Counselling families with hereditary breast and ovarian cancer: a psychosocial perspective. *Journal of Genetic Counselling* **4**(3): 219-32.

Royak-Schaler, R. and Benderly, B.K. 1992. *Challenging the Breast Cancer Legacy: A Program of Emotional Support and Medical Care for Women at Risk*. New York: Harper-Collins.

Schatzkin, A., Goldstein, A. and Freedman, L.S. 1995. What does it mean to be a cancer gene carrier? Problems in establishing causality from the molecular genetics of cancer. *Journal of the National Cancer Institute* **87**(15): 1126–30.

Schneider, K.A. 1994. *Counselling about Cancer: Strategies for Genetic Counsellors.* Supported by a grant from the Jane Engelberg Memorial Fund and supplied by the NSGC, Wallingford, PA.

Schneider, K.A. and Marnane, D. 1995. Is directiveness in cancer risk counselling ever appropriate? *Journal of Genetic Counselling* 4(4): 333–4.

Skolnick, M. 1996. Commentary on the ASCO statement on genetic testing for cancer susceptibility. *Journal of Clinical Oncology* 14(5): 1737–8.

Smith, K.R. and Croyle, R.T. 1995. Attitudes toward genetic testing for colon cancer risk. *American Journal of Public Health* 85(10): 1435–8.

Sorensen, J.R. 1993. Genetic counselling: values that have mattered. In *Prescribing Our Future: Ethical Challenges in Genetic Counselling*, ed. D.M. Bartels, B.S. LeRoy and A.L. Caplan, pp. 3–14. New York: Aldine de Gruyter.

Spiegel, D. 1992. Effects of psychosocial support on patients with metastatic breast cancer. *Journal of Psychosocial Oncology* 10(2): 113–20.

Stefanek, M.E. 1995. Bilateral prophylactic mastectomy: issues and concerns. *Journal of the National Cancer Institute Monograph* No. 17: *Hereditary Breast-Ovarian, and Colon Cancer.*

Struewing, J.P., Lerman, C., Kase, R.G., Giambarresi, T.R. and Tucker, M.A. 1995. Anticipated uptake and impact of genetic testing in hereditary breast and ovarian cancer families. *Cancer Epidemiology Biomarkers and Prevention* 4 169–73.

US Bureau of Census. 1990. Data obtained from the US 1990 Census of Population and Housing. Summary Tape file 1A and 3A.

US Bureau of Census. 1992. *Population Projections of the United States, by Age, Race, Sex, and Hispanic Origin: 1992–2050.* P25-1092. US Government Printing Office, Washington, DC.

Visco, F.M. and the National Breast Cancer Coalition. 1996. Commentary on the ASCO statement on genetic testing for cancer susceptibility. *Journal of Clinical Oncology* 14(5): 1737.

Weil, J. and Mittman, I. 1993. A teaching framework for cross-cultural genetic counselling. *Journal of Genetic Counselling* 2(3): 159–69.

Wellisch, D.K., Gritz, E.R., Schain, W., Wang, H.J. and Siaw, J. 1992. Psychological functioning of daughters of breast cancer patients. Part II. Characterizing the distressed daughters of the breast cancer patient. *Psychosomatics* 33(2):171–9.

Williams, T.T. 1991. *Refuge.* New York: Random House.

6

Cancer genetics in primary care

GENE FEDER and MICHAEL MODELL

Summary

The role of family doctors in offering genetic counselling and arranging cancer screening for individuals who may have a genetic cancer susceptibility is discussed in this chapter. In the UK, the general practitioner (GP) is the central figure in the provision of health care, and the UK system is briefly described. The potential workload for the GP is discussed, by considering the number of susceptible individuals in an average practice. The extent of involvement of the GP is discussed. Some of the ethical dilemmas that may arise in general practice are considered.

Introduction

This chapter examines the potential role of family doctors in integrating cancer genetics into clinical practice. To some extent family doctors already address genetic aspects of health. Their involvement is most marked in pre-conception and antenatal screening programmes, but also extends to the recognition, via family histories, of individuals at risk of the premature development of specific cancers, cardiovascular disease, or diabetes. Using the example of UK general practice, we start by discussing family practice as a site for genetic screening and counselling and examine issues emerging from the application of genetic knowledge in antenatal care, that can help us to understand the potential implication of cancer genetics for family practice. We consider the family tree as a key tool for identifying people at genetic risk. We then address the implications for family practice of a growing number of screening tests. A negative result may be very reassuring, but a positive result could have uncertain clinical value, may cause psychological damage to individuals and may be used to discriminate against them. We examine the educational needs of the family doctor in a fast-moving scientific field, and finally discuss methods of enhancing communication between primary care and cancer genetic services.

Family practice as a site for genetics counselling/screening

Family doctors and clinical geneticists are the only two groups of physicians with a specific remit to care for *families* rather than just individuals. The function of family physicians varies internationally and between rural and urban areas. They are only able to play a key role in genetic screening and counselling if their national health service is underpinned by a comprehensive system of primary care, as in the UK, the Netherlands, and Scandinavia. A key role is unlikely if either family medicine is relatively uncommon, as in the USA, China or developing countries, or people have routine direct access to specialists, or can consult several different family physicians each practicing separately from the other, as in Germany, France, and other European countries.

This chapter is grounded in our experience of the UK system of primary care, although many of the issues we raise will be relevant to other systems. The main objectives of UK general practice are to provide primary health care that is available and acceptable to the whole population and to refer appropriately to secondary care. It has a long tradition of involvement in national screening programmes. In the UK, GPs are generalists, doctors of first contact who set no limits to the type of health or social problems which patients can present. In recent years the prevention of ill health and surveillance of individuals with chronic disease have become increasingly important components of their work. GPs therefore have a key role in identifying and counselling people at risk of developing specific diseases.

Over 95% of the UK population are registered with one of over 33,000 GPs. Most practice in groups of four or five, increasingly as members of a team of health workers, including practice nurses and other professionals including generic counsellors. They accept responsibility for a defined list of patients from a restricted locality, in urban areas only extending over a few square miles. GPs see patients on average four times a year. They frequently look after several members of a family, who may live in the same house or neighbourhood for decades, and as a result develop a close relationship with many of their patients. This increases the GPs' respect for patient autonomy and acceptance of the need to negotiate acceptable solutions to problems – key concepts of genetic counselling. From the perspective of the population, it is the GPs *not* the hospital specialists, who provide personal and continuing care. Even specialist areas like obstetrics and management of serious chronic disease are usually shared between GP and specialist. It is therefore the responsibility of the specialist to inform the referring physician about the outcome of hospital admissions and visits to out-patient clinics.

First-hand family information is usually more accessible from general practice than from hospital records. GP records gradually accumulate data as the years go by and follow patients when they change practices. They contain GPs' notes of consultations, reports from other health professionals and hospitals, and records of investigations. Although in some practices, records from the same family are filed together, GP medical records are in general an underused and under-researched resource for identifying family patterns of disease. British practices increasingly use computers for the storage of patient clinical data and for surveillance of target groups (e.g. patients with diabetes or coronary heart disease). Availability of the computer during the consultation provides access to decision support programmes. These may be particularly useful in genetic counselling, and in helping estimate specific risks and probabilities for individual patients as part of a baseline evaluation (Harris and Harris, 1995).

Rapidly expanding medical knowledge and expertise has led to increasing specialization by health professionals. In hospitals, 'organ' or specific disease specialists have replaced GPs, inevitably leading to fragmentation of secondary care, with the exception of health care for children and the elderly. At the same time, research has confirmed the relationship between ill health and psychological, social and environmental factors. It follows that there is a need for a primary care doctor who is an expert in managing the health care of his specific patients in their particular social and psychological context (Orton, 1994). This need leads to the most important difference between a specialist and family physician. Namely, to remain competent, specialists must focus on maintaining their expertise in a restricted area. Family doctors remain generalists in order to respond to all problems brought to them and assess undifferentiated illness. They must be experts in early diagnosis and being able to identify individuals with a serious illness who consult with common symptoms. They are the link between the community and hospital, facilitating the most effective use of expensive hospital resources by appropriate referral to the correct specialist.

In the UK, a person registering with a GP is expected to attend for an introductory consultation with the doctor or nurse, during which brief details of the personal, past and family history are recorded, and act as an *aide-mémoire* at future consultations. This registration consultation, and even more relevant, family planning and consultations at the start of pregnancy, present an ideal opportunity to construct a brief family tree (Modell and Modell, 1992). This will need to be updated every few years.

Current 'genetic' practice within family medicine

Consultations related to reproduction are important in UK general practice and in family medicine in all parts of the world. Reproductive and related services, include provision of family planning, preconception advice and antenatal care. Genetic antenatal screening has two components.

Firstly, the identification of *sporadic disorders*, such as chromosomal and neural tube defects and other congenital abnormalities. These can only be screened for in pregnancy. Screening for an increased risk of Down syndrome and, increasingly, routine fetal anomaly scanning are now part of the antenatal programme in the UK and involve the GP in discussing the tests and their implications with the mother-to-be.

Secondly, the identification of *single gene disorders*. Screening for carriers of recessively inherited disorders is a widely accepted part of hospital-based antenatal screening programmes in the UK. Carrier couples have a 1:4 risk of an affected fetus in every pregnancy. Antenatal screening for haemoglobin disorders is integrated into the health system, and screening for cystic fibrosis is becoming established in Scotland and likely to develop elsewhere. There is increasing interest in screening for these disorders in primary care (Modell, 1993) because identification of 'at risk' couples before conception, or when the pregnancy is first reported to the GP (on average four weeks before the first hospital antenatal appointment), provides the maximum opportunity for these couples to consider their reproductive options. These include, not having children, accepting the risk of an affected child, or prenatal identification of the fetus's genotype.

Identification of carrier couples during pregnancy is not ideal. It is likely to lead to hurried counselling and a rushed decision whether or not to proceed with prenatal testing, often in mid-pregnancy. Amniocentesis, even if the result is normal, has adverse psychological effects on women that can persist after birth (Marteau, 1992).

Cancer genetics: a general practice strategy

Identification of people at risk – the family tree

The construction of a family tree is a key strategy for identifying people 'at risk' of a genetic problem. However, to make the task simple and quick, primary care workers need to be provided with tools, such as a simple computer template for drawing up a family tree, plus the recognized symbols and lists of genetic risk factors. The potential value of constructing a family tree is a fertile area of general practice research.

In some practices, the family tree is already extensively used as a shorthand method of highlighting past events of both emotional and genetic significance, and to help in understanding the dynamics of the family. There is seldom an obvious inherited late-onset disease, but it is often noted that families have more than their fair share of early-onset cancer or heart disease. The effect of a past history of a malignancy will be to increase the GPs' understanding of patients' anxieties and perhaps lower their threshold for investigating symptoms suggestive of a serious disease relevant to their family history.

Progression from taking this type of family history to construction of a simple pedigree is the key to increasing the involvement of the family doctor in community genetics. This pedigree will usually only need to include first degree relatives, unless genetic disease is suspected in a family member.

The aim of the primary care family tree is to:

● Document the family pattern of illness with the objective of highlighting susceptibility to premature onset of serious disease.
● Identify people with a family history that indicates that they may carry an X-linked or recessively inherited disease that confers a reproductive genetic risk.
● Identify people who would benefit from referral to a clinical geneticist.
● Identify relatives of patients with a known genetic disorder who may benefit from information and surveillance.

Potential workload

The average practice contains about 10,000 registered people. Newly diagnosed cancers are relatively unusual in day-to-day practice (Table 6.1), and a large practice is likely to contain only one or two families

Table 6.1. *Estimates of the incidence of new cancers in practice of 10,000 people in the UK*

Breast	5–10 a year
Breast (under the age of 30)	< 1 every 2 years
Lung	5–10 a year
Colon and rectum	3–4 a year
Stomach	1–2 a year
Ovary	1–2 every 2 years
Thyroid	1 every 7 years

Source: Adapted from Hodgson and Maher 1993

with an identified inherited cancer syndrome. Approximately 25/1000 patients will have a significant family history of breast, colon, ovarian or uterine cancer (Austoker, 1995). Initially, they will be the ones who will be offered genetic testing. However, genetic disease occurs in clusters, because relatives have a high risk of carrying the mutated gene. For example, first degree relatives of *BRCA1* mutation carriers will be at a 50% risk of also being carriers. Males, despite usually being unaffected, may pass the mutated copy of the gene onto their daughters. Thus the identification of one patient with inherited breast cancer means that the family doctor may be involved in counselling several female and male members of the family on his list. This also applies to other malignancies and as new gene loci are identified, potential workload will inevitably increase.

Women have an estimated 1:12 lifetime risk of developing breast cancer (Hodgson and Maher, 1993). It is thought that an inherited susceptibility accounts for 5% of all breast cancers and up to 25% of early-onset cases – less than one new case per GP every five years. Such estimates can give a false impression that heritable cancer susceptibility is too rare to be important for the family doctor. However, a practice contains many women who have already been treated for breast cancer, and they could also benefit from family studies. It has been estimated that one in 833 British women carry a mutated allele of *BRCA1* (Eeles, 1996). Therefore, a practice of 10,000 (5000 women) may include six carriers with a > 80% lifetime risk of developing breast and/or ovarian cancer (Ford et al., 1995). The number will be higher if the practice has a higher proportion of particular ethnic groups with a higher carrier prevalence, such as Ashkenazi Jews, where approximately 1% of the population may carry mutated alleles of *BRCA1* (Struewing et al., 1995).

Ethical dilemmas for family practitioners
DNA testing

Genetic testing is slowly becoming integrated into primary care. Family doctors' experience in offering genetic services in the context of reproduction appears to make them more willing to offer pre-symptomatic tests for adult onset diseases than their hospital (internist) or psychiatric colleagues (Geller et al., 1993). They are also becoming increasingly familiar with ethical issues of genetic testing. These include obtaining informed consent, confidentiality, informing a fit person of a health risk to themselves or a member of their present or future family, risk assessment and making difficult choices with respect to prenatal diagnosis and selective abortion. With reproductive genetic screening there may be problems of confidentiality around informing close relatives of newly identified carriers of their increased risk of carrying the disease in question. Thus, there are ethical aspects of antenatal screening within primary care that also apply to any extension of genetic testing. Survey and focus group studies of family physicians in the US showed that they were sceptical about the goals of full disclosure and non-directiveness, which are core values of counselling within clinical genetics (Geller and Holzman, 1995). British GPs may be less sceptical, but haemoglobinopathy screening tests unrelated to a pregnancy may be opportunistically requested with other blood tests without prior discussion with patients. GPs, in a study of cystic fibrosis screening in practice antenatal care, were concerned about the nature of informed consent by pregnant women and recognized that increased consultation time was needed for counselling (Harris et al., 1993). Over 100 distinct *BRCA1* mutations have been detected (Eeles, 1996) generally making screening impractical unless the mutation in the family has been delineated. A negative result in a woman in a family with a specific mutation does not mean that she cannot carry a *BRCA1* mutation, as there could possibly be a mutation on the other side of the family which has not been tested for.

DNA screening

The essential difference between 'reproductive' genetic screening and adult cancer genetic screening must be recognized and false parallels avoided. In the former the presenting person is fit, and testing is aimed at maximizing the possibility of the birth of a healthy baby; in the latter it is aimed at identifying risk of later disease in the presenting patient. As long as GPs offer genetic testing to small target groups on the basis of a family history (e.g. women with a significant family history of breast cancer), specific informed consent can be obtained, as for haemoglobino-pathy screening in pregnancy. But genetic screening for cancer and other adult onset diseases could eventually be extended from testing an individual with a strong family history to population screening, i.e. offering a test to all adults. This prospect, unlike reproductive screening, is some way in the future. Elias and Annas (1994) raise the possibility of 'generic' consent for screening, analogous to consent for a physical examination, which would be a fundamentally different model of genetic testing from that developed hitherto in antenatal care (Harris and Harris, 1995).

Discrimination

The use of genetic data by outside bodies who do not have the best interests of individual patients as a priority, needs to be addressed by GPs (Van McCrary et al., 1993). Precedents exist within current practice in the management of HIV test results. In the UK, many family doctors declined to divulge to insurance companies whether or not their patients had undergone HIV testing (Billings et al., 1992). This may lead to the non-recording of certain results, which could extend to genetic testing. In Belgium, France, and Norway the use of genetic information by life and medical insurance companies is prevented by law, which removes pressure from family physicians to hide the results of genetic testing on behalf of their patients. New Hampshire and a growing number of other American states have recently enacted legislation that prohibits employers from soliciting, requiring or administering genetic tests as a condition of employment. These issues are discussed in more detail in Chapter 3.

Uncertain outcomes

The explosion of information about genetic susceptibility to cancer is, in the foreseeable future, unlikely to be accompanied by evidence of clinical usefulness. For example, until we have trials evaluating possible preventive or treatment regimens for women with the *BRCA1* gene, their GP (and breast cancer specialist!) will not know which strategy will make a difference to their life expectancy and quality of life. Once the *BRCA1* gene is identified in a woman, it is likely that, at least in countries that have a comprehensive family doctor service, she will want to discuss her options with her family doctor as well as the breast cancer specialist.

Primary care guidelines for the management of women with a family history of breast cancer include criteria for selecting women who may be candidates for detection of deleterious genes, but acknowledge that increased surveillance of affected women may not necessarily reduce breast cancer mortality (Hoskins et al., 1995). Family physicians, particularly in the US, already deal with women who have had these tests in the context of research studies. Now, in spite of protests from the American Society of Human Genetics and the National Breast Cancer Coalition, a *BRCA1* gene test is being offered on a commercial basis in the US to women from ethnic groups at higher risk of carrying this gene (Mcarthy, 1996). Ethnic-specific tests are also available non-commercially in Canada (Rosenblatt et al., 1996). Family doctors may not have control over the use of these tests in their patients.

Commercial pressures to induce people to be tested for cancer susceptibility genes result in patients approaching their family physicians for information about, or referral for, the tests in countries where access to specialist care and testing is controlled by primary care. Where there is direct access to specialist clinical genetic services, family physicians will be presented with the *fait accompli* of test results. In either case, they will have to address the issues arising from cancer genetics testing long before there is evidence on effective management of patients with 'deleterious' genes, and deal with the psychological impact on patients who learn they are at high risk of malignancy (Kash et al., 1992).

What does the family physician need to know?

Family doctors will not become experts in cancer risk assessment. However, experienced family doctors should be able to manage the increasingly common situation of a woman requesting advice because of a family history of cancer of the breast and a vague knowledge from the media that 'it may be inherited'. They should also be aware of the indications for referral for an expert genetic opinion. This, of course, also applies to other common malignancies, such as cancer of the colon. Postgraduate training and continuing medical education for general practice has not kept pace with the current or future scope of genetics in clinical practice. This will have to change if family practice is to be able to provide truly comprehensive primary health care in the area of cancer genetics. Returning again to the example of breast cancer, it is possible to tentatively characterize necessary knowledge for the family doctor (Table 6.2).

Table 6.2. *Core knowledge for the family doctor (breast cancer)*

- It is a common disease, occurring in about 9% of British women during a lifetime.
- Most breast cancer is not inherited. However, in a small number of families there is a dominant pattern of inheritance, when children of the affected proband, here presumed to be a gene carrier, have a 50% chance of carrying the gene, and a high risk of developing the disease. When the mutant gene can be identified 'at risk' family members can often be definitively diagnosed by DNA studies.
- Clinical geneticists are often able to give a relatively accurate assessment of risk.
- Because breast cancer is common, it is not unusual for an affected proband to have a positive family history, for example of one post-menopausal affected relative. The female relatives of these women may only have a slightly increased risk of developing the disease and do not necessarily need to be referred unless they are particularly concerned.
- There may be genetic implications if a young woman develops breast cancer, even if there is a negative family history. She may be the first member of the family to present with a *BRCA1* or *BRCA2* mutation-related malignancy. Not all women with hereditary breast cancer have a positive family history.
- Indications for early referral for a geneticist's opinion include women with a first degree relative with ovarian cancer, more than one first degree relative affected by cancer of the breast especially if that malignancy developed before the age of 50

Communication between specialist and family doctor

Care shared between the specialist and the referring family doctor provides the opportunity for the optimum management of an individual who has been informed that she is at an increased risk of developing a malignancy – extremely stressful information. This requires good communication from the clinical geneticist back to the family doctor who would expect to receive specific information about their patient (Table 6.3).

The patient is very likely to come to the family doctor for advice following the hospital appointment, and the doctor must be provided with enough information to be able to continue counselling. Ideally the specialist should also provide the patient and family with written information as soon as the situation is clear. Future discussions are likely to be more fruitful if the family has had time to read and absorb information and thus to decide on the questions they wish to be answered. Discussions with family doctors are likely to cover a much wider area than surveillance or prophylaxis and will overlap with clinic consultations. The doctor may well have interacted with the family at their home or in the

Table 6.3: *Information from specialist to family doctor*

- What the patient has been told and how they reacted.
- The results of genetic tests. Is the help of the family doctor required to explain the need for testing other family members? NB The patient has the right to withold test results from any third party, including the family doctor.
- An assessment of the life-time risk of the disease developing.
- Which other family members are likely to be at risk.
- Management options – for example, increased surveillance, prophylactic surgery, and chemoprevention (should any drugs or behaviours be avoided).
- Follow-up arrangements.

consulting rooms in different circumstances, regarding the birth of a child, the severe illness of an elderly relative, redundancy or a change of job. These experiences may well provide them with insight into how best to help this particular family in times of stress or crisis. Many of the issues highlighted in Table 6.4 are common to primary or secondary care counselling of people with identified cancer susceptibility genes.

Finally, the case of Inga illustrates the problems that can arise if a patient is not under the care of a generalist who has an overview of a patient's problems and needs, provides continuing care and is in a position to co-ordinate the services provided by other health professionals.

Inga was aged 42, married with three young children when she arrived in the UK from Germany. She had a distant relationship with her family doctor and considered herself as under the care of 'the specialists'. Her mother had died at the age of 41 from cancer of the uterus. The mother had also suffered from cancer of the colon as had two of her sisters. Inga herself had had a malignant colonic polyp removed three years earlier, and had been told to have yearly colonoscopies. The surgeon she saw in the UK did not consider

Table 6.4. *Family doctor counselling for people at high genetic risk for cancer*

- Providing information in a manner that can be understood by the patient.
- Discussing the management options and the time-scale of making decisions.
- Discussing the insurance and employment implications.
- Ensuring that genetic information is clearly recorded in the family doctor's records (with consent of the patient).
- Maintenance of confidentiality. Informing other family members, if the patient agrees, although traditionally this is left to the patient.

annual surveillance to be necessary, and suggested biennial examinations. Unfortunately she developed subacute intestinal obstruction from a recurrence 18 months later. Shortly after this second operation she saw a geneticist who suggested a pelvic ultrasound because of the family history. The letter with the ultrasound appointment never arrived and Inga, not having been warned about symptoms of a possible problem, did not realize the significance of prolonged periods with intermenstrual bleeding. Invasive cancer of the uterus was diagnosed 18 months later, following a routine visit to the bowel surgeon.

Ideally if her family doctor had developed a good relationship with Inga, it would have been known that she had a remarkable family history of cancer of the colon and uterus. This would have lead to discussing with her which symptoms may indicate a possible serious problem, what would be the ideal gap between colonoscopies and referral to the *appropriate* surgeon. The doctor would be aware of the psychological benefits of annual surveillance, would have ensured that the ultrasound appointment arrived promptly and referred early for intermenstrual bleeding.

References

Austoker, J. 1995. Cancer prevention in primary care. Current trends and some prospects for the future II. *British Medical Journal* **309**: 517–20.

Billings, P.R., Kohn, M.A., de Cueva, M., Beckwith, J., Alper, J.S. and Natowicz, M.R. 1992 *American Journal of Human Genetics* **50**: 476–82.

Eeles, R. 1996. Testing for the breast cancer predisposition gene, *BRCA1*. *British Medical Journal* **313**: 572.

Elias, S. and Annas, G. 1994. Generic consent for genetic screening. *New England Journal of Medicine* **330**: 1611–13.

Ford, D., Easton, D.F. and Peto, J. 1995. Estimates of the gene frequency of BRCA1 and its contribution to breast and ovarian cancer incidence. *American Journal of Human Genetics* **57**: 1457–62.

Geller, G. and Holzman, N.A. 1995. A qualitative assessment of primary care physicians' perceptions about the ethical and social implications of offering genetic testing. *Qualitative Health Research* **5**: 9–167.

Geller, G., Tambor, E.S., Chase, G.A., Hofman, K.A., Faden, R.R. and Holtzman, N.A. 1993. Incorporation of genetics in primary care practice: will physicians do the counselling and will they be directive? *Archives of Family Medicine* **2**: 1119–25.

Harris, R. and Harris, H. 1995. Primary care for patients at genetic risk. *British Medical Journal* **311**: 579–80.

Harris, H., Scotcher, D., Hartley, N., Wallace, A., Craufurd, D. and Harris, R. 1993. Cystic fibrosis carrier testing in early pregnancy by general practitioners. *British Medical Journal* **306**: 1580–3.

Hodgson S.V. and Maher, E.R. 1993. *A Practical Guide to Human Cancer Genetics*. Cambridge: Cambridge University Press.

Hoskins, K.F., Stopfer, J.E., Calzone, K.A., Merajver, S.D., Rebbeck, T.R., Garber, J.E. and Weber, B.L. 1995. Assessment and counselling for women with a family history of breast cancer: a guide for clinicians. *JAMA* **273**: 577–85

Kash, K.M., Holland, J.C. Halper, M.S. and Miller, D.G. 1992. Psychological distress and surveillance behaviors of women with a family history of breast cancer. *Journal of the National Cancer Institute* **84**(1): 24–30

Marteau, T. 1992. Psychological effects of having amniocentesis: are these due to the procedure, the risk or the behaviour? *Journal of Psychosomatic Research* **36**: 395–402.

Mcarthy, M. 1996. US lab starts breast-cancer-gene screening. *Lancet* **347**: 1033.

Modell, M. 1993. Screening for carriers of cystic fibrosis – a general practitioner's perspective. *British Medical Journal* **307**: 849–52.

Modell, B. and Modell, M. 1992. *Toward a Healthy Baby: Congenital Disorders and the New Genetics in Primary Health Care.* Oxford: Oxford University Press.

Orton, P. 1994. Shared Care [Primary Care Tomorrow]. *Lancet* **344**: 1413–15.

Rosenblatt, D.S., Foulkes, W.D. and Narod, S.A. 1996. Genetic screening for breast cancer. *New England Journal of Medicine* **334**: 1200.

Struewing, J.P., Abeliovich, D., Peretz, T. et al. 1995. The carrier frequency of the 185dekAG mutation is approximately 1% in Ashkenazi Jewish individuals. *Nature Genetics* **11**: 198–200.

Van McCrary, S., Allen, B., Moseley, R., Crandall, L.A., Ostrer, J., Curry, R.W., Dewar, M.A. and Nye, D. 1993. Ethical and practical implications of the human genome initiative for family medicine. *Archives of Family Medicine* **2**: 1158–63.

7

Genetic epidemiologic approaches to finding genes that influence susceptibility to cancer

PAMELA ST. JEAN and NICHOLAS SCHORK

Summary

This chapter reviews the motivation and basic strategy behind gene mapping techniques that take advantage of modern molecular genetic tools. This approach often requires large samples of related individuals and the accommodation of, or acknowledgment that, factors other than the one investigated at the time may contribute to disease and, hence, are typically implemented in large-scale epidemiologic investigations. Two complementary biologically-motivated strategies that are rooted in this approach – the whole genome search and the candidate gene approach – are contrasted in this review, as are the two primary statistical strategies used to identify and characterize the effect of genes with related individuals: pedigree-based linkage analysis methods and allele sharing methods. Examples of published gene mapping studies that use this approach are listed in an effort to acquaint the interested reader with relevant investigations. In addition, a critical discussion of the problems that plague gene mapping studies of the type described is given, as are recommendations for combating these problems. Finally, a discussion of the utility of large cancer registries in gene mapping studies is offered to foster greater emphasis on their creation, support and use.

Introduction

The Human Genome Project (HGP) and related genetics research initiatives have placed a major emphasis on elucidating the role of genetic factors in disease. To support this emphasis, the HGP has facilitated the development of tools and resources that might lend themselves to relevant studies. For example, a major goal of the HGP is the construction of genetic and physical maps of each of the 24 human chromosomes (Jordan, 1992). One outcome of such constructions has been the production of high resolution genetic linkage maps that basically consist of laboratory tools that one can use to examine 'landmark' spots along different chromosomes and determine the relationship between these landmark regions and disease. Investigations of the association and/or 'linkage' of these landmark spots (known as 'marker loci') with a trait or disease in an effort to identify regions of chromosomes likely to encode mutations or DNA variants which influence that trait or disease are often referred to as 'gene mapping' studies. This review will focus on the motivation, theory and practices of such studies as they relate to cancer.

Cancer and genetics

Cancer is hypothesized to arise either through acquired somatic mutations, the result of heritable germline mutations, or a combination of both. Somatic mutations are those mutations which occur in any cell not destined to become a germ cell and, therefore, are not transmissible to future generations. Many types of cancer such as Wilms' tumour (Breslow, 1993) appear to be primarily due to the acquisition of somatic mutations (see Chapter 19). One tool for mapping somatic mutations has been to compare genetic material in tumour versus normal tissue within an individual and to look for somatic allele loss in tumours. Although work in the area of somatic cell damage and cancer is legion, our discussion will not focus on somatic mutations, but will be limited to discussing analytical methods, and their limitations, in detecting transmissible germline mutations through gene mapping techniques.

A primer on transmission genetics

In humans, nuclear DNA is linearly organized into 23 pairs of chromosomes. The collective genetic material associated with all chromosomes is termed a genome. Twenty-two of the chromosome pairs are autosomal (i.e. common to both sexes) while the remaining two chromosomes determine an individual's sex. One of each pair of chromosomes is maternally inherited, the other being inherited from the father. The chromosomes that make up a pair are termed homologs.

Most cell divisions occur through a process known as mitosis resulting in the formation of daughter cells which are identical to each other and to the parental cell from which they arose. These cells are diploid meaning they contain both members of a chromosome pair. Germ cell division, meiosis, is different in that the resulting daughter cells (egg or sperm) are haploid containing only one member from each chromosome pair. In meiosis there is an independent assortment of chromosomes, such that only one of each chromosomal pair is present in the daughter cell. Upon fertilization, the haploid germ cells unite thereby restoring the diploid number of chromosomes.

Genes are units of heredity responsible for inherited characteristics. A locus (plural loci) refers to a specific position on a chromosome or genome and includes both genes as well as regions of DNA of unknown function. A locus may sometimes show variation between individuals and the variants at a particular locus are called alleles. A polymorphic locus is one in which the most common allele occurs at a frequency of 95% or less in the population (Ott, 1991). A number of polymorphic loci along the human genome have been detected as a result of the HGP and related initiatives. These identified loci, or 'marker loci', collectively offer a 'map' of the human genome. Figure 7.1 depicts a hypothetical chromosome segment with the position of inter and intragenic DNA markers identified. The term genotype refers to the combination of alleles at a locus across two homologous chromosomes. Genotypes composed of alleles of the same type are called homozygous and genotypes composed of alleles of different types are called heterozygous.

During meiosis, homologous chromosomes pair up and exchange genetic material. This exchange of material, called recombination, results in chromosomes that differ from each of the two parental chromosomes. The recombination fraction, θ, is the probability that a gamete produced by a parent is a recombinant between two loci. Genetic distance is often measured in centiMorgans (cM) with 1 cM roughly corresponding to a θ of 0.01 (1% recombination). The points of exchange, called chiasmata, occur roughly every 50 cM (an average chromosome being approximately 150 cM long). The closer two loci are to each other, the less chance there is that a recombination will occur between them. When there is less than a 50% chance the loci will recombine, the loci are said to be linked. A θ close to 0 implies the two loci are tightly linked and highly likely to cosegregate or be transmitted together while a θ of 0.5 implies the two loci are segregating independently of one another (i.e. they are unlinked).

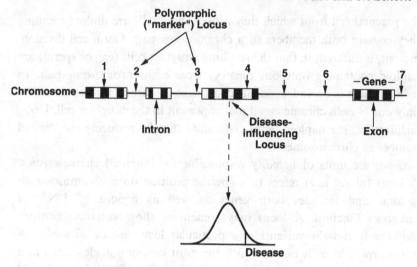

Figure 7.1. Graphical representation of the placement of genes and DNA markers. The horizontal line represents a segment of a chromosome (or genome). The boxes represent genes, or stretches of DNA that encode biologically functional information. The shaded segments of the genes represent exons or the coding segments of a gene, whereas the non-shaded segments denote introns or possibly inert filler or non-coding segments of a gene. The arrows represent the positions of DNA markers. Note that some of these markers might be within genes (e.g. markers 1 and 4), exons (marker 1), or introns (marker 4), while the majority reside in the intergenic regions of the genome (markers 2, 3, 5, 6 and 7), and that at some points it is possible to have multiple markers reside in an intergenic segment (markers 5 and 6).

Basic techniques for detecting disease genes

Two basic methods are used to localize disease genes to specific chromosomal regions. These methods trace cosegregation and recombination patterns within pedigrees and assess allele sharing between pairs of relatives. In the next section we will describe both of these methods along with their limitations. To begin with, however, we will discuss two complementary approaches that are at the heart of gene mapping studies – the candidate gene approach and genome-wide searches using anonymous markers. Candidate genes are genes whose biological functions (or disruption thereof) may be of relevance to the disease under consideration. Such genes may be identified through model organism studies and human evolutionary homolog comparisons, knowledge of the expression pattern of the gene, or through knowledge of some biological product influenced by the gene that is known to be implicated in the disease process. We will return to candidate gene studies later.

Unlike the candidate gene approach, genome-wide searches do not assume prior knowledge of the gene(s) involved in the disease process. Genome scans work by tracing the inheritance of variants (i.e. alleles) at landmark spots (i.e. marker loci) on the genome to draw inferences about the putative trait-influencing loci that reside near those landmark spots. Most marker loci have no known function. However, candidate loci may be included among the marker loci in such studies. The marker may be a restriction fragment length polymorphism (RFLP), although most of the newer markers being developed are derived from highly variable tandem repeat sequences such as dinucleotide or tetranucleotide repeats. With the initiation of the HGP and related initiatives such as Généthon (Weissenbach et al., 1992; Gyapay et al., 1994) and the Cooperative Human Linkage Center, CHLC (Buetow et al., 1994; Murray et al., 1994), the number of highly polymorphic DNA markers identified has increased at an exponential rate. By having a number of such marker loci (whose relative order or physical location is known) and having an appropriate sample of individuals who have been genotyped at these markers, it is possible to test whether various regions along the genome show evidence of linkage or association to the trait under investigation. The power of such gene mapping studies may be increased by using markers that are more closely spaced and which are highly polymorphic, as this maximizes the amount of information one can extract from various positions along the genome. Since most markers are biologically inert, they can only be used to provide an estimate of the approximate position of relevant disease or trait-influencing loci. Once linkage or association is detected then additional methods such as positional cloning must be employed to actually identify the disease gene and its relevant mutations (Collins, 1995)

Tracing the inheritance of marker loci within families in an effort to draw inferences about the location of putative disease loci is often done in one of two ways. The first method involves tracing cosegregation and recombination phenomena between observed marker locus alleles and putative (unobserved) trait locus alleles among large families or pedigrees. The second method involves examining the degree to which related individuals affected by a disease share alleles at a particular locus or across multiple loci. Each of these methods is discussed below.

Linkage analysis within pedigrees

Linkage analysis within pedigrees works by tracing the transmission and cosegregation of alleles which can be observed (i.e. at a marker locus) with the hypothetical alleles at a locus that controls a disease. Assumptions about the number and nature of the alleles (i.e. is one dominant to the others?) as well as the distance of the hypothetical locus from the marker locus must be made. Figures 7.2 and 7.3 offer a

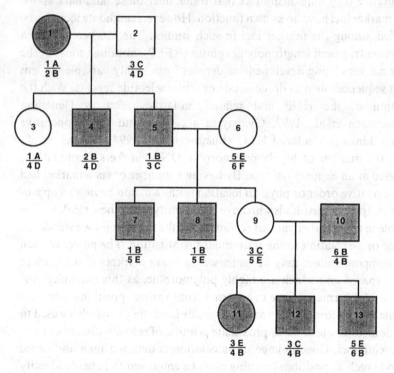

Figure 7.2. Graphical representation of the segregation of linked marker locus alleles with disease locus alleles. Circles denote females and squares denote males. Shading denotes diseased individuals. Segregation of alleles at two linked loci are portrayed: a number locus (whose variants or alleles are denoted by numbers) which is the linked marker locus and a letter locus which represents the disease influencing locus. The B allele is taken to be fully penetrant and dominant to all other alleles and hence induces disease unequivocally and without fail. The line between the two alleles possessed by each individual denotes phase information. Thus, for example, person 4 inherited the 2 and B alleles from his mother and the 4 and D alleles from his father. Since the 2 and B alleles and the 4 and D alleses were on the same chromosomes within the mother and father, respectively, no recombination between the number and letter loci took place in the meiotic events leading to the formation of the gametes passed on to individual 4. This is not the case for person 5, in which the 1 and B alleles transmitted from the mother represent a recombination event. Note that disease alleles can enter into a pedigree through a marry-in (e.g. person 10). Such phenomena often confound the tracing of co-segregation and recombination events within pedigrees, since their is no clear-cut single line of descent for disease alleles.

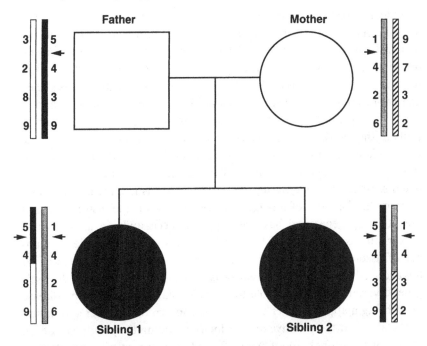

Figure 7.3. Graphical representation of the transmission of alleles at multiple linked loci within a nuclear family. The numbers represent alleles at four different loci. The different shading patterns within the rectangular bars represent the chromosome pairs within the father and mother. The arrow denotes the location of a disease locus which induces disease only when two copies of a deleterious allele are present (e.g. the disease allele is recessive). The two offspring are both affected because they were transmitted segments of parental chromosomes that harbored the disease allele. Recombination events are denoted by the mixture of shading within the offspring chromosomes and reflect chromosomal segments that recombined within the parents during meiosis. Note that the marker alleles are not fully informative at some loci. For example, the bottom locus for the father was homozygous for the 9 allele, making it impossible to distinguish which chromosome the 9 allele transmitted to his offspring came from. However, by using the neighbouring marker loci one could probabilistically assess which chromosome such alleles came from by taking recombination into account. Thus for sibling 2, the fact that the 9 allele at the bottom locus was transmitted along with the 5, 4, and 3 alleles at the neighbouring loci suggests that the 9 allele was inherited from the darkened chromosome from the father. If only marker alleles were observed (i.e. we did not have shading patterns denoting chromosomal segments and their origin in parents) and the distance between the bottom locus and the neighbouring loci was small, thus making recombination between the loci improbable, then it could be *inferred* that the 9 allele at the bottom locus originated from the chromosome that harboured the 5, 4, and 3 alleles.

graphical depiction of the segregation and recombination principles behind linkage analysis. If, in a linkage analysis setting, one can conclude that little, if any, recombination would have had to occur between the observed marker alleles and the hypothetical disease locus alleles given the pattern of transmission for the marker alleles and the disease, then one could infer that a disease locus is likely to reside near the marker locus. If a great deal of recombination would have had to occur to explain the marker locus alleles and disease transmission, then one would likely test for linkage at another locus. Evidence for a lack of recombination – and hence linkage between the marker locus and a putative disease locus – is typically captured in a statistic known as the 'lod' score or the *log od*ds of linkage. Linkage analysis is the historic method used to map genes and has been applied successfully in a number of cancer studies (see Tables 7.1 through 7.5). As suggested earlier, a number of assumptions are required to conduct traditional pedigree-based linkage analysis. First and foremost is that the majority of the disease's genetic variance is attributable to a single, major locus (i.e. the disease locus being mapped). Other assumptions concern the number and nature of the alleles at the putative disease locus including the *penetrance* of the alleles, or the probability of being affected given a particular genotype at the putative disease locus. When the mode of inheritance is not clear, something that is likely to be the case for a complex disease like cancer, a researcher will often select a few predetermined models under which the analyses will be conducted.

As noted earlier, a measure of the extent of linkage is given by the lod score, the base 10 logarithm of the likelihood ratio comparing the hypothesis of linkage ($\theta < 0.5$) with the null hypothesis of free recombination ($\theta = 0.5$) between the marker and hypothetical disease loci. For standard pedigree-based linkage analyses a lod score greater than 3.3 should be considered evidence for linkage (Lander and Schork, 1994; Lander and Kruglyak, 1995). Once evidence for linkage is found, one could genotype pedigree members at additional loci near the marker(s) showing linkage in an effort to find stronger evidence for linkage and thereby refine the location of the disease locus.

Since many diseases of contemporary interest do not follow simple mendelian patterns of inheritance, it is extremely likely that the genetic model specified in a pedigree-based linkage analysis will not be correct. The effect of model misspecification can be dramatic depending on how badly the model is misspecified (Clerget-Darpoux et al., 1986). To avoid some of the problems inherent in model-based methods such as this,

Table 7.1. *Skin neoplasia linkage studies*

Neoplasia type	Reference	Comments
Familial atypical multiple mole-melanoma (FAMM)	Bale et al. (1989b)	Multipoint linkage analysis indicated gene for cutaneous malignant melanoma/dysplastic nevus (CMM/DN) was located on 1p36 between D1S47 and PND
	van Haeringen et al. (1989), Cannon-Albright et al. (1990), Nancarrow et al. (1992)	Reported evidence against linkage of CMM/DN to 1p36
	Goldstein et al. (1993)	Analyzed 7 new families as well as updated versions of 6 families described in Bale et al. (1989b). Evidence for linkage of CMM to 1p as well as evidence for genetic heterogeneity.
	Cannon-Albright et al. (1992), Nancarrow et al. (1993)	Evidence of linkage of melanoma to 9p21. Dysplastic nevi were not considered part of the phenotype
	Bergman et al. (1994)	In 7 Dutch families FAMMM was linked to 9p21 and excluded from 1p
	Goldstein et al. (1994)	Considered CMM/DN as combined trait and found evidence of linkage to 9p as well as evidence for heterogeneity
Nevoid basal cell carcinoma (NBCC)	Gailani et al. (1992)	Cosegregation of markers on 9q31 with NBCC
Neurofibromatosis type 1 (NF1)	Barker et al. (1987), Seizinger et al. (1987)	Evidence of linkage of NF1 to 17q
	Goldgar et al. (1989)	Refinement of linkage of NF1 to proximal 17q (pHHH202-NF1-EW206)
Bazex–Dupré–Christol syndrome	Vabres et al. (1995)	Evidence of linkage to Xq24-q27

Table 7.2. *Multiple endocrine neoplasia linkage studies*

Neoplasia type	Reference	Comments
Multiple endocrine neoplasia type 1 (MEN1)	Larsson et al. (1988), Thakker et al. (1989), Bale et al. (1989a), Nakamura et al. (1989)	MEN1 localized to pericentromeric region of 11 (11q12-q13)
Hereditary hyperparathyroidism and prolactinoma (MEN1$_{BURIN}$)	Petty et al. (1994)	Phenotypically similar to MEN1 but lacks pancreatic islet tumours. MEN1$_{BURIN}$ maps to same region as MEN1 and may represent intralocus heterogeneity
Multiple endocrine neoplasia type 2A (MEN2A)	Mathew et al. (1987)	MEN2A linked to pericentromeric region of chromosome 10
Multiple endocrine neoplasia type 2B (MEN2B)	Gardner et al. (1993) Lairmore et al. (1991)	Mapping of MEN2A refined to 10q11.2 MEN2B mapped to pericentromeric region of chromosome 10

Table 7.3. *Breast cancer linkage studies*

Cancer type	Reference	Comments
Early onset breast–ovarian cancer	Hall et al. (1990; Narod et al. (1991)	Linkage to 17q21
	Easton et al. (1993)	Breast Cancer Linkage Consortium reported evidence that *BRCA1* lay between D17S588 and D17S250. An estimated 100% of breast–ovarian cancer families and 45% of families without ovarian cancer were linked to *BRCA1* under the genetic model used in the analysis
	Narod et al. (1995a)	76% of 145 breast–ovarian cancer families linked to *BRCA1*. Families with male breast cancer were not linked to *BRCA1*
Early onset breast cancer not linked to *BRCA1*	Wooster et al. (1994)	*BRCA2* mapped to 13q12-q13. High risk of early onset breast cancer but not ovarian cancer
	Narod et al. (1995b)	Seven of the 10 breast–ovarian cancer families (Narod et al., 1995a) with lod-scores < −0.80 with markers flanking *BRCA1* showed positive linkage to *BRCA2*

Table 7.4. *Colon cancer linkage studies*

Cancer type	Reference	Comments
Familial adenomatous polypopsis (FAP)	Bodmer et al. (1987); Leppert et al. (1987)	Linkage between gene for FAP (designated APC) and pC11p11 (D5S71) located at 5q21-q22
	Nakamura et al. (1988)	Refinement of linkage distal to D5S71; no evidence of genetic heterogeneity between FAP and Gardner syndrome (GS)
	Leppert et al. (1990)	Family with variable number of adenomatous polyps linked to same area of 5q as FAP and GS
Hereditary nonpolyposis colorectal cancer (HNPCC)	Peltomaki et al. (1993)	Linkage of HNPCC to D2S123 on 2p15-16 in two large families
	Green et al. (1994)	One of 7 Canadian families showed strong evidence of linkage to the 2p HNPCC locus designated COCA1.
	Lindblom et al. (1993), Tännergard et al. (1994)	Three HNPCC families linked to 3p23-p21
	Nyström-Lahti et al. (1994)	Finnish families linked to 3p in a 1 cM interval between D3S1561 and D3S1298 with evidence of a single ancestral mutation

Table 7.5. *Miscellaneous neoplasia linkage studies*

Cancer type	Reference	Comments
Retinoblastoma (RB)	Sparkes et al. (1983)	**RB** linked to esterase-D on 13q14 ($Z = 3.50$, $\theta = 0.0$)
	Scheffer et al. (1989)	Flanking and intragenic RB1 markers were used to estimate frequency of non-penetrant mutations
Ataxia-telangiectasia (A-T)	Gatti et al. (1988); Foroud et al. (1991)	Localization of A-T gene to 11q23.
Neurofibromatosis type 2 (NF2)	Wertelecki et al. (1988)	NF2 mapped to 22q11.1-q13.1
von Hippel-Lindau disease (VHL)	Seizinger et al. (1988); Maher et al. (1990); Hosoe et al. (1990)	VHL linked to RAF1 on 3p25-26
	Richards et al. (1993)	Mapping refined to D3S1250-VHL-D3S18
Familial platelet disorder with propensity to develop AML	Legare et al. (1995)	Platelet disorder mapped to 21q22.1-22.2
Focal palmoplantar keratoderma with oesophageal cancer	Kelsell et al. (1995)	Linkage to 17q24

many investigators are relying more on allele sharing methods which are less reliant on modeling the actions of the putative disease alleles.

Allele-sharing methods

Allele-sharing methods take advantage of the simple intuition that phenotypically similar pairs of relatives are more likely to share genetic material at relevant loci than phenotypically dissimilar individuals. The analytical procedures for allele-sharing methods are relatively straightforward. For each relative pair, measures of phenotypic similarity and genotypic similarity are computed. If an association between the measure of phenotypic similarity and genotypic similarity is found, then one could infer that the genetic material in the vicinity of the locus used to define genotypic similarity encodes variants or alleles which influence the trait in question. This strategy can be simplified by taking only concordant relative pairs (e.g. siblings both afflicted with cancer) and determining if these pairs share alleles more often than expected under random mendelian expectation. The two most commonly used measures of allele sharing are the number of alleles shared *identical-by-state* (IBS) and the number of alleles shared *identical-by-descent* (IBD). Alleles IBS are merely alleles that are alike in kind. Alleles IBD have been transmitted to a pair of relatives from a common ancestor. Thus, IBD implies IBS, but not vice versa (Figure 7.2). IBD measures require parental information, whereas IBS measures do not. For example, under the null hypothesis of no linkage the probability that sibling pairs share 0, 1 or 2 alleles IBD is 0.25, 0.50 and 0.25, respectively. One could then test if (in siblings) the probability of sharing 2 alleles IBD is greater than 25% or whether they share 1 marker allele greater than 50% of the time.

Since the goal of genetic analysis, and allele sharing methods in particular, is to investigate the *transmission* of deleterious or trait-influencing genetic material, IBD measures are more reliable than IBS measures. This is especially the case if there is a very frequent allele at the marker locus under investigation, since relative pairs may share that allele merely because it is frequent in the population, not because it was transmitted to them along with a specific trait influencing allele at a neighbouring locus. When it is difficult to resolve IBD status because parents are homozygous for a particular allele, neighbouring marker alleles can be used to investigate 'haplotype' transmission or sequence of alleles at the marker loci.

Several points need to be made regarding allele sharing methods. Firstly, no underlying genetic model is assumed so one need not worry about model misspecification. Secondly, IBS methods are generally less powerful than IBD methods and are also very sensitive to knowledge of allele frequencies in the population at large. The more polymorphic a marker locus is, the more likely IBS information computed at the marker approximates the IBD information for the marker. In IBS analysis, allele frequency information must be included and if one mistakenly assumes that an allele is less frequent than it really is, the false positive rate may be increased. Thirdly, if a marker locus is not near the actual disease locus, IBD/IBS sharing at the marker locus will not provide a good estimate of IBD/IBS sharing at the disease locus. Fourthly, as emphasized previously, unlike linkage analysis within pedigrees, one may look at a sample of relative pairs composed entirely of affecteds and simply compare the frequency of alleles or regions (if using multiple loci) of shared IBD or IBS with what would be expected under the null hypothesis of no linkage. If the deviation from expected is significant, one can infer that this region may harbour the disease locus. Finally, in a recent paper, Lustbader, Rebbeck and Buetow (1995) suggest that incorporating tumour loss of heterozygosity data in cancer studies can improve marker allele similarity measures in normal tissue leading to an increase in power to reject linkage. They caution that this method is only applicable to cancers arising through the 'model of recessive oncogenesis'.

Case control and general candidate gene analysis

Tests of candidate genes, alleles, or mutations can be conducted easily. One either examines the greater frequency of the allele among affected as opposed to unaffected individuals, or looks for the greater-than-expected transmission of the specific allele to affected offspring (Terwilliger and Ott, 1992; Schaid and Sommer, 1993; Spielman et al., 1993).

Problems encountered in genetic analysis

The approaches described in the previous section are not without their problems. We discuss some of these problems below, and where possible, make suggestions as to how to overcome them.

Reduced penetrance and phenocopies

Many diseases exhibit *reduced or incomplete penetrance* whereby some individuals who carry the disease causing gene are unaffected. This suggests that other genetic or environmental factors may also contribute to the pathogenesis of the disease. In many diseases penetrance increases with advancing age. For example, in women carrying a mutation at the *BRCA1* locus, the probability of being affected with breast cancer is 55%, 73% and 87% by ages 40, 50 and 70, respectively (Ford et al., 1994). If one assumes a disease is fully penetrant when it is not, then it becomes difficult to tell if an individual is unaffected because she or he does not carry the disease allele or is simply non-penetrant at that point in time. The power to detect linkage will be reduced and the recombination fraction, θ, will tend to be overestimated, suggesting a greater distance between marker and disease locus. One way to deal with reduced penetrance is to include a penetrance parameter in the linkage analysis that would allow for differences in penetrance by sex and/or age. Another method is to carry out an affecteds-only analysis using either allele-sharing methods or linkage analysis within pedigrees as described in Terwilliger and Ott (1994).

Another problem plaguing genetic analysis that is similar to reduced penetrance involves the presence of *phenocopies,* in which some individuals with the disease have it because of non-genetic factors. An example of this might be lung cancer due to cigarette smoking rather than to an inherited gene. Many diseases are influenced by strong environmental components and, thus, determining whether an individual's disease is due to his or her genotype, environmental exposure or a combination of both can be difficult. As with reduced penetrance, the inclusion of phenocopies in a study will reduce the power to find linkage and will result in an overestimate of θ. Often genetic cases of disease have an earlier age-at-onset than is seen with phenocopies, thus, restricting analysis to families with early age-at-onset, which may aid in detecting linkage.

Genetic (locus) heterogeneity and epistasis

Mutations in more than one gene may lead to the same (or similar) phenotype. When mutations at different loci can cause a disease independently of one another *locus heterogeneity* is said to exist. As an example, in hereditary nonpolyposis colorectal cancer (HNPCC) linkage has been demonstrated to the short arms of both chromosomes 2 and 3 (Peltomaki et al., 1993; Lindblom et al., 1993; Green et al., 1994; Tånnergard et al.,

1994; Nyström-Lahti et al., 1994). Locus heterogeneity makes gene mapping more difficult since a genetic region may segregate with the disease in some families but not in others. One can use tests to detect heterogeneity. The HOMOG program (Ott, 1991) conducts two different tests to this end. One of these involves a test for homogeneity given linkage and the other tests for linkage given heterogeneity. A different phenomenon, known as *allelic heterogeneity*, in which more than one disease causing allele exists at the same locus, tends not to affect linkage analyses, but it is important when attempts are made to identify the mutations that actually cause (or are causally related to) a disease.

When the interaction of two or more different loci are required for the disease to be occur *epistasis* is said to be present. As with locus heterogeneity, epistasis can hamper gene mapping studies as one does not often have prior information as to the number or nature of the interaction of genes involved in producing the disease. No reliable tests exist for the detection of epistasis, although Schork et al. (1993) provide some methods. As of now, the only means to address this problem are to use methods which are powerful enough to detect the association between one of a number of genes leading to the disease and the disease itself. Ghosh and Collins (1996) suggest that using an affecteds-only method might increase the power to detect epistatic loci.

Pleiotropy

A locus which leads to multiple phenotypic endpoints is said to be acting *pleiotropically*. As an example, the *BRCA1* gene has been implicated in ovarian as well as breast cancer (Easton et al., 1993). Pleiotropy has not been explored in depth in linkage analysis contexts. Recent work by Jiang and Zeng (1995), however, suggests that including information on multiple traits together in an analysis leads to increased power in detecting a pleiotropic locus, but only under certain conditions.

Other genetic mechanisms

In recent years, genetic mechanisms beyond autosomal and sex-linked loci have been found to influence disease. These mechanisms include genomic imprinting, mitochondrial inheritance and trinucleotide repeat expansions. These mechanisms may account for non-mendelian patterns of inheritance seen in many diseases. Their accommodation in linkage settings, although not unprecedented (see Schork and Guo, 1993), has not been pursued seriously.

The use of cancer registries in genetic epidemiological studies

Cancer registries can provide a valuable resource in the genetic analysis of cancer. They provide for the identification of probands (index cases). These probands can be used in case/control association studies as well as being used to identify families enriched for multiple affected relatives that can in turn be used in linkage and/or association studies. If a registry provides information such as age-at-diagnosis, area of residence or origin, cancer site, or presence of other cancers, then a researcher may identify potentially homogeneous subgroups of patients (and families), which are likely to be more informative in association and linkage studies than a random collection of families.

There are three main kinds of cancer registries: (1) those which are population based; (2) those which are hospital-based; and (3) those which are limited to a particular type of cancer (see Tables 7.6 and 7.7). Population-based cancer registries are usually representative of the population from which they are drawn and may be used in a variety of ways for both genetic and epidemiological analyses. For example, population registries may be used to identify cases for case/control studies as well as to identify cancer proband families for use in linkage analyses. They may also be used for more traditional epidemiological studies such as identifying geographic differences in cancer prevalence, as well as evaluating cancer risk factors, survival patterns or treatment effectiveness. The SEER database in the US covers approximately 10% of the US population and encompasses individuals from different ethnic backgrounds as well as from different geographic areas (Ries et al., 1994). The Utah Population Database (UPDB) is distinctive in that it combines information from the Utah Cancer Registry and Utah death certificates with a genealogy database (Cannon-Albright et al., 1994). In approximately 36% of all cancer cases in Utah, genetic relationships can be established and examined and families with multiple affecteds may be identified. In a recent study, Slattery and Kerber (1994) used the UPDB to address the effect of cancer family history on the risk of developing colon cancer and concluded that colon cancer screening is warranted in individuals who have a first-degree relative with colon cancer and perhaps should be extended to those individuals with second- or third-degree relatives with colon cancer.

Cancer registries may also be hospital based or specific for a type of cancer. In the UK, several registries exist for familial adenomatous polyposis (FAP). These registries are particularly valuable in identifying can-

Table 7.6. *Population-based cancer registries*

Cancer registry	Reference	Comments
United States		
SEER (surveillance epidemiology and end results)	Ries et al. (1994)	Supported by National Cancer Institute since 1973. It includes 9 population-based registries and covers more than 10% of the US population. The Connecticut registry has been in existence since 1935
Utah Cancer Registry	Goldgar et al. (1993), Cannon-Albright et al. (1994)	Identification of cancer pedigrees by linking Utah Population Database with the registry
Europe		
Danish Cancer Registry	Parkin et al. (1992)	Initiated in 1942
Birmingham and West Midlands Cancer Registry – England and Wales		Established in 1936
Cancer Registry of Norway		Covers all of Norway and was initiated in 1952
Vas Registry – Hungary		Operational since 1952
Zaragoza Registry – Spain		Began in 1960
South American		
Cali Registry – Colombia	Parkin et al. (1992)	Operational since 1962
Asia		
Singapore Registry	Parkin et al. (1992)	Dates back to 1968
Miyagi Prefectual Cancer Registry – Japan		Began in 1951
Shanghai Registry		Established in 1963
Bombay Cancer Registry		Operational since 1963

Table 7.7. *Cancer registries by cancer type*

Cancer registry	Reference	Comments
UK Northern Region Polyposis registry	Burn et al. (1991)	Registry of FAP families established in 1987 in Northern England
Northern Ireland FAP registry	Campbell (1991)	Established in 1989
Polyposis Registry at St. Mark's Hospital, London	Bodmer et al. (1987)	Registry has existed for over 50 years. Families identified through this registry were used to localize FAP locus to chromosome 5
Health Care District of Modena, Italy	Ponz de Leon et al. (1993)	Colorectal cancer registry established in 1984 with the objective to identify and study families with HNPCC
National UK Coordinating Committee for Cancer Research Familial Ovarian Cancer Registry	Green et al. (1993)	Established in 1991 to identify women with at least two close relatives with ovarian cancer

Note: FAP: familial adenomatous polyposis; HNPCC: hereditary non-polyposis colorectal cancer.

cer families. The Polyposis Registry at St. Mark's Hospital, London was used to identify families that were then used to localize the FAP locus to chromosome 5 (Bodmer et al., 1987).

Conclusion

In this chapter we have tried to spell out, in as non-technical a way as possible, the principles and concepts behind modern genetic-epidemiological approaches towards the identification of genes influencing the susceptibility to cancer. We have tried to document many of the successes as these approaches have had by listing studies claiming to have identified cancer susceptibility loci. However, we have made explicit attempts to temper enthusiasm one might develop from such successes by pointing out the very overt problems that plague genetic-epidemiological analysis of complex traits like cancer. Although those problems are, in principle, capable of being overcome, this will only come about through an appropriate use of resources, such as cancer registries and modern molecular biology tools. It is our belief that the best way to advance the field of cancer genetics is to comment on what has been done, expose the shortcomings of the approaches used, make suggestions for correcting these shortcomings, and in this way ultimately inform and motivate a new breed of researcher to take things to the next step.

References

Bale, S.J., Bale, A.E., Stewart, K. et al. 1989a. Linkage analysis of multiple endocrine neoplasia type 1 with INT2 and other markers on chromosome 11. *Genomics* **4**: 320–2.

Bale S.J., Dracopoli N.C., Tucker, M.A. et al. 1989b. Mapping the gene for hereditary cutaneous malignant melanoma-dysplastic nevus to chromosome 1p. *New England Journal of Medicine* **320**: 1367–72.

Barker, D, Wright, E., Nguyen, K. et al. 1987. Gene for von Recklinghausen neurofibromatosis is in the pericentromeric region of chromosome 17. *Science* **236**: 1100–2.

Bergman, W., Gruis, N.A., Sandkuijl, L.A. and Frants, R.R. 1994. Genetics of seven Dutch familial atypical multiple mole-melanoma syndrome families: a review of linkage results including chromosomes 1 and 9. *Journal of Investigative Dermatology* **103**: 122S–125S.

Bodmer, W.F., Bailey, C.J., Bodmer, J. et al. 1987. Localization of the gene for familial adenomatous polyposis on chromosome 5. *Nature* **328**: 614–16.

Breslow, N. 1993. *Are All Bilateral Wilms Tumors Hereditary?* Technical Report No. 123. National Wilms' Tumor Study.

Buetow, K.H., Weber, J.L., Ludwigsen, S. et al. 1994. Integrated human genome-wide maps constructed using the CEPH reference panel. *Nature Genetics* **6**: 391–3.

Burn, J., Chapman, P., Delhanty, J. et al. 1991. The UK Northern Regional genetic register for familial adenomatous polyposis coli: use of age of onset, congenital hypertrophy of the retinal pigment epithelium, and DNA markers in risk calculation. *Journal of Medical Genetics* **28**: 289–96.

Campbell, W.J. 1991. Regional register for familial adenomatous polyposis. *British Journal of Surgery* **78**: 1511.

Cannon-Albright, L.A., Goldgar, D.E., Meyer, L.J. et al. 1992. Assignment of a locus for familial melanoma, MLM, to chromosome 9p13-p22. *Science* **258**: 1148–52.

Cannon-Albright, L.A., Goldgar D.E., Wright, E.C. et al. 1990. Evidence against the reported linkage of the cutaneous melanoma-dysplastic nevus syndrome locus to chromosome 1p36. *American Journal of Human Genetics* **46**: 912–8.

Cannon-Albright L.A., Thomas, A., Goldgar, D.E. et al. 1994. Familiality of cancer in Utah. *Cancer Research* **54**: 2378–85.

Clerget-Darpoux, F., Bonaïti-Pelliè, C. and Hochez, J. 1986. Effects of misspecifying genetic parameters in lod score analysis. *Biometrics* **42**: 393–9.

Collins, F.S. 1995. Positional cloning moves from perditional to traditional. *Nature Genetics* **9**: 347–50.

Easton, D.F., Bishop, D.T., Ford, D., Crockford, G.P. and the Breast Cancer Linkage Consortium. 1993. Genetic linkage analysis in familial breast cancer and ovarian cancer: results from 214 families. *American Journal of Human Genetics* **52**: 678–701.

Ford, D., Easton, D.E., Bishop, D.T., Narod, S.A., Goldgar, D.E. and the Breast Cancer Linkage Consortium. 1994. Risks of cancer in BRCA1-mutation carriers. *Lancet* **343**: 692–5.

Foroud, T., Wei, S., Ziv, Y. et al. 1991. Localization of an ataxia-telangiectasia locus to a 3-cM interval on chromosome 11q23: Linkage analysis of 111 families by an international consortium. *American Journal of Human Genetics* **49**: 1263–79.

Gailani, M.R., Bale, S.J., Leffell, D.J. et al. 1992. Developmental defects in Gorlin Syndrome related to a putative tumor suppressor gene on chromosome 9. *Cell* **69**: 111–17.

Gardner, E., Papi, L., Easton, D.F. et al. 1993. Genetic linkage studies map the multiple endocrine neoplasia type 2 loci to a small interval on chromosome 10q11.2. *Human Molecular Genetics* **2**: 241–6.

Gatti, R.A., Berkel, I., Boder, E. et al. 1988. Localization of an ataxia-telangiectasia gene to chromosome 11q22-23. *Nature* **336**: 577–80.

Ghosh, S. and Collins, F.S. 1996. The geneticist's approach to complex disease. *Annual Review of Medicine* **47**: 333–53.

Goldgar, D.E., Cannon-Albright, L.A., Oliphant, A. et al. 1993. Chromosome 17q linkage studies of 18 Utah breast cancer kindreds. *American Journal of Human Genetics* **52**: 743–8.

Goldgar, D.E., Green, P., Parry, D.M. and Mulvihill, J.J. 1989. Multipoint linkage analysis in neurofibromatosis type 1: An international collaboration. *American Journal of Human Genetics* **44**: 6–12.

Goldstein, A.M., Dracopoli, N.C., Engelstein, M., Fraser, M.C., Clark, W.H. and Tucker, M.A. 1994. Linkage of cutaneous malignant melanoma/dysplastic nevi to chromosome 9p, and evidence for genetic heterogeneity. *American Journal of Human Genetics* **54**: 489–96.

Goldstein, A.M., Dracopoli, N.C., Ho, E.C. et al. 1993. Further evidence for a locus for cutaneous malignant melanoma-dysplastic nevus (CMM/DN) on chromosome 1p, and evidence for genetic heterogeneity. *American Journal of Human Genetics* **52**: 537–50.

Green, J., Murton, F., Statham, H. 1993. Psychosocial issues raised by a familial ovarian cancer register. *Journal of Medical Genetics* **30**: 575–9.

Green, R.C., Narod, S.A., Morasse, J. et al. 1994. Hereditary nonpolyposis colon cancer: analysis of linkage to 2p15-16 places the COCA1 locus telomeric to D2S123 and reveals genetic heterogeneity in seven Canadian families. *American Journal of Human Genetics* **54**: 1067–77.

Gyapay, G., Morissette, J., Vignal, A. et al. 1994. The 1993–1994 Généthon human genetic linkage map. *Nature Genetics* **7**: 246–339.

Hall, J.M., Lee, M.K., Newman, B. et al. 1990. Linkage of early-onset familial breast cancer to chromosome 17q21. *Science* **250**: 1684–9.

Hosoe, S., Brauch, H., Latif, F. et al. 1990. Localization of the von Hippel-Lindau disease gene to a small region of chromosome 3. *Genomics* **8**: 6–40.

Jiang, C. and Zeng, Z.B. 1995. Multiple trait analysis of genetic mapping for quantitative trait loci. *Genetics* **140**: 1111–27.

Kelsell, D.P, Stevens, H.P., Bryant, S.P. et al. 1995. Genetic analysis of families with focal palmoplantar keratoderma with or without malignancy. *American Journal of Human Genetics* **57**: A24.

Jordan, E. 1992. The Human Genome Project: where did it come from, where is it going? *American Journal of Human Genetics* **51**: 1–6.

Lairmore, T.C., Howe, J.R., Korte, J.A. et al. 1991. Familial medullary thyroid carcinoma and multiple endocrine neoplasia type 2B map to the same region of chromosome 10 as multiple endocrine neoplasia type 2A. *Genomics* **9**: 181–92.

Lander, E. and Kruglyak, L. 1995. Genetic dissection of complex traits: guidelines for interpreting and reporting linkage results. *Nature Genetics* **11**: 241–7.

Lander, E.S. and Schork, N.J. 1994. Genetic dissection of complex traits. *Science* **265**: 2037–48.

Larsson, C, Skogseid, B., Öberg, K., Nakamura, Y. and Nordenskjöld, M. 1988. Multiple endocrine neoplasia type 1 gene maps to chromosome 11 and is lost in insulinoma. *Nature* **332**: 85–7.

Legare, R.D., Ho, C.Y., Otterud, B. et al. 1995. A familial platelet disorder with propensity to develop acute myeloid leukemia is linked to human chromosome 21q22.1-22.2. *American Journal of Human Genetics* **57**: A24.

Leppert M., Burt, R., Hughes, J.P. et al. 1990. Genetic analysis of an inherited predisposition to colon cancer in a family with a variable number of adenomatous polyps. *New England Journal of Medicine* **322**: 904–8.

Leppert, M., Dobbs, M., Scambler, P. et al. 1987. The gene for familial polyposis coli maps to the long arm of chromosome 5. *Science* **238**: 1411–13.

Lindblom, A., Tannergård, P., Werleius, B. and Nordenskjöld, M. 1993. Genetic mapping of a second locus predisposing to hereditary non-polyposis colon cancer. *Nature Genetics* **5**: 279–82.

Lustbader, E.D., Rebbeck, T.R. and Buetow, K.H. 1995. Using loss of heterozygosity data in affected pedigree member linkage tests. *Genetics Epidemiology* **12**: 339-50.

Maher, E.R., Bentley, E., Yates, J.R.W. et al. 1990. Mapping of Von Hippel-Lindau disease to chromosome 3p confirmed by genetic linkage analysis. *Journal of Neurological Science* **100**: 27–30.

Mathew, C.G.P, Chin, K.S., Easton, D.F. et al. 1987. A linked genetic marker for multiple endocrine neoplasia type 2A on chromosome 10. *Nature* **328**: 527–30.

Murray, J.C., Buetow, K.H., Weber, J.L. et al. 1994. A comprehensive human linkage map with centimorgan density. *Science* **265**: 2049–54.

Nakamura, Y., Larsson, C., Julier, C. et al. 1989. Localization of the genetic defect in multiple endocrine neoplasia type 1 within a small region of chromosome 11. *American Journal of Human Genetics* **44**: 751–5.

Nakamura, Y., Lathrop, M., Leppert, M. et al. 1988. Localization of the genetic defect in familial adenomatous polyposis within a small region of chromosome 5. *American Journal of Human Genetics* **43**: 638–44.

Nancarrow, D.J., Mann, G.J., Holland, E.A. et al. 1993. Confirmation of chromosome 9p linkage in familial melanoma. *American Journal of Human Genetics* **53**: 936–42.

Nancarrow, D.J., Walker, G.J., Weber, J.L., Walters, M.K., Palmer, J.M. and Hayward, N.K. 1992. Linkage mapping of melanoma (MLM) using 172 microsatellite markers. *Genomics* **14**: 939–47.

Narod, S.A., Feunteun, J, Lynch, H.T. et al. 1991. Familial breast–ovarian cancer locus on chromosome 17q21-q23. *Lancet* **338**: 82–3.

Narod, S., Ford, D., Devilee, P. et al. 1995b. Genetic heterogeneity of breast–ovarian cancer revisited. *American Journal of Human Genetics* **57**: 957.

Narod, S.A., Ford, D., Devilee, P. et al. 1995a. An evaluation of genetic heterogeneity in 145 breast-ovarian cancer families. *American Journal of Human Genetics* **56**: 254–64.

Nyström-Lahti, M., Sistonen, P., Mecklin, J.-P. et al. 1994. Close linkage to chromosome 3p and conservation of ancestral founding haplotype in hereditary nonpolyposis colorectal cancer families. *Proceedings of the National Academy of Sciences, USA* **91**: 6054–8.

Ott, J. 1991. *Analysis of Human Genetic Linkage*, 2nd edn. Baltimore: The Johns Hopkins University Press.

Parkin, D.M., Muir, C.S., Whelan, S.L., Gao, Y.T., Ferlay, J. and Powell, J. (Eds). 1992. *Cancer Incidence in Five Continents*, vol VI. IARC Publications No. 120. Lyon: International Agency for Research on Cancer.

Peltomaki, P., Aaltonen, L.A., Sistonen, P. et al. 1993. Genetic mapping of a locus predisposing to human colorectal cancer. *Science* **260**: 810–12.

Petty, E.M., Green, J.S., Marx, S.J., Taggart, R.T., Farid, N. and Bale, A.E. 1994. Mapping the gene for hereditary hyperparathyroidism and prolactinoma (MEN1$_{\text{BURIN}}$) to chromosome 11q: evidence for a founder effect in patients from Newfoundland. *American Journal of Human Genetics* **54**: 1060–6.

Ponz de Leon, M., Sassatelli, R., Benatti, P. and Roncucci, L. 1993. Identification of hereditary nonpolyposis colorectal cancer in the general population. *Cancer* **71**: 3493–501.

Richards, F.M., Maher, E.R., Latif, F. et al. 1993. Detailed genetic mapping of the von Hippel-Lindau disease tumour suppressor gene. *Journal of Medical Genetics* **30**: 104–7.

Ries, L.A.G., Miller, B.A., Hankey, B.F., Kosary, C.L., Harras, A. and Edwards, B.K. (eds.). 1994. *SEER Cancer Statistics Review, 1973:-1991: Tables and Graphs*, National Cancer Institute, NIH Publication No. 94-2789. Bethesda: National Institutes of Health.

Schaid, D.S. and Sommer, S.S. 1993. Genotype relative risks: methods for design and analysis of candidate-gene association studies. *American Journal of Human Genetics* **53**: 1114–26.

Scheffer, D., te Meerman G.J., Kruize Y.C.M. et al. 1989. Linkage analysis of families with hereditary retinoblastoma: Nonpenetrance of mutation, revealed by combined use of markers within and flanking the RB1 gene. *American Journal of Human Genetics* **45**: 252–60.

Schork, N.J., Boehnke, M., Terwilliger, J.D. and Ott, J. 1993. Two-trait-locus linkage analysis: a powerful strategy for mapping complex genetic traits. *American Journal of Human Genetics* **53**: 1127–36.

Schork, N.J. and Guo, S.W. 1993. Pedigree models for complex human traits involving the mitochondrial genome. *American Journal of Human Genetics* **53**: 1320–37.

Seizinger, B.R., Rouleau, G.A., Ozelius, L.J. et al. 1988. Von Hippel-Lindau disease maps to the region of chromosome 3 associated with renal cell carcinoma. *Nature* **332**: 268–9.

Seizinger, B.R., Rouleau, G.A, Ozelius, L.J. et al. 1987. Genetic linkage of von Recklinghausen neurofibromatosis to the nerve growth factor receptor gene. *Cell* **49**: 589–94.

Slattery, M.L. and Kerber, R.A. 1994. Family history of cancer and colon cancer risk: the Utah Population Database. *Journal of the National Cancer Institute* **86**: 1618–26.

Sparkes, R.S., Murphree, A.L., Lingua, R.W. et al. 1983. Gene for hereditary retinoblastoma assigned to human chromosome 13 by linkage to esterase D. *Science* **219**: 971–3.

Spielman, R.S., McGinnis, R.E. and Ewens, W.J. 1993. Transmission test for linkage disequilibrium: the insulin gene region and insulin-dependent diabetes mellitus (IDDM). *American Journal of Human Genetics* **52**: 506–16.

Tånnergard, P., Zabarovsky, E., Stanbridge, E., Nordenskjöld, M. and Lindblom, A. 1994. Sublocalization of a locus at 3p21.3-23 predisposing to hereditary nonpolyposis colon cancer. *Human Genetics* **94**: 210–14.

Terwilliger, J.D. and Ott, J. 1992. A haplotype-based 'haplotype relative risk' approach to detecting allelic associations. *Human Heredity* **42**: 337–46.

Terwilliger, J.D. and Ott, J. 1994. *Handbook of Genetic Linkage.* Baltimore: The Johns Hopkins University Press.

Thakker, R.V., Bouloux, P., Wooding, C. et al. 1989. Association of parathyroid tumors in multiple endocrine neoplasia type 1 with loss of alleles on chromosome 11. *New England Journal of Medicine* **321**: 218–24.

Vabres, P., Lacombe, D., Rabinowitz, L.G. et al. 1995. The gene for Bazex-Dupré-Christol syndrome maps to chromosome Xq. *Journal of Investigative Dermatology* **105**: 87–91.

van Haeringen, A., Bergman, W., Nelen, M.R. et al. 1989. Exclusion of the dysplastic nevus syndrome (DNS) locus from the short arm of chromosome 1 by linkage studies in Dutch families. *Genomics* **5**: 61–4.

Weissenbach, J., Gyapay, G., Dib, C., et al. 1992. A second-generation linkage map of the human genome. *Nature* **359**: 794–801.

Wertelecki W., Rouleau, G.A., Superneau, D.W. et al. 1988. Neurofibromatosis 2: clinical and DNA linkage studies of a large kindred. *New England Journal of Medicine* **319**: 278–83.

Wooster, R., Neuhausen S.L., Mangion J. et al. 1994. Localization of a breast cancer susceptibility gene, BRCA2, to chromosome 13q12-13. *Science* **265**: 2088-90.

8
Mutation detection

LOUISE HOSKING, KARIN AU and PHILIPPE
SANSÉAU

Summary

Following the identification of cancer susceptibility genes, a major issue
for both researchers and diagnostic laboratories is how to find all the
mutations in the gene in question. As the authors point out, there is no
one ideal method. In this chapter each of the commonly used methods is
reviewed, with the technical aspects explained and their strengths and
weaknesses considered. Finally, there is a discussion of DNA chip-
based diagnostics, which are likely finally to replace all other forms of
mutation detection in the next decade or so. The authors note a word of
caution – how much will the chip technology cost and will it lead to
centralization?

Introduction

With the identification of an increasing number of disease-related genes
in cancer, finding mutations in nucleic acid sequences is becoming one of
the most important fields in molecular biology today. In most cases
mutation detection techniques are used to incriminate a candidate
cDNA for a particular disease and to screen for alleles at known loci
for diagnostic purposes.

Often mutation detection techniques are separated into two distinct
groups. The first consists of methods to identify unknown mutations,
the second to uncover known mutations mainly for diagnostic purposes.
Some techniques, such as direct sequencing, can be used in both groups.
With the advent of the polymerase chain reaction (PCR; Mullis and
Faloona, 1987) several new methods have been developed in recent

Table 8.1. *Starting biological material for mutation analysis – mRNA versus genomic DNA*

	mRNA	Genomic DNA
Advantages	No need to know gene structure	No need to know the tissue distribution of the gene
	Fewer PCR reactions	Mutations in splice site junctions can be detected
	For autosomal recessive and X-linked traits	For autosomal dominant traits
Disadvantages	Gene may not be represented in accessible tissues	Need to know the gene structure (introns and exons)
	Only mutations in the coding sequence are detected	More PCR reactions needed since only exons are amplified

years. More recently, a new range of enzymes such as resolvases or mismatch repair enzymes have been used to detect mutations.

Since the choice of techniques is increasing all the time the most appropriate method is influenced by the laboratory resources available, the biological material (mRNA and/or genomic DNA), the expected nature of the mutation, the size of the gene to analyse and the sensitivity required.

For clarity in this review, mutation detection methods will be divided into techniques identifying large changes, PCR-based, and other enzyme-based techniques. Lastly, a new approach – the GeneChip technology developed by Affymetrix (Santa Clara, California, USA) – will be discussed.

Choice of biological material

mRNA and genomic DNA are the two materials of choice to carry out mutation detection. The advantages and disadvantages of both materials are described in Table 8.1. mRNA can be used to scan large stretches of sequence as no introns are present and therefore fewer PCR reactions are needed. The candidate gene must be expressed in the tissue used to prepare the mRNA. In recessive autosomal and X-linked traits, mRNA is the material of choice since the analysis of one allele is sufficient. Genomic DNA is the first choice for autosomal dominant traits where both alleles are equally represented. Analysing the gene using genomic DNA requires more PCR reactions and the intron/exon structure to be known.

Identification of large changes

Fluorescence in situ hybridization

Large alterations (in the megabase range) can be identified using cytogenetic methods such as fluorescence in situ hybridization (FISH; Wolstenholme and Burn, 1992). This technology is particularly valuable for the diagnostic detection of deletions, duplications and loss of heterozygosity (LOH) in tumour samples (Taylor et al., 1993).

Southern blot hybridization

Southern blot hybridization is one of the oldest methods for mutation detection (Southern, 1975). The main advantages of this technique are its simplicity and robustness. In addition, the knowledge of the nucleic acid sequence or the intron/exon structure of the candidate gene is not necessary. Major changes such as deletions and insertions can be detected by modifications in the pattern or intensities of the bands in blots after autoradiography. Moreover, point mutations may be detectable if mutations affect an endonuclease restriction site.

PCR-based methods

The most popular mutation detection techniques rely on PCR amplification of the starting genomic DNA or mRNA prior to analysis. Most of the following methods are used to detect the most common type of mutation – single-base alterations.

Single-strand conformation polymorphism (SSCP) analysis

SSCP analysis, one of the most widely used simple methods of mutation detection, was first described by Orita et al. (1989). The analysis exploits differential mobilities of single DNA strands under non-denaturing polyacrylamide gel electrophoresis. Using this technique, mutations can be localized to a small region of DNA (generally around 200 bp) but not defined exactly, with an efficiency around 80%. Briefly, sequences of interest are amplified by specific primers in a simple PCR reaction. Normally the amplicon is radiolabelled by the incorporation of ^{32}P or ^{35}S dCTP for subsequent visualization, although results can also be obtained by ethidium bromide or silver staining of the gel. Reaction products are heat denatured and then single strands are separated using non-denaturing gel electrophoresis. As the single strands run through the gel they may take up different secondary conformations which will migrate at different rates (Figure 8.1). A homozygote can be seen as two bands on a gel and a heterozygote as four bands. Differences between wild type and mutant DNA as small as a single

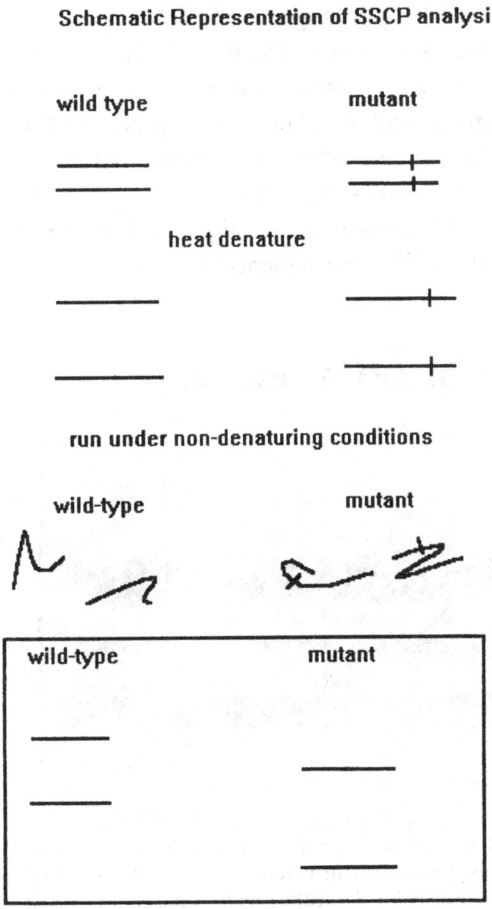

Figure 8.1. Schematic representation of single-strand conformation polymorphism (SSCP) analysis. A change in the SSCP leads to a difference in the mobility of the DNA molecules in the gel.

base change can result in different mobilities of the DNA strands
(Figure 8.2). The DNA gel is then dried and the mutant band excized.
The DNA can be re-solubilized and then sequenced to identify the
sequence change giving rise to the band shift. Alternatively, the PCR
reaction can be sequenced directly. The main advantages of the technique are the simplicity and sensitivity for small amplicons. However,
SSCP analysis does not necessarily pick up all mutations. A greater
rate of detection can be obtained by combining two or more different
sets of physical conditions (e.g. temperature, ionic strength, voltage,
acrylamide concentration). MDE-hydrolink gel is particularly good
for separating the different alleles of DNA strands up to 800 bp
long, although generally when looking at longer length DNA fragments
the rate of mutation detection goes down. SSCP analysis has been
applied with great success to mutation detection in large disease associated genes such as the breast and ovarian cancer gene, *BRCA1*
(Friedman et al., 1994; Hosking et al., 1995). This gene contains 24
exons with mutations occurring across the whole coding sequence,
and therefore lends itself well to a scanning technique such as SSCP
that will localize the mutations in different patients.

SSCP analysis of BRCA1 exon 23

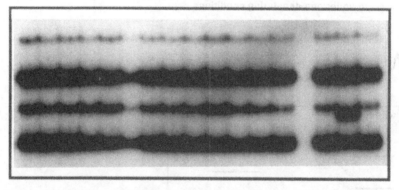

Figure 8.2. Single-strand conformation polymorphism analysis of *BRCA1* exon
23 in ovarian tumour sample. Exon 23 was amplified using flanking intronic
primers in a ^{32}P incorporation polymerase chain reaction. Single DNA strands
were separated under non-denaturing MDE-hydrolink gel electrophoresis. The
gel was dried onto paper and exposed to autoradiographic film at −70 °C, over-
night. A clear band shift is demonstrated in the tumour sample in lane 16 indicating the presence of a DNA mutation.

Denaturing gradient gel electrophoresis (DGGE)

Like SSCP, electrophoretic migration differences between mutant and wild-type DNA is the basis of the DGGE technique (Fischer and Lerman, 1983). An amplicon of the gene of interest is fractionated through a gradient of increasing concentrations of a denaturing agent such as urea or formamide. The two strands begin to melt at the denaturant concentration equal to its melting temperature. The presence of a single base substitution is sufficient to alter the melting profile of an amplicon compared to wild-type DNA (Figure 8.3). The use of heteroduplex molecules between wild-type and mutant DNA increases the sensitivity of the method – this could be as high as 98% for products up to 600 base pairs (bp) in size (Grompe, 1993; Guldberg et al., 1993). This is particularly the case if the mutation is located in a domain with a relatively low melting temperature. It is of great importance to have GC-clamp (Myers et al., 1985a) attached to one primer to ensure that the amplicon has a low dissociation temperature. Various softwares have been developed for the placement of oligos, the design of clamps and the prediction of melting profiles.

DGGE is a scanning method and the precise location and nature of the mutation has to been determined by an additional technique such as direct sequencing of the amplicon.

Chemical mismatch cleavage (CMC)

In CMC, both the detection and the localization of the mutation are possible (Cotton et al., 1988). DNA–DNA or DNA–RNA mutant/wild-type heteroduplex molecules are modified at the sites of mutations by chemical compounds such as hydroxylamine (mismatched cytosines) and osmium tetroxide (mispaired thymines). Then, the modified strand of the heteroduplex is cleaved by piperidine and the molecules are separated by size using denaturing PAGE and detected by autoradiography (Figure 8.4). The sensitivity of CMC is 100% when both wild-type and mutant DNA are labelled. Moreover fragments up to 1.8 kb in size can be scanned for mutations with a very high efficiency (Zheng et al., 1991). The main disadvantage of CMC is high toxicity of the chemical compounds used. However, recently non-isotopic detection methods have been developed for this purpose (Rowley et al., 1995; Green et al., 1996).

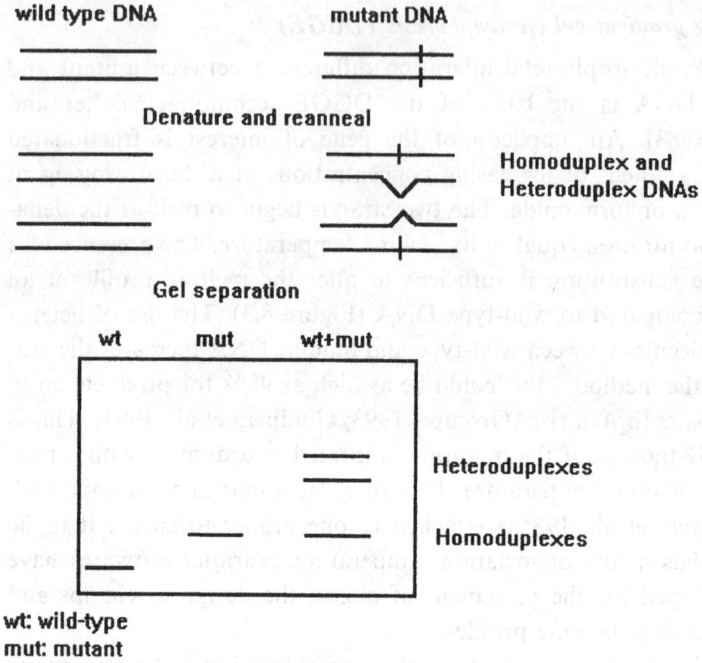

Figure 8.3. Schematic representation of denaturing gradient gel electrophoresis analysis. Polymerase chain reaction amplicons of wild type and mutant DNA are denatured and reannealed to generate homo- and heteroduplexes. A different melting point leads to differential mobility in a gel with a gradient of increasing concentration of denaturing agent.

Heteroduplex analysis (HA)

During a PCR reaction heteroduplex molecules can be formed in mutant and wild-type DNA. In polyacrylamide gels heteroduplexes with only a single base pair change can have a different mobility because of the conformational modifications in the double stranded DNA molecules. Different gel matrices are available for HA where mutant and wild type homo- and heteroduplexes are electrophoresed side by side. A sensitivity similar to SSCP for small PCR products (< 300 bp) has been described (Keen et al., 1991). The main attraction of this technique is its simplicity. The main disadvantage is the lack of 100% detection rate.

Direct Sequencing (DS)

Most methods of mutation detection will localize an area of the gene encompassing the mutation. DNA sequencing not only pinpoints the

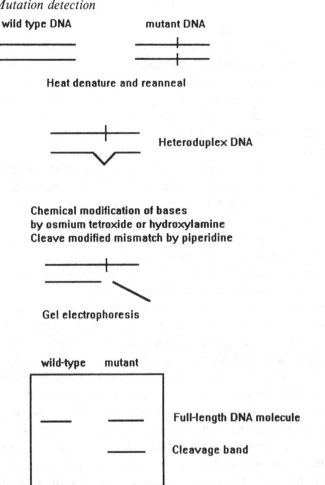

Figure 8.4. Schematic representation of chemical mismatch cleavage analysis. A heteroduplex between wild-type and mutant DNA is chemically modified and cleaved. The cleavage band is detected as an extra band in the gel.

exact location of the mutation but may give an indication as to what effect the mutation actually has on the encoded protein and therefore has enormous impact on gene functional studies and the subsequent understanding of tumour biology. Direct sequencing can also be used as a diagnostic procedure in cancer patients and their families when carrying known mutations. Both solid tumour and blood DNA are suitable substrates for this method, detecting not only hereditary mutations but also the presence of somatic ones. Most other technologies, with the exception of CMC, risk missing some mutations but with direct sequencing the sensitivity is nearly 100%. Directly sequencing entire genes has up to now been a very time consuming, expensive and laborious process. DNA sequencing is often used to complement other 'scanning' methods that localize the area of interest thus reducing the amount of DNA to be sequenced. However, as automation is constantly improving and technology advancing this may become the preferred method for detection of unknown mutations.

Direct sequencing is performed according to the principle of the Sanger dideoxy chain termination method (Sanger et al., 1977). Gene specific primers can be used to amplify the region of interest and the resultant PCR product can then be sequenced directly without the need for sub-cloning. There are numerous methods available for the preparation of DNA prior to direct single-stranded sequencing.

Single-stranded DNA molecules can then be sequenced by incorporating radiolabelled nucleotides into the DNA molecule and visualizing the products on a dried gel by exposure to autoradiographic film. More recently a modification of this method, cycle sequencing, has been used with great success (Rosenthal and Charnock-Jones, 1992). Only a small amount of template is needed for this reaction as the template is concurrently amplified using PCR and labelled with either a radiolabelled nucleotide or with fluorescently labelled dideoxy terminators. Each dideoxy terminator is labelled with a different fluorescent dye allowing the four termination products to be separated on the same lane of a sequencing gel, vastly increasing the number of samples that can be analysed simultaneously. Computer software accompanying this methodology allows the high throughput automated analysis of a large number of DNA samples.

Enzyme-based mutation detection methods

RNAse cleavage

In this technique RNA–DNA heteroduplexes between a wild-type RNA and mutant DNA are subjected to RNAse cleavage. This enzyme will cleave single stranded RNA where a mismatch is present (Myers et al., 1985b). The digestion is analysed on a gel and the size of the cleavage band will indicate the position of the mismatch. Compared to CMC the technique is not very sensitive with a rate of mismatch detection around 60%.

Enzyme mismatch cleavage (EMC)

A resolvase, the T4 endonuclease VII, is the cornerstone of the EMC technique (Youil et al., 1995). Heteroduplex molecules of wild-type DNA and mutant DNA are cleaved by the enzyme within 6 bases 3' of a mismatch or a loop. This process allows the localization of the nucleotide change. Cleavage products are electrophoresed on 8% acrylamide-urea gels and detected by autoradiography since either the normal or mutant DNA is radioactively labelled (Youil and Cotton, 1996).

Mismatch repair enzyme cleavage (MREC)

The mismatch repair enzymes of *Escherichia coli* such as MutS can bind to mismatches of heteroduplex molecules of wild-type and mutant DNA (Lu and Tsu, 1991). The changes are cleaved by the enzyme and the DNA molecules subjected to electrophoresis on a denaturing gel. MutS can recognize deletions or mismatches of up to 4 bp, although C:C mismatches are not well recognized.

Cleavase fragment length polymorphism (CFLP)

A family of endonucleases has recently been identified by Third Wave Technologies Inc. (Madison, Wisconsin, USA) that can recognize folded hairpin-like sequence dependent structures formed by DNA strands after denaturation (Hayashi, 1991). One member of this family is cleavase that can identify DNA molecules differing by a single base change. After denaturation and cooling, DNA strands are cleaved by the enzyme and DNA fragments separated on denaturing polyacrylamide gels. A different pattern (or cleavage fingerprint) should be observed when comparing the wild-type and mutant DNA lanes (Figure 8.5). The method is very sensitive and can be used as a scanning technique for fragments up to 2 kb. In our hands the efficiency was 95% for amplicons up to 1 kb. This method is a good non-radioactive alternative to SSCP analysis.

In vitro synthesis techniques

Protein truncation test (PTT)

PTT or in vitro synthesized-protein assay (IVSPA) are similar procedures used to detect stop mutations in large genes such as the Duchenne

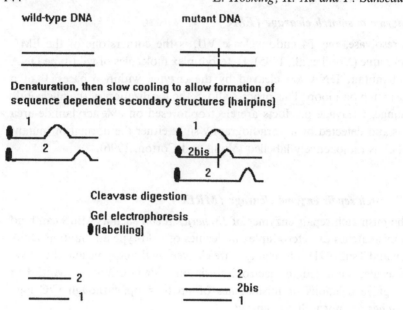

Figure 8.5. Schematic representation of the cleavage fragment length polymorph-ism mutation detection technique. After the formation of secondary structures the DNA molecules are cleaved at the base of the hairpins. DNA fragments that differ by as little as a single base pair will give a different fingerprint in a poly-acrylamide denaturing gel.

muscular dystrophy gene or the familial adenomatous polyposis gene (APC) (Powell et al., 1993; Roest et al., 1993). A schematic representa-tion of the method is described in Figure 8.6. Briefly, RNA (PTT and IVSPA) or genomic DNA (IVSPA) samples from the patients are reverse transcribed (for RNA) and amplified by PCR. A T7 promoter sequence and a consensus sequence for an eukaryotic translation initia-tion sequence are directly introduced in the primers, or introduced in nested oligos used in a second PCR reaction. These modifications allow the coupled in vitro transcription/translation of the PCR amplicons. Translation products are visualized on SDS-polyacrylamide gels. Short proteins will immediately indicate stop mutations in the gene of interest. Since two alleles, one mutated and one normal, can be ampli-fied in the PCR reaction, the latter can provide the positive internal control. Nevertheless, controls also have to be included to confirm that both alleles are amplified.

The main advantages of the method are the ability to analyse long stretches of coding sequence and its simplicity. PTT has been extensively

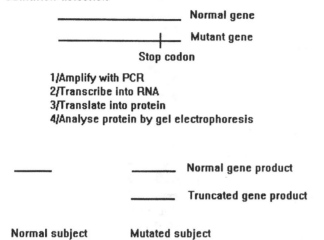

Figure 8.6. Schematic representation of the protein truncation test (PTT) (Powell et al., 1993). The stop codon in the mutant gene generates a shorter product after in vitro synthesis and analysis by gel electrophoresis.

used to characterize mutations in large cancer-related genes such as *BRCA1* (Hogervorst et al., 1995) and more recently the ataxia telangiectasia gene, *ATM* (FitzGerald et al., 1997).

DNA chip technology

The GeneChip technology developed by the biotechnology company Affymetrix offers an attractive new alternative towards screening patient DNA samples for large numbers of known mutations simultaneously. In this method, samples are analysed by hybridization to high density arrays (tens of thousands per square cm) of oligonucleotides attached to a silicon surface (Fodor et al., 1991). These oligonucleotides are designed to interrogate the DNA sequences of specific known genes of interest with high redundancy. The sequence of each nucleotide at every position on the chip is known.

DNA chip assays typically involve the following steps (Figure 8.7):

(1) Amplification of sequences of interest from genomic DNA or mRNA, fragmentation of the amplicons into a size optimal for efficient hybridization, and incorporation of fluorescent label into the sample.

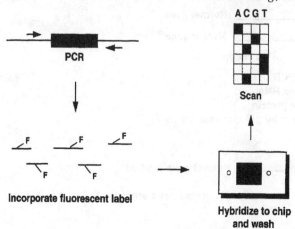

Figure 8.7. Schematic representation of the chip technology. Polymerase chain reaction (PCR) fragments of the gene of interest are labelled and hybridized on the gene-chip. A fluorescent reader scans the chip to detect changes in the sequence.

(2) Hybridization of the labelled sample to the chip followed by washing under stringent conditions.
(3) Scanning of the chip with instrumentation that calls the sequence of the sample based upon the intensity of fluorescent label hybridized to each position on the chip.

The application of the chip technology towards the detection of germline mutations in *BRCA1* has recently been reported (Hacia et al., 1996). Moreover, DNA chips can also be used to monitor expression levels, and research is currently underway at Affymetrix to apply DNA chip technology toward the measurement of expression levels of a variety of cancer-related genes.

Conclusions

The ideal mutation detection technique should be simple, cheap, 100% efficient, reproducible, automatable, not gene type dependent and applicable for analysing large DNA fragments. However, despite the rapid development of new mutation detection techniques the 'one best' method has yet to be described. In most cases, the choice of method for the detection of known mutations will depend upon the resources (biological and technical material) available in the laboratory and the characteristics of the gene to analyse. When looking for unknown mutations in a large gene it may be appropriate to combine two methods – for example a scanning technique such as SSCP or DGGE to localize the area containing the mutation, followed by direct sequencing to identify it. Commonly used techniques involving incorporation of radio-labelled nucleotides, for example, SSCP or CMC, are being replaced in favour of non-radioactive alternatives or enzyme-based techniques such as mismatch repair enzymes.

The future of mutation detection for diagnostic purposes is very likely to see the advent of large scale scanning methods. DNA microchip technology developed by Affymetrix seems especially attractive for diagnostic purposes. Already an HIV chip, which contains the proteases and reverse transcriptases genes, is commercially available and a p53 chip is underway. Recently, Francis Collins and colleagues have reported the screening for known mutations in the breast cancer gene, *BRCA1*, using Affymetrix technology – 14 out of 15 heterozygous changes in exon 11 of the gene were detected (Hacia et al., 1996). An advantage of the chip technology is the highly automated, high throughput analysis that inevitably leads to greater speed of mutation detection. One of the main disadvantages is the cost involved in chip construction and the material necessary for the detection of the signals. Many small institutions may be unable to afford such technology.

However, as with many other techniques, advancing technology and improved computer support will ultimately lead to the more rapid detection of disease-associated mutations.

Acknowledgements

The authors would like to thank Karen Lewis for technical assistance.

References

Cotton, R.G., Rodrigues, N.R. and Campbell, R.D. 1988. Reactivity of cytosine and thymine in single-base-pair mismatches with hydroxylamine and osmium tetroxide and its application to the study of mutations. *Proceedings of the National Academy of Sciences, USA* **85**: 4397–1.

Fischer, S.G. and Lerman, L.S. 1983. DNA fragments differing by single base-pair substitutions are separated in denaturing gradient gel. *Proceedings of the National Academy of Sciences, USA,* **80**: 1579–83

FitzGerald, M.G., Bean, J.M., Hedge, S.R. et al. 1997. Heterozygous ATM mutations do not contribute to early onset of breast cancer. *Nature Genetics* **15**: 307–10.

Fodor, S.P., Read, J.L., Pirrung, M.C., Stryer, L., Lu, A.T. and Solas, D. 1991. Light-directed spatially adrdressable parallel chemical synthesis. *Science* **251**: 767–73.

Friedman, L.S., Ostermeyer, E.A., Szabo, C.I., Dowd, P., Lynch, E.D., Rowell, S.E. and King, M.C. 1994. Confirmation of *BRCA1* by analysis of germline mutations linked to breast and ovarian cancer in ten families. *Nature Genetics* **8**: 399–404.

Green, P.M., Rowley, G., Saad, S. and Giannelli, F. 1996) In *Laboratory Protocols for Mutation Detection*, 1st edn. ed. U. Landegren, pp. 61–4. Oxford: Oxford University Press.

Grompe, M. 1993. The rapid detection of unknown mutations in nucleic acids. *Nature Genetics* **5**: 111–17.

Guldberg, P., Henriksen, K.F. and Guttler, F. 1993. Molecular analysis of phenylketonuria in Denmark: 99% of the mutations detected by denaturing gradient gel electrophoresis. *Genomics* **17**: 141–6.

Hayashi, K. 1991. PCR–SSCP: A simple and sensitive method for detection of mutations in genomic DNA. *PCR Methods and Applications* **1**: 34–8.

Hacia, J.G., Brody, L.C., Chee, M.S., Fodor, S.P. and Collins, F.S. 1996. Detection of heterozygous mutations in *BRCA1* using high density oligonucleotide arrays and two-color fluorescence analysis. *Nature Genetics* **14**: 441–9.

Hogervorst, F.B.L., Cornelis, R.S., Bout, M. et al. 1995. Rapid detection of *BRCA1* mutations by the protein truncation test. *Nature Genetics* **10**: 208–12.

Hosking, L.K., Trowsdale, J., Nicolai, H. et al. 1995. A somatic *BRCA1* mutation in an ovarian tumour. *Nature Genetics* **9**: 343–4.

Keen, J., Lester, D., Inglehearn, C., Curtis, A. and Bhattacharya, S. 1991. Rapid detection of single base mismatches as heteroduplexes on hydrolink gels. *Trends in Genetics* **7**: 5.

Lu, A.L. and Tsu, I.-C. 1991. Detection of single DNA base mutations with mismatch repair enzymes. *Genomics* **14**: 249–55.

Mullis, K.B. and Faloona, F.A. 1987. Specific synthesis of DNA *in vitro* via a polymerase-catalysed chain reaction. In *Methods of Enzymology*, vol. 155, part F, ed. R. Wu, pp. 335–50. San Diego: Academic Press.

Myers, R.M., Fischer, S.G., Lerman, L.S. and Maniatis, T. 1985a. Nearly all single base substitutions in DNA fragments joined to a GC-clamp can be detected by denaturing gradient gel electrophoresis. *Nucleic Acids Research* **13**: 3131–45.

Myers, R.M., Larin, Z. and Maniatis, T. 1985b. Detection of single base substitutions by ribonuclease cleavage at mismatches in RNA:DNA duplexes. *Science* **230**: 1242–6.

Orita, M.Y., Suzuki, Y., Sekiya, T. and Hatashi, K. 1989. Detection of polymorphism of human DNA by gel electrophoresis as single-strand conformation polymorphism. *Proceedings of the National Academy of Sciences, USA* **86**: 2766–70.

Powell, S.M., Petersen, G.M., Krush, A.J., Booker, S., Jen, J., Giardeiello, F.M., Hamilton, S.R., Vogelstein, B. and Kinzler, K.W. 1993) Molecular diagnosis of familial adenomatous polyposis. *The New England Journal of Medicine* **329**: 1982–7.

Roest, P.A.M., Roberts, R.G., Sugino, S., van Ommen, G-J. B. and den Dunnen, J.T. 1993) Protein truncation test (PTT) for rapid detection of translation-terminating mutations. *Human Molecular Genetics* **2**: 1719–21.

Rosenthal, A. and Charnock-Jones, D.S. 1992. New protocols for DNA sequencing with dye terminators. *DNA Sequence* **3**: 61–4.

Rowley, G., Saad, S., Giannelli, F. and Green, P.M. 1995. Ultrarapid mutation detection by multiplex solid-phase chemical cleavage. *Genomics* **30**: 574–82.

Sanger, F., Nicklen, S. and Coulson, A.R. 1977. DNA sequencing with chain-terminating inhibitors. *Proceedings of the National Academy of Sciences USA* **74**: 5463–7.

Southern, E.M. 1975. Detection of specific sequences among DNA fragments separated by gel electrophoresis. *Journal of Molecular Biology* **98**: 503–17.

Taylor, C., Patel, K., Jones, T., Kiely, F., De Stavola, B.L. and Sheer, D. 1993. Diagnosis of Ewing's sarcoma and pheripheral neuroectodermal tumour based on the detection of t(11;22) using fluorescence in situ hybridization. *British Journal of Cancer* **67**: 128–33.

Wolstenholme, J. and Burn, J. 1992. The applications of cytogenetic investigations to clinical practice. In *Human Cytogenetics: A Practical Approach*, 2nd edn., vol.1, *Constitutional Analysis*: ed. D.E., Rooney and B.H. Czepulkowski, pp. 119–56. Oxford: IRL Press.

Youil, R., Kemper, B.W. and Cotton, R.G. 1995. Screening for mutations by enzyme mismatch cleavage with T4 endonuclease VII. *Proceedings of the National Academy of Sciences, USA* **92**: 87–91.

Youil, R. and Cotton, R.G. 1996. EMC-enzyme mismatch cleavage. In *Laboratory Protocols for Mutation Detection*, 1st edn., ed. U. Landegren, pp.65–8. Oxford: Oxford University Press.

Zheng, H., Hasty, P., Brenneman, M.A., et al. 1991. Fidelity of targeted recombination in human fibroblasts and murine embryonic stem cells. *Proceedings of the National Academy of Sciences, USA* **88**: 8067–71.

Part II

Hereditary contribution to cancer: site-by-site and special groups

9

Cancers of the digestive system

TAMAR FLANDERS and WILLIAM FOULKES

Summary

The commonest group of cancers in the world are those of the gastro-intestinal tract and associated organs. The hereditary contribution at the major sites is reviewed, starting with the oropharynx and working downwards. Descriptive epidemiological studies are introduced, followed by the genetic epidemiology of cancer at the relevant site. The contribution of various syndromes to the incidence of specific cancers is considered and where relevant, data from laboratory investigations are reviewed. The major inherited cancer syndromes are also briefly discussed. Tables have been used to summarize some key findings.

Introduction

The hereditary contribution to cancers of the digestive system varies from very large (small intestinal cancer) to the minimal (hepatocellular carcinoma) but overall, cancers of the gastrointestinal tract form a considerable proportion of all hereditary cancers. Following descriptions of families with either remarkable phenotypes or large numbers of gastrointestinal cancers, or both, it became clear that some forms of colorectal cancer could be inherited in an autosomal dominant fashion. Some highly penetrant genes that predispose to intestinal cancer have been identified. More recently, the genetic contribution to pancreatic, oesophageal, and head and neck cancer has been recognized, and in some cases may be influenced by individual differences in the ability to metabolize the products of tobacco.

Squamous cell carcinoma of the head and neck

This carcinoma is an important cause of morbidity and mortality throughout the world, but particularly in developing countries (Pisani et al., 1993). Susceptibility to cancer of the upper airways is discussed in Chapter 17. Here the genetic component of oropharyngeal cancer is discussed. Tobacco and alcohol are clearly the most important risk factors for oropharyngeal cancer. The areas of highest incidence are areas where consumption of alcohol, tobacco or both is highest, for example in southern Brazil (Parkin et al., 1993). Three studies have demonstrated elevated relative risks for oropharyngeal cancer in association with a family history of head and neck cancer. Interestingly, the significantly elevated relative risks for head and neck cancer (including laryngeal cancer) were all in the same range – 3.5 (Copper et al., 1995), 3.65 (Foulkes et al., 1995) and 3.79 (Foulkes et al., 1996). The numbers of affecteds were too small in these studies to distinguish the effect of a family history of cancer at different head and neck sites. One case-control study in the US showed no effect of family history on risk of oropharyngeal cancer (Day et al., 1993), but there were some ethnic differences in risk, despite controlling for differences in alcohol and tobacco consumption.

Nasopharyngeal carcinoma

In a similar fashion to squamous cell carcinoma of the head and neck, nasopharyngeal cancer does not appear to have a strong familial component. However, family history of nasopharyngeal cancer has been shown to confer some increased risk. For instance, an increased incidence of this malignancy occurs among relatives of Cantonese Chinese affected with nasopharyngeal cancer. An investigation of 750 families of nasophayrngeal carcinoma patients, ascertained from the National Taiwan University Hospital determined a relative risk of 4.3 ($p < 0.001$) for the disease among siblings of affected probands (Wang et al., 1995). A similar study of Alaskan Eskimo nasopharyngeal cancer patients revealed a relative risk of 2.73 ($p < 0.001$) for the same cancer among siblings with the cancer (Ireland et al., 1988).

A number of instances of familial clustering of nasopharyngeal carcinoma have been reported (Table 9.1). Table 9.1 shows that most familial cases are not associated with other cancers, except the virus-related salivary gland tumours seen in the Inuit of Canada and Greenland. Coffin et al. (1991) described a large American kindred with five cases of naso-

Table 9.1. *Familial nasopharyngeal cancer (NPC): case reports**

Family number	Number of individuals reported in pedigree	Number of NPC cases (number of affected generations)	Other cancers (number of cases if > 1)	References
1	4	2(2)	none	Jung, 1965
2	4	4(2)	none	Jung, 1965
3	12	2 (twins)	none	Nevo et al. (1971)
4	21	9(3)	none	Ho, 1972
5	3	3(1)	none	Williams and de-The (1974)
6	44	3(1)	none	Brown et al. (1976)
7	24	2(1)	Burkitt's lymphoma (3), multiple myeloma, acute lymphoblastic leukemia	Joncas et al. (1976)
8	68	4(3)	primary site unknown, pancreas	Lanier et al. (1979)
9	13	4(1)	stomach	Gajwani et al. (1980)
10	8	3(1)	prostate, bowel	Fischer et al. (1984)
11	165	5(3)	melanoma, lymphoma, tongue squamous cell carcinoma (2), colon, bilateral breast	Coffin et al. (1991)
12	12	3(1)	basal cell carcinoma (double primary with NPC)	Levine et al. (1992)
13		2(1)	none	Albeck et al. (1993)
14		3(2)	salivary gland	Albeck et al. (1993)
15		2(2)	none	Albeck et al. (1993)
16		2(1)	salivary gland	Albeck et al. (1993)
17		2(1)	none	Albeck et al. (1993)
18		2(2)	cervix, brain tumour	Albeck et al. (1993)
19		3(1)	none	Albeck et al. (1993)

*Defined as 2 or more cases of NPC.

pharyngeal carcinoma and six other malignancies (Table 9.1, family 11). All 31 family members tested had antibodies to Epstein Barr virus but had no evidence of acute infection. Epstein Barr virus infection is regarded as an essential prerequisite for the development of nasopharyngeal carcinoma. The HLA haplotype of A1-B37-DR6 was associated with this and other cancers in this family; the relative risk of nasopharyngeal carcinoma for family members with this haplotype was 13.67 ($p < 0.01$), however linkage to a HLA locus was not identified.

Susceptibility to cancer in this family was transmitted in an apparently autosomal codominant fashion. There is some evidence that this malignancy is associated with Burkitt's lymphoma, related to Epstein Barr virus infection (Williams and de-The, 1974; Joncas et al., 1976; Li, 1976). Based on a study of affected sibling pairs, a relative risk as high as 21 of nasopharyngeal carcinoma was associated with a gene (or genes) closely linked to the HLA locus (Lu et al., 1990).

Oesophagus

Epidemiology

In the US, oesophageal cancer occurs at a rate of 2.7 per 100,000 (Miller et al., 1992). This malignancy is four times more common among males. The epidemiology of oesophageal cancer has been studied extensively in certain areas of China, Iran, and Japan, where there is a high incidence of the disease. Dietary factors are probably paramount, but family history of cancer is among the risk factors identified.

Malignant tumours were the leading cause of death between 1959 and 1983 in Linxian county in the Henan province of China. Oesophageal cancer accounts for approximately 64 % of cancer deaths in this region (Lu et al., 1985). A segregation analysis of 221 high-risk nuclear families from the Yaocun Commune in Linxian revealed the presence of a putative autosomal recessive gene predisposing to oesophageal malignancies at a frequency of 19% in this population (Carter et al., 1992). An investigation of 640 oesophageal cancer patients from Linxian revealed that a family history of any kind of cancer was associated with an increased risk of oesophageal cancer (odds ratio 1.4, 95% confidence interval (CI) 1.1–1.8) (Guo et al., 1994). Case control studies in other Chinese provinces identified an increased risk in association with family history of oesophageal cancer; relative risks of 2.68 ($p < 0.001$) and 2.00 ($p < 0.005$) were demonstrated in studies done in two counties in Jiangsu province (Li, 1982). In Yangcheng county, Shanxi Province, the overall relative rate for oesophageal cancer death comparing positive to negative family history was significantly increased for males but not for females (males: 2.17, $p < 0.001$; females: 1.05, not significant) (Hu et al., 1992). The authors suggest that this gender difference may be due to unreported or misclassified female cases of oesophageal cancer. For instance, females tended to be less likely than males to report symptoms, so that for females, causes of death were often classified as 'stomach disease', 'wasting', or 'unknown'.

A high incidence of oesophageal cancer in the Turkoman population in the Caspian Littoral of northern Iran has been reported. Of the Turkoman oesophageal cancer patients in this high-risk region 47% reported a positive family history of the disease, compared with only 2% among non-Turkomans (Ghadirian, 1985). One family from Sabsevar, Iran is particularly interesting – 13 members in three generations were diagnosed with oesophageal cancer (Pour and Ghadirian, 1974). The likely mode of inheritance in this kindred may well be complex as there is much consanguinity.

An epidemiological study examining multiple occurrence of carcinoma of the upper aerodigestive tract associated with oesophageal cancer among Japanese males revealed an increased risk of a second cancer of the upper aerodigestive tract in patients with oesophageal cancer (odds ratio 10, 95% CI 2.2–45.7) (Morita et al., 1994).

Inherited cancer syndromes with susceptibility to oesophageal cancer

Tylosis

Focal palmoplantar keratoderma (tylosis), now referred to as palmoplantar ectodermal dysplasia type III, is an extremely rare autosomal dominant skin disease characterized by hyperkeratosis of the palms and soles. An association between tylosis and carcinoma of the oesophagus was reported in 1957 in a large kindred from Liverpool, denoted family 'S' (Howel-Evans et al., 1958). Analysis of family 'S' continues to date; 25 of 89 tylotic members in six generations have been diagnosed with oesophageal cancer (Ellis et al., 1994). Tylotic members of this family have a 92% probability of developing cancer by age 70 (Shine and Allison, 1966). Genetic linkage studies of this kindred located a putative tylosis oesophageal cancer gene (*TOC*) in the 17q23-qter region between D17S929 and D17S802, telomeric to the keratin 16 gene (Risk et al., 1994).

Most of the literature on oesophageal cancer with tylosis is limited to the Liverpool kindred, however two additional kindreds with this association have recently been reported, both showing linkage to markers at the 17q23-qter locus. The first is an extensive family from the American Midwest with 92 tylotic members, 21 of whom have died of cancer of the oesophagus to date (Stevens et al., 1996a). Unlike the Liverpool kindred, there was one case of oesophageal cancer without tylosis in the US kindred. Tylotic members of this family have a 40% chance of developing oesophageal cancer before the age of 70. The second is a smaller German kindred who may be ancestrally related to the Liverpool kindred (Hennies et al., 1995). The association between tylosis and oesophageal malignancy has also been observed in several smaller kindreds (Shine and Allison, 1966; Ritter and Petersen, 1976; Yesudian et al., 1980). In addition, tylosis without oesophageal cancer has been observed in a large kindred in the Orkney islands (Muir, 1978). Thus it appears that there are two distinct forms of tylosis caused by mutations in two different genes – one type has a variable age of onset and is associated with oesophageal cancer, while the other is diagnosed within the first year of life and is not associated with cancer. Other than the presence or absence of associated malignancy, there is little clinical difference between the two forms. Other cancers have been observed in association with punctate palmoplantar keratoderma, a similar disease (see below) (Bennion and Patterson, 1984b; Stevens et al., 1996b). It is probably advisable to screen individuals with tylosis annually by oesophagoscopy with biopsy. The presence of dysplasia on biopsy is an indication for oesophagectomy.

Barrett's oesophagus

Barrett's oesophagus is defined as a columnar epithelium-lined distal oesophagus, often related to gastro-oesophageal reflux. Based on a review of 121 cases of adenocarcinoma associated with Barrett's oesophagus reported in the English medical literature, the incidence of oesophageal malignancy is approximately 10% in this condition (Sjogren and Johnson, 1983). There is a very rare familial form of Barrett's oesophagus, also associated with adenocarcinoma, which appears to be transmitted in an autosomal dominant fashion (Table 9.2).

Stomach

Epidemiology

The incidence of gastric cancer in the US is 3.7 per 100,000 (Miller,1992). The disease occurs twice as commonly in men as in women. In the Western world, the frequency of this cancer is decreasing, but it is increasing in developing countries (Parkin et al., 1988; Parkin et al., 1993). The bacterium, *Helicobacter pylori*, is a deteriminant of gastric cancer (Forman, 1996). There are long-standing epidemiological data showing

Table 9.2. *Barrett's oesophagus and adenocarcinoma*

Number of individuals reported in pedigree	Number of individuals with Barrett's oesophagus	Number of individuals with adenocarcinoma of the oesophagus	Other malignancies	Reference
43	4	1 (without Barrett's oesophagus)	colon, stomach (2 cases), prostate, leukaemia, uterus, breast	Crabb et al. (1985)
27	6	3 (with Barrett's oesophagus)	none	Jochem et al. (1992)
23	7	2 (with Barrett's oesophagus)	none	Eng et al. (1993)

blood group A as a risk factor for gastric cancer, contrasting with the blood group (O) seen to be a risk factor for duodenal ulcer (McConnell, 1966). It has been confirmed in a large cohort study that there is a significantly lower incidence of gastric cancer in those who have previously been diagnosed with duodenal ulcers (relative risk 0.6, 95% CI 0.4–0.7) (Hansson et al., 1996). Screening for gastric cancer in the general population has been applied in Japan, but there are no controlled trials that show convincing benefit from this procedure (Pisani and Parkin, 1996).

In support of the extensive early findings on blood group, two case-control studies of gastric cancer in northern Italy indicate that genetic factors may play a role in the pathogenesis of this malignancy. The first investigated 154 gastric cancer patients in the health care district of Modena and reported a threefold increased risk of the disease among first-degree relatives of affected individuals (odds ratio 3.14, $p < 0.01$); this risk was highest among siblings (odds ratio 4.33, $p < 0.02$) (Zanghieri et al., 1990). The second assessed 628 patients and calculated relative risks of stomach cancer for parents (2.5, 95% CI 1.7–3.6) and siblings (2.8, 95% CI 1.5–3.5) of affected individuals (La Vecchia et al., 1992). Based on these data, the authors calculated that approximately 8% of stomach cancers could be explained by familial factors.

The finding of simultaneous gastric cancer in monozygotic twins provides additional evidence for a genetic component of this disease (Table 9.3, family 13) (Matsukura et al., 1988). The first twin was diagnosed with type 3 advanced gastric cancer at the age of 47 and died three years later. His identical twin brother developed type 1 early gastric cancer at age 50, underwent subtotal gastrectomy, and was healthy five years later. In a Greek family, gastric cancer was reported in both parents and their two offspring (Table 9.3, family 14) (Triantafillidis et al., 1993).

Gastric cancer in inherited cancer-predisposing syndromes

Stomach cancer is seldom seen in hereditary cancer syndromes in Western populations, whereas it is more commonly a feature of cancer syndromes in Asian countries.

Hereditary nonpolyposis colorectal cancer (HNPCC) (Table 9.4)

Based on 23 HNPCC kindreds, Lynch et al., (1991a) estimated a relative risk of 4.1 ($p < 0.001$) of gastric cancer in individuals with HNPCC (see Table 9.7). In fact, an excess of gastric cancer was reported in Warthin's original description of family 'G', the first report of a kindred

Table 9.3. *Familial gastric cancer: case reports**

Family number	Number of individuals reported in pedigree	Number of gastric cancer cases (number of affected generations)	Other cancers (number of cases if > 1)	References
1	6	6(2)	none	Maimon and Zinninger (1953)
2	9	8(2)	none	Paulsen cited by Maimon and Zinninger (1953)
3	11	8(3)	none	Bateman cited by Maimon and Zinninger (1953)
4	147	5(1)	melanoma, rectum, carcinoma, site not specified (3)	Woolf and Gardner cited by Maimon and Zinninger (1953)
5	21	3(1)	skin, colon (3), ovary, carcinoma, site not specified (7)	Bargen, May and Griffin cited by Maimon and Zinninger (1953)
6	75	13(4)	rectum (2 double primary with gastric), breast	Macklin (1960)
7	290	4(2)	leukaemia, pancreas, colon, nose (2), breast (3, 1 double primary with lip), lung, skin, lip (2, 1 double primary with breast)	Woolf and Isaacson (1961)
8	53	4(2)	breast	Woolf and Isaacson (1961)
9	87	4(2)	breast, colon, AML, spleen, lymphoma, brain	Woolf and Isaacson (1961)
10	319	5(2)	uterus, colon, breast	Woolf and Isaacson (1961)
11	306	5(2)	colon, throat, sarcoma, breast (2)	Woolf and Isaacson (1961)
12	30	5(2)	colon	Farinati et al. (1987)
13	7	2 (monozygotic twins)	none	Matsukura et al. (1988)
14	6	4(2)	none	Triantafillidis et al. (1993)

*Defined as two or more cases of gastric cancer.

Table 9.4. *Characteristics of three hereditary cancer syndromes with dominant inheritance and prominent gastrointestinal features*

Characteristic	FAP	HNPCC	Peutz–Jeghers Syndrome
Age of onset	commonly teenage years	average 45 years at diagnosis of first CRC	early: intussception due to small bowel hamartomas, also perioral pigmented lesions
Location of colon cancer	anywhere (malignant transformation of adenomas)	most commonly proximal colon	can develop in hamartomas in large bowel
Extracolonic cancer sites	duodenum, Ampulla of Vater, pancreas, thyroid, brain, hepatoblastoma	endometrium, ovary, stomach, small bowel, pancreas, kidney, urinary tract	breast, duodenum, small bowel, uterus, pancreas, cervix (adenoma malignum), testicle, ovary
Colonic polyps	hundreds to thousands, tubular adenomatous type	few adenomas, often tubulovillous or villous	hamartomatous type
Other clinical features	congenital hypertrophy of the retinal pigment epithelium (CHRPE); gastroduodenal polyposis; desmoid tumours; epidermoid cysts; osteomas (characteristically of the mandible); impacted teeth; dentigenous cysts; supernumerary and unerupted teeth; exocytoses of the skull, digits, and long bones; cortical thickening	none	melanin spots on lips and buccal mucosa; multiple polyps of the entire gastrointestinal tract, urinary tract, and nasal mucosa; benign sex cord tumours of ovary

Variants	Gardner Syndrome Attenuated APC Turcot (clinical features included above)	Muir–Torre Syndrome (includes cutaneous manifestations such as sebaceous hyperplasia, adenoma, and carcinoma, with keratoacanthoma and basal cell carcinoma)	
Mode of inheritance	autosomal dominant, close to 100% penetrance	autosomal dominant, incomplete penetrance (~ 80%)	autosomal dominant, high penetrance
Genes	*APC*	*hMSH2* *hMLH1* *PMS1* *PMS2*	not known (localised to 19p)
Management	yearly sigmoidoscopy from second decade, upper GI endoscopy for affected individuals, rectal surveillance after ileorectal anastomosis	biennial colonoscopy from age 20-25, prophylactic colectomy in affected individuals, surveillance for endometrial cancer	regular upper and lower GI endoscopy and screening for extraintestinal tumours

Note: FAP: familial adenomatous polyposis; HNPCC: hereditary nonpolyposis colorectal cancer; CRC: colorectal cancer.

with HNPCC. Since then, this malignancy has been observed in many HNPCC kindreds (Lynch et al., 1988) Family 5 in Table 9.3 may represent one such family. In one notable kindred, gastric cancer was observed in six members (Cristofaro et al., 1987). In 10 HNPCC families from the Creighton University Hereditary Cancer Institute, 13 (4%) of 116 HNPCC patients had cancer of the stomach, compared with an estimated 2% incidence of this malignancy in the general population (Fitzgibbons et al., 1987). Based on 193 putative HNPCC gene carriers, the cumulative life-time risk for gastric cancer was 18.9% (Aarnio et al., 1995). It appears that those who carried mutations in the mismatch repair gene, *hMSH2* (see below) may have a higher risk for gastric cancer than *hMLH1* gene carriers (relative risk 19.3, 95% CI 6.2–59.9 versus *non-significantly increased risk*). *Upper gastrointestinal endoscopy may be indicated in some HNPCC kindreds, but there have been no controlled trials.*

Familial adenomatous polyposis (FAP) (Table 9.4)

A sevenfold increased risk of gastric cancer associated with FAP was calculated based on an investigation of 72 Korean FAP patients (standardized incidence ratio 6.9, 95% CI 1.4–20.1, $p < 0.05$) (Park et al., 1992). This may be directly related to the high incidence of gastric cancer among Koreans, as reports in non-Asian ethnic groups do not demonstrate an increased risk of gastric cancer in FAP (Watanabe et al., 1978; Jagelman et al., 1988; Spigelman et al., 1989b; Offerhaus et al., 1992). Gastric polyposis (hyperplastic polyps and adenomas) has been reported to occur in anywhere from 8 to 100% of FAP patients (Ranzi et al., 1981; Gahtan et al., 1989) but this does not result in an increased risk of gastric cancer for these individuals. Fundic gland polyposis has also been reported to occur as a separate entity in non-FAP patients (Iida et al., 1984; Tsuchikame et al., 1993). Screening of the upper gastrointestinal tract is indicated in affected individuals, but the appropriate screening interval is not established.

Generalized juvenile gastrointestinal polyposis

Yoshida et al. (1988) reported a family with four cases of gastric cancer – three were associated with gastrointestinal polyposis and the fourth was associated with generalized juvenile gastrointestinal polyposis, a variant of juvenile polyposis. Other malignancies diagnosed in this kindred included two rectal carcinomas (one associated with polyposis) and two hepatic cancers.

Familial gastric polyposis

This disease, distinct from FAP, was first described by dos Santos and Magalhães (1980) based on the observation of two kindreds with gastric polyposis and adenocarcinoma of the stomach (Seruca et al., 1991). In one family, two brothers of a proband with gastric polyposis died of adenocarcinoma of the stomach. In the other, there were 10 cases of gastric polyposis over three generations, and six cases of gastric cancer, inherited in an autosomal dominant fashion. No colorectal lesions or extra gastric malignancies were observed in any of the family members examined.

Ataxia-telangiectasia

This syndrome features an increased risk of cancer at numerous sites (Swift et al., 1990). Haerer et al. (1969) described a family in which 5 of 12 siblings had ataxia-telangiectasia. Two of these were also diagnosed with gastric adenocarcinoma. Data from this and other studies are insufficient to determine whether there is a significantly increased risk of stomach cancer in ataxia-telangiectasia.

Cowden disease and Peutz–Jeghers syndrome

Gastrointestinal neoplasms commonly seen in Cowden disease tend to be benign. Gastric polyposis was identified in three of four unrelated Cowden patients examined by Hizawa et al. (1994). However, gastric malignancy has also been reported in this syndrome. Hamby et al. (1995) described a Cowden disease patient who was diagnosed with gastric carcinoma. The patient also had bilateral invasive ductal adenocarcinoma of the breasts, follicular adenoma of the thyroid, hyperplastic gastric polyps, and over 100 nonadenomatous colonic polyps. The gene for Cowden disease has now been identified (see below and Chapter 10). Cancer of the stomach is the fourth most common malignancy seen in Peutz–Jeghers syndrome (Table 9.4) (Konishi et al., 1987), and therefore it is advisable to offer upper gastrointestinal endoscopy. The interval may depend on the age of the patient, and whether any gastric lesions were present on the last endoscopy.

Duodenum and small bowel

The duodenum and small bowel are uncommon sites of carcinoma in virtually all parts of the world. The presence of duodenal, jejunal, or ileal cancer may indicate genetic susceptibility to HNPCC, or less commonly, FAP or Peutz–Jeghers syndrome.

Small bowel cancer in hereditary syndromes

FAP, HNPCC and Peutz–Jeghers syndrome

Duodenal polyps have been reported to occur in anywhere between 10 and 93% of FAP patients (Kurtz et al., 1987). The relative risk of duodenal cancer in FAP is over 300, however the absolute life-time risk is 3.0% (Giardiello and Offerhaus, 1995). The relative risk for cancer of the small bowel in HNPCC may be similarly high at 290 (Vasen et al., 1996; Lynch et al., 1991a). Among 293 putative HNPCC gene carriers from Finland, there were three cases (1%) of small bowel cancer (Aarnio et al., 1995). Mecklin and Jarvinen (1991) also reported five cases (1%) of small bowel cancer among 472 affected members from 40 HNPCC kindreds.

Based on a review of the literature on cancers associated with Peutz–Jeghers syndrome, the duodenum was the second commonest site of malignancy (after the large bowel) (Konishi et al., 1987). There were 10 reported cases of duodenal cancer in this syndrome. Six of these cancers arose in Peutz–Jeghers syndrome polyps. Interestingly, nine of the ten reported cases were observed in Western populations, compared with only one Japanese case.

Liver

Liver cancers are of two main types – the childhood hepatoblastoma, sometimes seen in association with specific inherited cancer syndromes, and the much more common hepatoma or hepatocellular carcinoma occurring in US adults at a rate of 2 per 100,000 (Miller et al., 1992). This cancer has a worldwide distribution that overlaps with that of endemic Hepatitis B virus (HBV) infection, which is the most important risk factor. There were approximately 300,000 new cases of hepatocellular cancer worldwide in 1985, making it the sixth commonest cancer in the world. Nearly 45% of the world's cases occur in China (Parkin et al., 1993). Aflatoxin exposure is an important risk factor, and alcoholic cirrhosis also increases the risk of hepatocellular carcinoma. Individuals with hereditary haemachromatosis are at increased risk of hepatoma.

Genetic conditions conferring increased risk of hepatoblastoma

FAP

Based on an investigation of 197 pedigrees with FAP, the relative risk of developing hepatoblastoma was 847 (95% CI 320–2168) (Giardiello et al., 1991b), but the absolute life-time risk was only 1.6% (Giardiello and Offerhaus, 1995). To date, 32 cases of hepatoblastoma in FAP have been reported in the medical literature (Garber et al., 1988; LeSher et al., 1989; Giardiello et al., 1991b; Hughes and Michels, 1992).

Kurahashi et al. (1995) investigated the status of the *APC* gene in 11 cases of hepatoblastoma. None of the cases reported family history of FAP. In one case, genetic alterations were identified in both APC alleles. A de novo germline G → T transversion was identified at the intron 3-exon 4 junction splice site of one of the alleles, and there was loss of heterozygosity at this locus in the tumour. No germline or somatic mutations of APC were found in the remaining 10 tumours. Other conditions conferring increased risk include the overgrowth syndromes such as Beckwith–Wiedemann, Sotos, Bannayan–Riley–Ruvalcaba and to a lesser extent, Weaver and Marshall Smith syndromes (Hodgson and Maher, 1993). Recently, mutations in *PTEN*, responsible for Cowden disease (see Chapter 10) have been reported in kindreds with Bannayan–Riley syndrome (Marsh et al., 1997).

Type 1a glycogen storage disease

Hepatoblastoma is a rare complication of type 1a glycogen storage disease, a deficiency of glucose-6-phosphatase leading to increased glycogen concentrations in the liver, kidneys, and intestine. For example, there has been a report of hepatoblastoma in two siblings with this disease (Ito et al., 1987).

Hepatocellular carcinoma

Familial aggregation

A high incidence of hepatocellular carcinoma is observed among Alaskan natives. Alberts et al. (1991) described a clustering of this tumour in five Alaskan native families. There was a total of 15 hepatocellular carcinomas in these kindreds. The authors also reviewed the literature on familial clustering of hepatocellular carcinoma; a total of 86 cases from 33 families were reported. HBV status was not available for all the reported kindreds, however 34 (90%) of 38 patients were seropositive for HBsAg. Chronic HBV infection is a known risk factor for hepatocellular carcinoma (Beasley and Hwang, 1984), although the mechanism for this is not well-defined; it may be related to patterns of transmission of the virus, genetic factors influencing host response to HBV, or other genetic factors which predispose to hepatocellular carcinoma (reviewed in Alberts et al., 1991). It is not clear whether the increased incidence of cancer in these kindreds is due to genetic factors in an area of endemic HBV infection or whether it is purely a chance clustering of familial chronic HBV infection.

Multiple primaries

There is also a high incidence of hepatocellular carcinoma in Japan. Multiple primary tumours are common with hepatocellular carcinoma – 27 (9.2%) of 293 Japanese patients with this cancer were found to have second malignancies; 24 of these had triple primaries. Tumours observed in these patients included eight gastric, four uterine, and four colon cancers (Miyanaga et al., 1989). In those with multiple primary hepatomas, there is molecular evidence that the some of the tumours share clonal origins, and hence are not true multiple primaries (Muto et al., 1996). If this is confirmed, then the presence of multiple hepatocellular carcinomas in a person might not imply an increased likelihood of a hereditary component to the disease.

Genetic predispositions to hepatocellular carcinoma

Haemochromatosis

Hepatocellular carcinoma was the leading cause of death among 44 Italian hereditary haemochromatosis patients (Fargion et al., 1992). Of the total study population of 212 patients, 25 developed this cancer. In another series of 163 hereditary haematochromatosis patients, Strohmeyer et al. (1988) reported a mortality ratio of 219 (95% CI for observed deaths 9.1–24.8) for hepatic cancer (13 hepatocellular carcinomas, 3 carcinomas of the intrahepatic bile duct). A similar result was found in 208 cases of hereditary haematochromatosis – a relative risk of 240 (95% CI 138–390) was calculated for hepatocellular carcinoma in this disease (Bradbear et al., 1985).

Cirrhosis of the liver is most likely the primary mechanism in the development of malignancy in hereditary haematochromatosis; no hepatocellular carcinomas developed in non-cirrhotic livers (Strohmeyer et al., 1988; Fargion et al., 1992). In fact, although the annual incidence of hepatocellular carcinoma in Farigion's series was higher than that reported in the general population, it was similar to the annual rate among patients with cirrhosis of different aetiologies. Other risk factors for hepatocellular carcinoma in hereditary haematochromatosis include age (relative risk 13.3, 95% CI 3.6–48.7 in hereditary haematochromatosis patients over the age of 55) and HBsAg (relative risk 4.9, 95% CI 1.3–18.5); a non-significant relative risk of 2.3 (95% CI 1.0–5.1) was associated with alcohol abuse (Yao et al., 1977). Now that a gene, *HLA-H*, conferring susceptibility to hereditary haemochromatosis has been identified (Feder et al., 1996) it may be possible in the future to detect homozygotes before signs of liver disease develop and intervene appropriately with phlebotomy before iron overload becomes apparent.

FAP and HNPCC

Hepatocellular carcinoma is rare in FAP and HNPCC but has been documented in several kindreds (Weinberger et al., 1981; Zeze et al., 1983; Larferla et al., 1988). There is a fivefold increased risk of cancers of the hepatobiliary system in HNPCC (relative risk 4.9, $p < 0.05$) (Table 9.7) (Lynch et al., 1991a).

Hereditary tyrosinaemia and other inborn errors of metabolism

Hereditary tyrosinaemia is an inborn error of metabolism characterized by increased levels of tyrosine in the plasma and urine, often associated with hepatic and renal dysfunction. Hepatocellular carcinoma may complicate this disease, probably due to the toxic effect of tyrosine or one of its metabolites. A review of the literature on chronic hereditary tyrosinaemia and hepatocellular carcinoma show that there were 16 (37%) cases of carcinoma in a total of 43 hereditary tyrosinaemia patients who survived beyond two years of age (Weinberg et al., 1976). More recently, hepatic cancer was observed in two of seven children over the age of two, both in association with cirrhosis (Russo and O'Regan, 1990).

From a study of acute hepatic porphyria among Finnish patients, there was a significantly elevated risk of hepatocellular carcinoma associated with this disorder (relative risk 61, 95% CI 18–145) (Kauppinen and Mustajoki, 1988). This does not appear to be associated with cirrhosis. A similar result was reported from Sweden: 11 cases of hepatocellular carcinoma were found among 206 patients with acute intermittent porphyria, diagnosed on the basis of increased levels of porphobilinogen in urine (Lithner and Wetterberg, 1984). This was highly significant. Previous diseases of 83 patients with hepatocellular carcinoma were investigated by Hardell et al. (1984). Porphyria cutanea tarda and acute intermittent porphyria were reported by 7.2% and 3.6% of these patients, respectively. No controls reported these inborn errors. The authors also described two acute intermittent porphyria pedigrees in which two and three family members, respectively, had both acute intermittent porphyria and hepatocellular carcinoma (Bengtsson and Hardell, 1986). Germanaud et al. (1994) described a 54-year-old woman with familial porphyria variegata who developed hepatocellular carcinoma, a rarer association. Since porphyrias are characterized by an impairment of the detoxification mechanism, the most probable explanation for their association with hepatocellular carcinoma is an accumulation of carcinogenic substances.

Hepatocellular carcinoma is also a feature of glycogen storage disease type 1a, discussed above. Malignant hepatoma was reported in a 14-year-old boy with glycogen storage disease type 1a (Zangeneh et al., 1969). Liver biopsies several years prior to the cancer diagnosis revealed benign adenomatous nodules. The patient's brother, who was also suffering from severe glycogen storage disease type 1a, was suspected of having hepatoma. The relationship between the metabolic abnormality in this disease and the malignant degeneration of benign adenomatous nodules after several years is not entirely clear, but glycogen build-up in hepatic cells may trigger neoproliferation (Howell et al., 1976).

Fanconi anaemia

Both hepatocellular carcinoma and fibrolamellar carcinoma of the liver have been reported in persons with Fanconi Anaemia. It is believed that the most likely explanation for this occurrence is the androgenic therapy used to treat these patients (LeBrun et al., 1991; Linares et al., 1991), but this remains conjectural.

Pancreato-biliary tract

Epidemiology

There were approximately 185,000 cases of pancreatic cancer worldwide in 1985 (Parkin et al., 1993). This number represents 2.4% of all cancers. The age-adjusted incidence of this disease is highest in the developed world and appears to be increasing slightly (Parkin et al., 1988, 1993). Cigarette smoking is the most consistent risk factor for pancreatic adenocarcinoma.

Genetic epidemiology

A study of 362 cases of pancreatic adenocarcinoma and 1408 hospital controls from northern Italy demonstrated an adjusted relative risk of 2.8

(95% CI 1.3–6.3) for pancreatic adenocarcinoma in association with a family history of this cancer in first-degree relatives (Fernandez et al., 1994). A study of francophone Montrealers found that 7.8% of cases but only 0.6% of controls reported a family history of pancreatic cancer (Ghadirian et al., 1991). Further questioning of individuals with familial pancreatic adenocarcinoma did not reveal any environmental exposure differences between the cases and matched controls. An elevated risk for pancreatic cancer was also reported for individuals with a close relative with any cancer (odds ratio 1.86, 95% CI 1.42–2.44) (Falk et al., 1988). Persons with close relatives with pancreatic cancer had a higher risk (odds ratio 5.25, 95% CI 2.08–13.2). A population-based study of familial cancer based on the Utah Population Database found a familial relative risk of 1.25 for pancreatic cancer (Goldgar et al., 1994). However, this elevated risk was not significant. A study of second primary tumours following diagnosis of colon cancer, based on the Utah Cancer Registry, revealed a standardized incidence ratio of 2.38 (95% CI 1.32–4.30) for pancreatic cancer (Slattery et al., 1995).

Case series

Several case series of families with three or more affected members support the hypothesis that genetic factors are an important determinant of risk (reviewed in Flanders and Foulkes, 1996). Some of these clusterings may be explained by known genes such as *CDKN2A* (see below and chapter 14), *BRCA1* and *BRCA2* (see below and Chapter 10). Lynch et al. (1995; 1992; 1990) have described a number of pancreatic cancer-prone kindreds. In many of the families, the disease was present in two consecutive generations; the pattern of cancer occurrence in these families appears to be consistent with an autosomal dominant mode of inheritance. Screening for pancreatic cancer in the general population is not recommended. In high-risk families, ultrasound, endoscopy or magnetic resonance imaging may have a role, but none of these has been evaluated.

Inherited cancer syndromes and pancreatic cancer

Familial atypical mole-multiple melanoma (FAMMM)

Pancreatic adenocarcinoma is probably the second commonest cancer FAMMM families (see Chapter 14). The observed/expected ratio for the frequency of pancreatic cancer among 200 individuals from nine FAMMM families was 13.4 ($p < 0.001$) (Bergman et al., 1990). In several chromosome 9p-linked FAMMM families, a mutation in the cell cycle inhibitor gene *CDKN2A* has been found to co-segregate with both melanoma and pancreatic adenocarcinoma (Hussussian et al., 1994; Goldstein et al., 1995; Gruis et al., 1995). By contrast, in some families, most persons with cancer have pancreatic or other gastrointestinal malignancies rather than melanoma (Whelan et al., 1995). Whether or not there is a true excess of pancreatic cancer in FAMMM pedigrees, or whether some or all of the excess might be explained by biased ascertainment is not yet resolved.

Familial breast and ovarian cancer syndromes

Pancreatic adenocarcinoma is seen in some breast cancer families accounted for by *BRCA1* and *BRCA2* mutations (Simard et al., 1994; Tonin et al., 1995); *BRCA1* and *BRCA2* families are characterized by an excess of ovarian cancer and male breast cancer, respectively (Phelan et al., 1996) (see Chapter 10). In these families, some persons with pancreatic cancer have inherited the at-risk haplotype and therefore it is likely that the pancreatic adenocarcinoma seen in these individuals is accounted for by *BRCA1* or *BRCA2* mutations. An investigation of 15 Swedish kindreds with *BRCA1* mutations revealed two cases of pancreatic cancer (diagnosed at ages 54 and 42), both of which had inherited the at-risk haplotype (Johannsson et al., 1996). Four out of seven Canadian families with known *BRCA2* mutations have at least one case of pancreatic cancer (Phelan et al., 1996) and pancreatic cancer may be a feature of Jewish breast cancer families (Tonin et al., 1996). Three out of seven male breast cancer pedigrees from Iceland contain one or more cases of pancreatic or biliary tract cancer (Arason et al., 1993). In Iceland, there is a significant excess (relative risk 1.66) of pancreatic cancer in the male first degree relatives of women with breast cancer (Tulinius et al., 1994). Most, if not all, Icelandic breast cancer families can be accounted for by a founder mutation in *BRCA2* (Thorlacius et al., 1996).

HNPCC

Pancreatic cancer is included in the tumour spectrum of HNPCC, but it is not certain whether the excess number of cases seen is a chance finding (Watson and Lynch, 1993). Lynch et al. (1991a) reported a relative risk of 1.4 ($p < 0.05$) for pancreatic cancer in HNPCC. In a study of 40 Finnish HNPCC kindreds, 6 of 293 putative gene carriers with clinically or histologically documented cancer had pancreatic carcinoma (Aarnio et al., 1995). The cumulative risk for biliary tract cancer, including pancreatic cancer, by age 80, was 17.5% in HNPCC gene carriers (Table 9.7).

Conversely, an investigation of 22 Dutch HNPCC families identified no cases of pancreatic cancer among 148 cancer patients (Vasen et al., 1989). Lynch has described a number of HNPCC kindreds with at least one individual diagnosed with pancreatic cancer (Lynch et al., 1988; Lynch et al., 1991a,b). In the most notable of these, one case of pancreatic cancer was seen in three of the five affected generations (Lynch et al., 1985). The average age at diagnoses of this tumour in the family was 56.3 years, which is younger than the average age in the US population.

Peutz–Jeghers syndrome, FAP and Li–Fraumeni syndrome

In 1986, Bowlby (1986) described a 15-year-old male with Peutz–Jeghers syndrome who died of pancreatic adenocarcinoma. In the 'Harrisburg family', one of the original Peutz–Jeghers syndrome families described in 1949, one man died of pancreatic adenocarcinoma at the age of 69 (Foley et al., 1988). Of 31 Peutz–Jeghers syndrome patients from 13 unrelated kindreds, 15 (48%) developed cancer and four had adenocarcinoma of the pancreas (Giardiello et al., 1987). In another study, 16 (22%) of 72 Peutz–Jeghers syndrome patients developed cancer (Spigelman et al., 1989a).

In a study of 197 FAP pedigrees, a relative risk of 4.46 (95% CI 1.2–11.4) for pancreatic adenocarcinoma was found in patients with the syndrome (Giardiello et al., 1993). Adenocarcinoma of the pancreas is occasionally seen in Li–Fraumeni syndrome (Strong et al., 1987). In a study of 24 Li–Fraumeni kindreds, one case of pancreatic cancer diagnosed before age 55 was seen in each of three families, and two cases were seen in a fourth (Li et al., 1988).

Ataxia-telangiectasia

A number of studies investigating the incidence of cancer in the relatives of patients with ataxia-telangiectasia report an association of pancreatic adenocarcinoma associated with the syndrome (Sholman and Swift, 1972; Narita and Takagi, 1984; Swift et al., 1987; Pippard et al., 1988), but few studies demonstrated the statistical significance of their findings.

Hereditary pancreatitis

Two cases of pancreatic cancer were reported in one family with hereditary pancreatitis, an autosomal dominant condition (Davidson et al., 1968). Kattwinkel et al. (1973) described another hereditary pancreatitis kindred in which there was one case of pancreatic cancer. However, in the two other hereditary pancreatitis families reported in the same paper, there were no confirmed cases of pancreatic malignancy. A recent international study of 248 individuals with hereditary pancreatitis has demonstrated a standardized incidence ratio of 53 (95% CI 23–105) for pancreatic cancer and a risk of pancreatic cancer to age 70 of 40%, with a higher risk for paternal inheritance. Although there may be ascertainment biases, there was no increased risk for cancer at other sites (Lowenfels et al., 1997). Mutations in the cationic trypsinogen gene responsible for hereditary pancreatitis (Whitcomb et al., 1996) were found in all 30 members of the international cohort so far studied.

Large bowel

Epidemiology

Colorectal cancer is one of the commonest causes of cancer death in the Western world. The highest age-adjusted incidence rates are seen in North American males (48.2 per 100,000), whereas the lowest rates are seen in West Africa (2.5 per 100,000 in men and women) (Parkin et al., 1993). While dietary factors have been implicated as risk factors, it has been difficult to pinpoint exactly which food items or micronutrients might be playing an important role in the promotion of or protection from these cancers. From an analytical epidemiology perspective, colon and rectal cancers are often treated separately, as the risk factors differ somewhat, but discussion of large bowel cancers will not be specifically subdivided here.

Colorectal cancer and inheritance

Non-syndromic familial colorectal cancer

Colorectal cancer has a strong familial component (Table 9.5). It is a feature of several hereditary cancer syndromes described below, but is also observed in a number of families unrelated to any known syndrome or predisposing genes. The clustering of colorectal cancer in these kindreds may be due to chance, to unmapped genes, or to a combination of environmental and genetic factors. For example, Ghadirian et al. (1993) described a kindred in which seven siblings were diagnosed with colorectal cancer at an average age of 64 years. There was no evidence of FAP in this family.

Lewis et al. (1996) performed linkage analysis of the four HNPCC genes, as well as DCC, APC, and TP53, in 10 kindreds ascertained from the Utah Cancer Registry based on the total number of colorectal cancer cases. In one kindred with early-onset colorectal cancer with high penetrance typical of HNPCC, the disease was linked to the mismatch repair gene, *hMSH2* on chromosome 2p (see below). None of the remaining families showed linkage to any of the candidate genes tested. Age of onset was higher and penetrance was lower in these families than in the HNPCC-linked family.

FAP

FAP has been recognized for over 100 years. In the UK, FAP accounts for about 1% of all colorectal cancer. The cardinal feature of FAP is the autosomal dominant inheritance of a propensity to develop hundreds to thousands of tubular adenomas throughout the large intestine, usually detectable by sigmoidoscopy before age 35. Malignant change is usually seen by the fifth decade if prophylactic surgery is not undertaken (Bussey, 1975). Extraintestinal features are common (Table 9.4). Following identification of a cytogenetic deletion in a man with Gardner syndrome (now accepted to be part of the FAP phenotype) the gene for FAP, *APC*, was linked to chromosome 5q21(Bodmer et al., 1987) and later identified (Groden et al., 1991) (Figure 9.1a). As the phenotype may differ from one individual to another both within a family or from different families with the same mutation, it has been of interest to determine any correlations between mutation position and risk of colorectal and other cancers – i.e. the genotype–phenotype relationship. There is some evidence for a relationship between mutation position and the severity of the colorectal phenotype. However, the strongest relationship between mutation position and phenotype is seen with congenital hypertrophy of the retinal pigment epithelium (CHRPE). Nearly all affected individuals from families with mutations before exon 9 in *APC* do not show CHRPE (Figure 9.1b). Because the variability in colorectal phenotype cannot be explained entirely by the mutation type and site, it has been suggested that other modifying genes may be acting. For example, germline mutation of the secretory phospholipase A_2 gene, *Pla2g2a*, in the murine model for FAP results in a marked increase in the number of colonic polyps. It was therefore hypothesized that mutation of a human homologue of this gene might be responsible for attenuated APC, a less severe variant of FAP (Spirio et al., 1993). Three members of this gene family were examined in 67 attenuated APC patients, however no mutations were found to correspond to a specific phenotype (Spirio et al., 1996).

Table 9.5. *Relative risk (RR) of colorectal cancer (CRC) in first-degree relatives of persons with colorectal cancer*

Study population	N	Exclusion criteria	RR (significance)	Reference
Mormons who died of CRC in Utah 1931–51	763	multiple polyposis	3.3 ($p < 0.01$)	Woolf (1958)
CRC patients, Tumour Registry, University Hospital, Columbus, Ohio	145		2.9	Macklin (1960)
St Mark's Hospital, London, CRC patients	209		3.5 ($p < 0.01$)	Lovett (1976)
Aberdeen group of hospitals, Scotland, consecutive CRC patients	50	diseases known to predispose to CRC	8/50 CRC patients with affected first degree relatives versus 1/50 among controls ($p = 0.03$)	Duncan and Kyle (1982)
Consecutive CRC patients 1979–83	170	FAP, HNPCC	6.3 ($p < 0.001$)	Maire et al. (1984)
Residents of Butler and Colfax counties, Nebraska, CRC diagnosis 1970–77	86		colon: 3.72 (95% CI 1.40–9.85) rectum: 15.90 (95% CI 3.79–66.7)	Pickle et al. (1984)
Oncology service, Tel Aviv area CRC patients	148		1.93 ($p < 0.05$) Ashkenazim: 1.15 ($p < 0.01$) non-Ashkenazim: 4.12 ($p < 0.001$) age: <65: 2.02 ($p < 0.05$) >65: 1.65 ($p < 0.05$)	Rozen et al. (1987b)

Population	n	Condition	Result	Reference
Asymptomatic adults (aged 35–70) having one first degree relative with CRC	417		3.1 ($p = 0.06$)	Rozen et al. (1987a)
National Institute for Cancer Research, Genoa, consecutive patients with CRC	414	FAP	2.36 (95% CI 1.54–3.60)	Bonelli et al. (1988)
Histologically confirmed new cases of CRC diagnosed 1980–81, residents of Melbourne	702	ulcerative colitis, FAP	2.13 (1.53–2.96)	Kune et al. (1989)
Health Care District of Modena, registered CRC patients 1984–1986	389		7.5 ($p < 0.001$)	Ponz de Leon et al. (1989)
Consecutive patients treated for primary CRC, Leeds UK	100	history of APC	4.6	Stephenson et al. (1991)
Danish Cancer Registry, all CRC patients diagnosed before age 60	1524	parents no longer living in Denmark after 1943	mothers: 1.62 (95% CI 1.31–2.01) fathers: 1.87 (95% CI 1.54–2.27) age < 50 (mothers and fathers): 5.52 (95% CI 2.65–10.2)	Søndergaard et al. (1991)
Réseau Inter-Hospitalier de Cancérologie de l'Université de Montréal, all colon cancer patients aged 35–79 1989–92	332		96 (28.9%) cases with FHx 19 (4%) controls with FHx $p < 0.05$	Ghadirian et al. (1993)

(continued)

Table 9.5. (cont.)

Study population	N	Exclusion criteria	RR (significance)	Reference
Australian residents diagnosed with CRC 1985–86	523	ulcerative colitis, Crohn disease, FAP, HNPCC, referral because of family history of colorectal neoplasm	2.1 (95% CI 1.4-3.1, $p = 0.001$) if proband <45 years at diagnosis: 3.7 (95% CI 1.5–9.1, $p = 0.001$)	St.John et al. (1993)
Hospitals in the Greater Milan area	766 (colon) 454 (rectum)		colon: 2.3 (95% CI 1.6–3.4) rectum: 1.7 (95% CI 1.1–2.7)	La Vecchia et al. (1992)
Female nurses, aged 30–55, male health professionals, aged 40–75	463	previous cancer, ulcerative colitis, FAP, previous colonoscopy/ sigmoidoscopy, previous adenoma	all ages, both sexes: 1.72 (95% CI 1.34–2.19) age breakdown: 30-44: 5.37 (1.98–17.4) 45-49: 3.85 (1.93–7.68) 50-54: 2.54 (1.45–4.46) 55-59: 1.66 (1.00–2.78) 60-64: 1.35 (0.81–2.25) 65-69: 1.09 (0.52–2.28) 70+: 1.00 (0.36–2.79)	(Fuchs et al. (1994)
Yorkshire Cancer Registry patients diagnosed with CRC before age 45	65		total: 5.21 ($p < 0.0001$) males: 2.08 ($p = 0.13$) females: 9.69 ($p < 0.0001$)	Hall et al. (1994a)

Utah population database, patients with first primary colon cancer	1244 men 1229 women		men: 2.15 (95% CI 1.73–2.66) women: 1.78 (95% CI 1.05–2.70)	Slattery and Kerber (1994)
Colorectal Tumour Registry of Modena (1984–86), Cancer Registry of Ragusa (1988-90)	Modena: 299 Ragusa: 121		Modena: 4.48 (95% CI 2.84–7.07) Ragusa: 5.74 (95% CI 2.29–14.4)	Modica et al. (1995)
Residents of Côte d'Or, France aged 30-79 with family history of CRC	171	FAP, HNPCC, inflammatory bowel disease	1.9 (95% CI 1.1–3.5, $p < 0.05$)	Boutron et al. (1995)

Note: FAP: familial adenomatous polyposis; HNPCC: hereditary nonpolyposis colorectal cancer; CI: confidence interval.

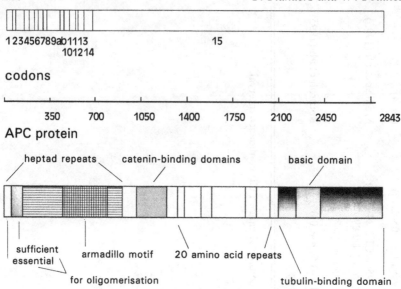

Figure 9.1(a). A diagrammatic representation of APC cDNA and protein. The numbers below the 'boxes' refer to the exons, using the nomenclature of Groden et al., 1991. The APC protein is shown below the codons. The putative motifs encoded by the gene are illustrated. The heptad repeat (apolar–X–X–apolar–X–X–X) is present in eight regions between codon 6 and codon 897. Another motif, armadillo, is seen within this region. The semi-conserved 20 amino acid motif F*VE*TP*CFSR*SSLSSLS is repeated at rough multiples of 50 amino acids, starting at amino acid 1262. The carboxy region contains a large 200 amino acid basic motif.

Turcot syndrome is an extremely rare disease characterized by colorectal adenomatous polyposis (although the number of polyps is variable) and malignancies of the central nervous system (generally medulloblastomas and glioblastomas). There is some uncertainty surrounding the mode of inheritance of this syndrome – there have been reports of both autosomal dominant and autosomal recessive patterns. Germline mutations of both the *APC* gene and of the mismatch repair genes associated with HNPCC have been found in patients from different families with Turcot syndrome. Interestingly, phenotypic characteristics of FAP are observed in Turcot kindreds with *APC* mutations. Similarly, most families with germline mutations in mismatch repair genes display clinical characteristics of HNPCC. Molecular genetic analysis of tumours from these families revealed replication errors typical of mismatch repair gene mutations (Hamilton et al., 1995).

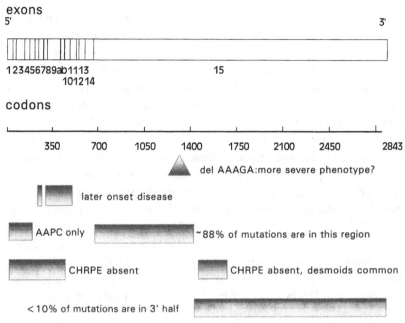

Figure 9.1(b). A diagrammatic representation of APC cDNA and genotype–phenotype correlations. The top two parts of the figure are as for Figure 9.1(a). The bottom part shows the genotype–phenotype correlations that are currently known. CHRPE: congenital hypertrophy of the retinal pigment epithelium; AAPC: attenuated APC; del AAAGA: the common 5 base pair deletion at codon 1309 (ΔAAAGA[1309], 1309delAAAGA). Mutations in this region may be associated with more severe rectal disease. The blocked area showing 88% of mutations is from data in a cumulative study of mutations (Nagase and Nakamura, 1993).

HNPCC

The syndrome of HNPCC is a dominantly inherited predisposition to early-onset cancer at colonic and extracolonic sites without profuse colonic polyposis. Minimum criteria for the diagnosis of HNPCC, established by the International Collaborative Group on HNPCC are: (1) three or more relatives with colorectal cancer, one of whom is a first-degree relative of the other two; (2) colorectal cancer involving at least two generations; (3) at least one case of colorectal cancer diagnosed before the age of 50; and (4) FAP excluded (Vasen et al., 1991). Newer, so-called 'Bethesda criteria' include other cancer sites. The prevalence of HNPCC is uncertain, but is probably responsible for about 2–5% of all colorectal cancer (Table 9.6) . A typical HNPCC pedigree is shown in Figure 9.2.

To date, four genes in which mutations can cause HNPCC have been identified, *hMSH2* on chromosome 2, *hMLH1* on chromosome 3, and *hPMS1* and *hPMS2*. It is estimated that the former two genes account for 90% of HNPCC cases (Liu et al., 1996). These four genes encode proteins involved in the repair of DNA mismatches. Polymerase chain reaction amplification of microsatellite DNA from individuals with this syndrome reveals extra bands in tumour compared with normal DNA samples. In other words, HNPCC tumours generally show microsatellite instability. This was subsequently found to be due to germline mutations in mismatch repair genes. These mutations result in a replication error repair (RER+) phenotype with sites of instability throughout the genome. This phenotype is present in over 80% of colorectal tumours from HNPCC kindreds (Aaltonen et al., 1994), but only 17% of sporadic tumours (Lothe et al., 1993). Liu et al. (1995) found that 58% of colorectal tumours in persons under the age of 35 were RER+. Moreover, Aaltonen et al. (1994) found that 8 (57%) of 14 colorectal adenomas associated with HNPCC were RER+, while only 1 (3%) of 33 of sporadic colorectal adenomas was RER+.

In a study of 130 HNPCC-like kindreds seen in London, UK, the relative risk of death from colon cancer in the first-degree relatives of probands with colon cancer was 5.6 for males and 15.2 for females (both $p < 0.001$) (Itoh et al. 1990). Confirmed carriers of a mutated HNPCC gene, *hMLH1* or *hMSH2*, may have a life-time risk as high as 92% of developing colorectal cancer (CRC) (Vasen et al., 1996). An investigation of 193 putative HNPCC gene carriers in the Finnish HNPCC Registry, revealed a life-time cumulative risk of colorectal cancer in HNPCC of 78.4% (Aarnio et al., 1995).

Colorectal cancers associated with HNPCC tend to be RER+, poorly differentiated, diploid, LOH-poor, *TP53* mutation-negative, with mucinous characteristics and lymphocytic infiltration (Lynch et al., 1993). Individuals from *hMHL1*-associated HNPCC kindreds tend to have better survival rates than those with sporadic colorectal carcinoma. This was determined in a study of 175 colorectal carcinoma patients from 39 HNPCC families diagnosed under the age of 65 (Sankila et al., 1996). One hundred and twenty of these were from kindreds with proven germline *hMLH1* mutations. Five-year cumulative relative survival rates for HNPCC versus sporadic colorectal carcinoma patients were 65% (95% CI 57–72) and 44% (95% CI 43–45), respectively. The better survival may in part (or in whole) be attributable to the RER+ phenotype since individuals with RER+ tumours without obvious germline

Table 9.6. *Prevalence of hereditary non-polyposis colorectal cancer (HNPCC)*

Study population	N	Exclusion criteria	% HNPCC	Reference
Finish Cancer Registry, all CRC patients diagnosed 1970–79, living in mid-Finland	468		3.8	Mecklin (1987)
All CRC patients diagnosed before age 55 in Northern Ireland, 1976–78	205	FAP	1–2	Kee and Collins (1991)
Alberta Cancer Registry, Tom Banks Cancer Centre, Calgary, CRC patients diagnosed before age 50, 1973–1987	318	cancer type other than adenocarcinoma, conditions known to predispose to CRC (FAP, inflammatory bowel disease, ureterosigmoidostomy)	3.1 (95% CI 1.6–5.3%)	Westlake et al. (1991)
Colon cancer registry (1984–88, Modena health care district, Italy	605		1.3	Mecklin et al. (1995)
All CRC patients in one clinic diagnosed 1990–91	406		Putative HNPCC: 7 Amsterdam Criteria: 0.7	Mecklin et al. (1995)

Note: CRC: colorectal cancer; FAP: familial adenomatous polyposis; CI: confidence interval

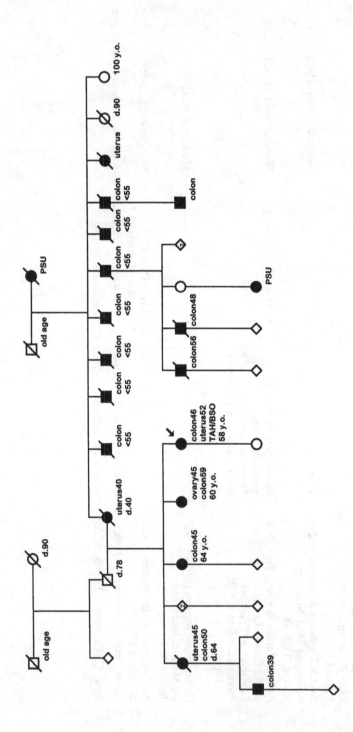

Figure 9.2 A typical multigeneration hereditary nonpolyposis colorectal cancer family. The proband is marked with an arrow. The numbers adjacent or below the cancer sites refer to the age at diagnosis. When preceded by d. the number is the age at death. When followed by y.o. the number is the current age. PSU: cancer, primary site unknown; TAH/BSO: total abdominal hysterectomy with bilateral salpingo-oophorectomy.

Table 9.7. *Extracolonic cancer risks in hereditary nonpolyposis colorectal cancer**

Site	RR	Cumulative risk to age 80 (%)
Endometrium	10	43
Ovary	3.5	9
Stomach	4.0	19
Small intestine	25-300	< 1
Hepatobiliary system	5.0	18
Kidney	3.5	not recorded separately to ureter
Ureter	22	< 5
Pancreas	1.5	not recorded separately to hepatobiliary

Note: Adapted from Lynch et al., 1991a; Watson and Lynch, 1993; Aarnio et al. 1995; Vasen et al., 1996.
*Risks vary from family to family and may differ with different mismatch repair gene mutations. RR: Relative risk.

mismatch repair gene mutations also have a better prognosis than expected (Bubb et al., 1996).

Germline mutations in *hMSH2* (Hall et al., 1994b) and *hMLH1* (Bapat et al., 1996) have been reported in families with Muir–Torre syndrome, a variant of HNPCC (Table 9.4; also see Chapter 15). It is unlikely that the phenotype variability seen can be explained by the type of mutation in the mismatch repair gene (see also Chapter 18), but is more likely to be the result of the action of other unknown genes. Some specific cancers, such as endometrial adenocarcinoma (relative risk, 10) and small bowel carcinoma (relative risk 25) are also common in HNPCC (Table 9.7).

Peutz–Jeghers syndrome, juvenile polyposis and other rare polyposis syndromes

Peutz–Jeghers syndrome is an autosomal dominant condition characterized by hamartomatous gastrointestinal polyps and mucocutaneous pigmentation (Table 9.4). Although hamartomatous polyps generally do not undergo malignant transformation, patients with this disease are at an increased risk of cancer at various sites in the digestive tract. From a study of 66 Peutz–Jeghers syndrome patients from the St. Mark's Polyposis Registry, the relative risk of death from gastrointestinal cancer in Peutz–Jeghers syndrome was 13 (95% CI 2.7–38.1) (Spigelman et al.,

1989a). A review of the literature on malignancy associated with Peutz–Jeghers syndrome listed the large bowel as the commonest site for malignancy (Konishi et al., 1987). Second most common was the duodenum, followed by the jejunum and the stomach. Using comparative genomic hybridization of hamartomas in one individual and subsequent linkage, a Peutz–Jeghers gene has been localized to chromosome 19p (Hemminki et al., 1997).

Juvenile polyposis is a rare condition characterized by the presence of numerous (50–100) histologically distinct polyps. These lesions occur throughout the gastrointestinal tract. The disease usually occurs sporadically, however there is a rare, autosomal dominantly inherited form. Hofting et al. investigated 262 cases of juvenile polyposis and found 98% of polyps in the colorectum, 13.6% in the stomach, 2.3% in the duodenum, and 6.5% in the jejunum and ileum (Desai et al., 1995). This condition is also associated with malignancy; in the same study, researchers identified a total of 48 (18%) cases of carcinoma occurring in the colorectum, stomach, small bowel, and pancreas. Colorectal cancer was diagnosed in 18 (21%) of 87 juvenile polyposis patients registered in the St. Mark's Polyposis Registry (Jass et al., 1988). Jarvinen et al. (1984) describe six members of one family with juvenile polyposis. Two developed colorectal adenocarcinoma and two others had severe adenomatous dysplasia in a juvenile polyp. In a retrospective study of the association between juvenile polyps and colorectal neoplasia, 20 of 57 patients with juvenile polyps had affected first-degree relatives (Giardiello et al., 1991a). This included two cases of colorectal adenocarcinoma, two cases of tubular adenoma separate from juvenile polyps, and four cases of adenomatous epithelium in juvenile polyps. In addition, the authors reviewed the literature on solitary and multiple juvenile polyps – carcinoma was observed in 3 of 8 and 20 of 39 cases, respectively. Rozen and Baratz (1982) described a mother and son with multiple juvenile colonic polyps. Although the polyps were not adenomas, some contained adenomatous-like elements. The mother developed metastatic adenocarcinoma of the large bowel, and the son subsequently underwent subtotal colectomy. The authors suggest that the family represents phenotype variation with features of both juvenile and adenomatous polyposis.

In the hereditary mixed polyposis syndrome (HMPS, reported in one family only), the polyps also contain elements of juvenile, adenomatous, as well as hamartomatous polyps. This syndrome is also autosomal dominantly inherited and is distinct from both FAP and juvenile polyposis.

Affected individuals develop atypical juvenile polyps, colonic adenomas, and colorectal carcinomas. Although many features of this syndrome resemble FAP, linkage to *APC* was ruled out. A genetic linkage analysis on 46 members of a large kindred with the disease located a putative HMPS locus on chromosome 6q between markers D6S468 and D6S310 (Thomas et al., 1996). In the colorectal allelotype of Vogelstein et al. (1989) 6q was the sixth commonest site of LOH (loss of heterozygosity), however there are no candidate colon cancer susceptibility genes in this region. LOH was seen in only 10 (13%) of 77 informative colon tumours in this HMPS kindred. Despite this finding, the responsible gene is likely to have tumour-suppressing functions.

A karyotype of a woman with multiple hyperplastic and mixed hyperplastic adenomatous polyps of the oesophagus, stomach and colorectum accompanying rectal cancer, showed a germline chromosomal inversion (3)(p12.2;q25.3) (Sasajima et al., 1993). This finding may implicate a locus on chromosome 3p in the aetiology of familial colorectal cancer, although the allelotype of sporadic colorectal cancer performed by Vogelstein revealed allelic deletions at 3p in only 20% of tumours (Vogelstein et al., 1989). A possible tumour suppressor gene, *FHIT* (see Chapter 11), at 3p14 does not appear to be the somatic target in colorectal cancer.

Cowden disease and other rare genodermatoses featuring colorectal cancer

Cowden disease, also known as multiple hamartoma syndrome, is a dominantly inherited disorder characterized by mucocutaneous lesions and malignancy, described above and also in Chapter 10. The commonest gastrointestinal manifestations in this condition are multiple hamartomatous polyps throughout the digestive tract, but primarily in the colon. These polyps are seen in approximatey 35% of Cowden disease cases, while adenocarcinoma of the colon and caecum, respectively, are reported in only 1% and 2% of cases (Starink et al., 1986). The two most common cancers seen are breast and thyroid. Other malignancies reported in this syndrome include uterine, ovarian, lung, squamous cell carcinoma, basal cell carcinoma, acute myelogenous leukemia, non-Hodgkin's lymphoma, cervix, bladder, melanoma, and liposarcoma of the arm (reviewed in Mallory, 1991). Linkage has recently been demonstrated between this disease and chromosome 10q22-23 (Nelen et al., 1996). The gene for Cowden disease, *PTEN*, has now been identified and missense and nonsense mutations have been reported in several kindreds (Liaw et al., 1997).

An extensive Irish kindred has been described in which punctate palmoplantar keratoderma is associated with a spectrum of malignancies that does not fit any known syndromic pattern (Stevens et al., 1996b). Of 49 individuals from this family affected with punctate palmoplantar keratoderma (inherited in an autosomal dominant fashion), 10 have been diagnosed with cancer. Six malignancies were observed among the 271 unaffected family members. Malignancies occurring in this kindred include carcinomas of the colon (three cases), breast (two cases), pancreas (two cases), lung, ovary, and renal cell carcinoma (two cases), transitional cell carcinoma of the bladder, leiomyosarcoma of the uterus, and Hodgkin's lymphoma (three cases). Six of these cancers were diagnosed before age 50. Another smaller family with a similar association was described by Bennion and Patterson (1984). Unlike focal palmoplantar keratoderma (associated with oesophageal cancer, see above), which has been mapped to chromosome 17q23-ter, the genetic mechanism for the association of this form of the disease with malignancy is not known; linkage to the known keratin gene clusters in the Irish pedigree was excluded (Kelsell et al., 1995).

Conclusion

Cancers of the gastrointestinal tract and related organs are the commonest cancers worldwide. It is increasingly evident that there is a genetic contribution to cancers at most of these sites. The largest hereditary component is probably seen in small bowel carcinoma, followed by large bowel carcinoma. Cancers of the pancreatobiliary tract are increasingly recognized as having a significant hereditary element, and stomach cancer has long been associated with blood group A. Cancers of the upper aerodigestive tract have strong environmental precipitants, but even in these cancers, there is some evidence for a genetic contribution. It is likely that polygenic and multifactorial models of adult cancers will be particularly applicable to gastrointestinal cancers, where diet is likely to play an important role.

References

Aaltonen, L.A., Peltomaki, P., Mecklin, J.P. et al. 1994. Replication errors in benign and malignant tumors from hereditary nonpolyposis colorectal cancer patients. *Cancer Research* **54**: 1645–8.

Aarnio, M., Mecklin, J.P., Aaltonen, L.A., Nystromlahti, M. and Jarvinen, H.J. 1995. Life-time risk of different cancers in Hereditary Non-polyposis Colorectal Cancer (HNPCC) syndrome. *International Journal of Cancer* **64**: 430–3.

Albeck, H., Bentzen, J., Ockelmann, H.H., Nielsen, N.H., Bretlau, P. and Hansen, H.S. 1993. Familial clusters of nasopharyngeal carcinoma and salivary gland carcinomas in Greenland natives. *Cancer* **72**: 196–200.

Alberts, S.R., Lanier, A.P., McMahon, B.J., Harpster, A., Bulkow, L.R., Heyward, W.L. and Murray, C. 1991. Clustering of hepatocellular carcinoma in Alaska Native families. *Genet Epidemiology* **8**: 127–39.

Arason, A., Barkardottir, R.B. and Egilsson, V. 1993. Linkage analysis of chromosome 17q markers and breast-ovarian cancer in Icelandic families, and possible relationship to prostatic cancer. *American Journal of Human Genetics* **52**: 711–17.

Bapat, B., Xia, L., Madlensky, L., Mitri, A., Tonin, P., Narod, S.A. and Gallinger, S. 1996. The genetic basis of Muir-Torre syndrome includes the hMLH1 locus. *American Journal of Human Genetics* **59**: 736–9.

Beasley, R.P. and Hwang, L.Y. 1984. Hepatocellular carcinoma and hepatitis B virus. *Seminars in Liver Disease* **4**: 113–21.

Bengtsson, N.O. and Hardell, L. 1986. Porphyrias, porphyrins and hepatocellular cancer. *British Journal of Cancer* **54**: 115–17.

Bennion, S.D. and Patterson, J.W. 1984. Keratosis punctata palmaris et plantaris and adenocarcinoma of the colon. A possible familial association of punctate keratoderma and gastrointestinal malignancy. *Journal of the American Academy of Dermatology* **10**: 587–91.

Bergman, W., Watson, P., de Jong, J., Lynch, H.T. and Fusaro, R.M. 1990. Systemic cancer and the FAMMM syndrome. *British Journal of Cancer* **61**: 932–6.

Bodmer, W.F., Bailey, C.J., Bodmer, J. et al. 1987. Localization of the gene for familial adenomatous polyposis on chromosome 5. *Nature* **328**: 614–16.

Bonelli, L., Martines, H., Conio, M., Bruzzi, P. and Aste, H. 1988. Family history of colorectal cancer as a risk factor for benign and malignant tumours of the large bowel. A case-control study. *International Journal of Cancer* **41**: 513–17.

Boutron, M.C., Faivre, J., Quipourt, V., Senesse, P. and Michiels, C. 1995. Family history of colorectal tumours and implications for the adenoma-carcinoma sequence: a case control study. *Gut* **37**: 830–4.

Bowlby, L.S. 1986. Pancreatic adenocarcinoma in an adolescent male with Peutz-Jeghers syndrome. *Human Pathology* **17**: 97–9.

Bradbear, R.A., Bain, C., Siskind, V. et al. 1985. Cohort study of internal malignancy in genetic hemochromatosis and other chronic nonalcoholic liver diseases. *Journal of the National Cancer Institute* **75**: 81–4.

Brown, T.M., Heath, C.W., Lang, R.M., Lee, S.K. and Whalley, B.W. 1976. Nasopharyngeal cancer in Bermuda. *Cancer* **37**: 1464–8.

Bubb, V.J., Curtis, L.J., Cunningham, C. et al. 1996. Microsatellite instability and the role of *hMSH2* in sporadic colorectal cancer. *Oncogene* **12**(12): 2641–9.

190   *T. Flanders and W. Foulkes*

Bussey, H.J. 1975. *Familial Polyposis Coli. Famiy Studies, Histopathology, Differential Diagnosis and Results of Treatment.* Baltimore: Johns Hopkins University Press.

Carter, C.L., Hu, N., Wu, M., Lin, P.Z., Murigande, C. and Bonney, G.E. 1992. Segregation analysis of esophageal cancer in 221 high-risk Chinese families. *Journal of the National Cancer Institute* **84**: 771–6.

Coffin, C.M., Rich, S.S. and Dehner, L.P. 1991. Familial aggregation of nasopharyngeal carcinoma and other malignancies. A clinicopathologic description. *Cancer* **68**: 1323–8.

Copper, M.P., Jovanovic, A., Nauta, J.J., Braakhuis, B.J., de Vries, N., van der Waal, I. and Snow, G.B. 1995. Role of genetic factors in the etiology of squamous cell carcinoma of the head and neck. *Archives of Otolaryngology Head and Neck Surgery* **121**: 157–60.

Crabb, D.W., Berk, M.A., Hall, T.R., Conneally, P.M., Biegel, A.A. and Lehman, G.A. 1985. Familial gastroesophageal reflux and development of Barrett's esophagus. *Annals of Internal Medicine* **103**: 52–4.

Cristofaro, G., Lynch, H.T., Caruso, M.L. et al. 1987. New phenotypic aspects in a family with Lynch syndrome II. *Cancer* **60**: 51–8.

Davidson, P., Costanza, D., Swieconek, J.A. and Harris, J.B. 1968. Hereditary pancreatitis. A kindred without gross aminoaciduria. *Annals of Internal Medicine* **68**: 88–96.

Day, G.L., Blot, W.J., Austin, D.F. et al. 1993. Racial differences in risk of oral and pharyngeal cancer: alcohol, tobacco, and other determinants. *Journal of the National Cancer Institute* **85**: 465–73.

Desai, D.C., Neale, K.F., Talbot, I.C., Hodgson, S.V. and Phillips, R.K. 1995. Juvenile polyposis. *British Journal of Surgery* **82**: 14–17.

dos Santos, J.G. and de Magalhães, J. 1980. Familial gastric polyposis. A new entity. *Journal de Génétique Humaine* **28**: 293–7.

Duncan, J.L. and Kyle, J. 1982. Family incidence of carcinoma of the colon and rectum in north-east Scotland. *Gut* **23**: 169–71.

Ellis, A., Field, J.K., Field, E.A. et al. 1994. Tylosis associated with carcinoma of the oesophagus and oral leukoplakia in a large Liverpool family–a review of six generations. *European Journal of Cancer and Oral Oncology* **30B**: 102–12.

Eng, C., Spechler, S.J., Ruben, R. and Li, F.P. 1993. Familial Barrett esophagus and adenocarcinoma of the gastroesophageal junction. *Cancer Epidemiology, Biomarkers and Prevention* **2**: 397–9.

Falk, R.T., Pickle, L.W., Fontham, E.T., Correa, P. and Fraumeni, J.F., Jr. 1988. Life-style risk factors for pancreatic cancer in Louisiana: a case-control study. *American Journal of Epidemiology* **128**: 324–36.

Fargion, S., Mandelli, C., Piperno, A. et al. 1992. Survival and prognostic factors in 212 Italian patients with genetic hemochromatosis. *Hepatology* **15**: 655–9.

Farinati, F., Cardin, F., Di Mario, F. et al. 1987. Genetic, dietary, and environmental factors in the pathogenesis of gastric cancer. Study of a high incidence family. *Italian Journal of Gastroenterology* **19**: 321–4.

Feder, J.N., Gnirke, A., Thomas, W. et al. 1996. A novel MHC class I-like gene is mutated in patients with hereditary haemochromatosis. *Nature Genetics* **13**: 399–408.

Fernandez, E., La Vecchia, C., D'Avanzo, B., Negri, E. and Franceschi, S. 1994. Family history and the risk of liver, gallbladder, and pancreatic cancer. *Cancer Epidemiology, Biomarkers and Prevention* **3**: 209–12.

Fischer, A., Fischer, G.O. and Cooper, E. 1984. Familial nasopharyngeal carcinoma. *Pathology* **16**: 23–4.

Fitzgibbons, R.J., Jr., Lynch, H.T., Stanislav, G.V. et al. 1987. Recognition and treatment of patients with hereditary nonpolyposis colon cancer (Lynch syndromes I and II). *Annals of Surgery* **206**: 289–95.

Flanders, T.Y. and Foulkes, W.D. 1996. Pancreatic adenocarcinoma – epidemiology and genetics. *Journal of Medical Genetics* **33**: 889–98.

Foley, T.R., McGarrity, T.J. and Abt, A.B. 1988. Peutz-Jeghers syndrome: a clinicopathologic survey of the 'Harrisburg family' with a 49-year follow-up. *Gastroenterology* **95**: 1535–40.

Forman, D. 1996. Helicobacter pylori and gastric cancer. *Scandinavian Journal of Gastroenterology (Supplement)* **214**: 31–43.

Foulkes, W.D., Brunet, J.S., Kowalski, L.P., Narod, S.A. and Franco, E.L. 1995. Family history of cancer is a risk factor for squamous cell carcinoma of the head and neck in Brazil – a case -control study. *International Journal of Cancer* **63**: 769–73.

Foulkes, W.D., Brunet, J.S., Sieh, W., Black, M.J., Shenouda, G. and Narod, S.A. 1996. Familial risks of squamous cell carcinoma of the head and neck: retrospective case-control study. *British Medical Journal* **313**: 716–21.

Fuchs, C.S., Giovannucci, E.L., Colditz, G.A., Hunter, D.J., Speizer, F.E. and Willett, W.C. 1994. A prospective study of family history and the risk of colorectal cancer. *New England Journal of Medicine* **331**: 1669–74.

Gahtan, V., Nochomovitz, L.E., Robinson, A.M., Garcia, V.F. and Smith, L.E. 1989. Gastroduodenal polyps in familial polyposis coli. *American Surgeon* **55**: 278–80.

Gajwani, B.W., Devereaux, J.M. and Beg, J.A. 1980. Familial clustering of nasopharyngeal carcinoma. *Cancer* **46**: 2325–7.

Garber, J.E., Li, F.P., Kingston, J.E. et al. 1988. Hepatoblastoma and familial adenomatous polyposis. *Journal of the National Cancer Institute* **80**: 1626–8.

Germanaud, J., Luthier, F., Causse, X., Kerdraon, R., Grossetti, D., Gargot, D. and Nordmann, Y. 1994. A case of association between hepatocellular carcinoma and porphyria variegata. *Scandinavian Journal of Gastroenterology* **29**: 671–2.

Ghadirian, P. 1985. Familial history of esophageal cancer. *Cancer* **56**: 2112–16.

Ghadirian, P., Boyle, P., Simard, A., Baillargeon, J., Maisonneuve, P. and Perret, C. 1991. Reported family aggregation of pancreatic cancer within a population-based case-control study in the Francophone community in Montreal, Canada. *International Journal of Pancreatology* **10**: 183–96.

Ghadirian, P., Cadotte, M., Lacroix, A., Baillargeon, J. and Perret, C. 1993. Colon cancer in seven siblings. *European Journal of Cancer* **29A**: 1553–6.

Giardiello, F.M., Welsh, S.B., Hamilton, S.R. et al. 1987. Increased risk of cancer in the Peutz-Jeghers syndrome. *New England Journal of Medicine* **316**: 1511–14.

Giardiello, F.M., Hamilton, S.R., Kern, S.E. et al. 1991a. Colorectal neoplasia in juvenile polyposis or juvenile polyps. *Archives of Diseases of Childhood* **66**: 971–5.

Giardiello, F.M., Offerhaus, G.J., Krush, A.J. et al. 1991b. Risk of hepatoblastoma in familial adenomatous polyposis. *Journal of Pediatrics* **119**: 766–8.

Giardiello, F.M., Offerhaus, G.J., Lee, D.H. et al. 1993. Increased risk of thyroid and pancreatic carcinoma in familial adenomatous polyposis. *Gut* **34**: 1394–6.

Giardiello, F.M. and Offerhaus, J.G. 1995. Phenotype and cancer risk of various polyposis syndromes. *European Journal of Cancer* **31A**: 1085–7.

Goldgar, D.E., Easton, D.F., Cannon-Albright, L.A. and Skolnick, M.H. 1994. Systematic population-based assessment of cancer risk in first-degree relatives of cancer probands. *Journal of the National Cancer Institute* **86**: 1600–8.

Goldstein, A.M., Fraser, M.C., Struewing, J.P. et al. 1995. Increased risk of pancreatic cancer in melanoma-prone kindreds with p16INK4 mutations. *New England Journal of Medicine* **333**: 970–4.

Groden, J., Thliveris, A., Samowitz, W. et al. 1991. Identification and characterization of the familial adenomatous polyposis coli gene. *Cell* **66**: 589–601.

Gruis, N.A., van der Velden, P.A., Sandkuijl, L.A. et al. 1995. Homozygotes for CDKN2 (p16) germline mutation in Dutch familial melanoma kindreds. *Nature Genetics* **10**: 351–3.

Guo, W., Blot, W.J., Li, J.Y. et al. 1994. A nested case-control study of oesophageal and stomach cancers in the Linxian nutrition intervention trial. *International Journal of Epidemiology* **23**: 444–50.

Haerer, A.F., Jackson, J.F. and Evers, C.G. 1969. Ataxia-telangiectasia with gastric adenocarcinoma. *JAMA* **210**: 1884–7.

Hall, N.R., Finan, P.J., Ward, B., Turner, G. and Bishop, D.T. 1994a. Genetic susceptibility to colorectal cancer in patients under 45 years of age. *British Journal of Surgery* **81**: 1485–9.

Hall, N.R., Murday, V.A., Chapman, P., Williams, M.A., Burn, J., Finan, P.J. and Bishop, D.T. 1994b. Genetic linkage in Muir-Torre syndrome to the same chromosomal region as cancer family syndrome. *European Journal of Cancer* **30A**: 180–2.

Hamby, L.S., Lee, E.Y. and Schwartz, R.W. 1995. Parathyroid adenoma and gastric carcinoma as manifestations of Cowden's disease. *Surgery* **118**: 115–17.

Hamilton, S.R., Liu, B., Parsons, R.E. et al. 1995. The molecular basis of Turcot's syndrome. *New England Journal of Medicine* **332**: 839–47.

Hansson, L.E., Nyren, O., Hsing, A.W. et al. 1996. The risk of stomach cancer in patients with gastric or duodenal ulcer disease. *New England Journal of Medicine* **335**: 242–9.

Hardell, L., Bengtsson, N.O., Jonsson, U., Eriksson, S. and Larsson, L.G. 1984. Aetiological aspects on primary liver cancer with special regard to alcohol, organic solvents and acute intermittent porphyria–an epidemiological investigation. *British Journal of Cancer* **50**: 389–97.

Hemminki, A., Tomlinson, I., Markie, D et al. 1997. Localization of a susceptibility locus for Peutz-Jeghers syndrome to 19p using comparative genomic hybridization and targeted linkage analysis. *Nature Genetics* **15**: 87–90.

Hennies, H.C., Hagedorn, M. and Reis, A. 1995. Palmoplantar keratoderma in association with carcinoma of the esophagus maps to chromosome 17q distal to the keratin gene cluster. *Genomics* **29**: 537–40.

Hizawa, K., Iida, M., Matsumoto, T., Kohrogi, N., Suekane, H., Yao, T. and Fujishima, M. 1994. Gastrointestinal manifestations of Cowden's disease. Report of four cases. *Journal of Clinical Gastroenterology* **18**: 13–18.

Ho, J.H. 1972. Nasopharyngeal carcinoma (NPC). *Advances in Cancer Research* **15**: 57–92.

Hodgson, S.V. and Maher, E. 1993. *A Practical Guide to Human Cancer Genetics*: Cambridge: CUP.

Howel-Evans, W., McConnell, R.B., Clarke, C.A. and Sheppard, P.M. 1958. Carcinoma of the oesophagus with keratosis palmaris et plantaris (tylosis). A study of two families. *Quarterly Journal of Medicine* **27**: 413–29.

Howell, R.R., Stevenson, R.E., Ben-Menachem, Y., Phyliky, R.L. and Berry, D.H. 1976. Hepatic adenomata with type 1 glycogen storage disease. *JAMA* **236**: 1481–4.

Hu, N., Dawsey, S.M., Wu, M. et al. 1992. Familial aggregation of oesophageal cancer in Yangcheng County, Shanxi Province, China. *International Journal of Epidemiology* **21**: 877–82.

Hughes, L.J. and Michels, V.V. 1992. Risk of hepatoblastoma in familial adenomatous polyposis. *American Journal of Medical Genetics* **43**: 1023–5.

Hussussian, C.J., Struewing, J.P., Goldstein, A.M. et al. 1994. Germline p16 mutations in familial melanoma. *Nature Genetics* **8**: 15–21.

Iida, M., Yao, T., Watanabe, H., Itoh, H. and Iwashita, A. 1984. Fundic gland polyposis in patients without familial adenomatosis coli: its incidence and clinical features. *Gastroenterology* **86**: 1437–42.

Ireland, B., Lanier, A.P., Knutson, L., Clift, S.E. and Harpster, A. 1988. Increased risk of cancer in siblings of Alaskan native patients with nasopharyngeal carcinoma. *International Journal of Epidemiology* **17**: 509–11.

Ito, E., Sato, Y., Kawauchi, K., Munakata, H., Kamata, Y., Yodono, H. and Yokoyama, M. 1987. Type 1a glycogen storage disease with hepatoblastoma in siblings. *Cancer* **59**: 1776–80.

Itoh, H., Houlston, R.S., Harocopos, C. and Slack, J. 1990. Risk of cancer death in first-degree relatives of patients with hereditary non-polyposis cancer syndrome (Lynch type II): a study of 130 kindreds in the United Kingdom. *British Journal of Surgery* **77**: 1367–70.

Jagelman, D.G., DeCosse, J.J. and Bussey, H.J. 1988. Upper gastrointestinal cancer in familial adenomatous polyposis. *Lancet* **1**: 1149–51.

Jarvinen, H. and Franssila, K.O. 1984. Familial juvenile polyposis coli; increased risk of colorectal cancer. *Gut* **25**: 792–800.

Jass, J.R., Williams, C.B., Bussey, H.J. and Morson, B.C. 1988. Juvenile polyposis-a precancerous condition. *Histopathology* **13**: 619–30.

Jochem, V.J., Fuerst, P.A. and Fromkes, J.J. 1992. Familial Barrett's esophagus associated with adenocarcinoma. *Gastroenterology* **102**: 1400–2.

Johannsson, O., Ostermeyer, E.A., Hakansson, S. et al. 1996. Founding BRCA1 mutations in hereditary breast and ovarian cancer in Southern Sweden. *American Journal of Human Genetics* **58**: 441–50.

Joncas, J.H., Rioux, E., Wastiaux, J.P., Leyritz, M., Robillard, L. and Menezes, J. 1976. Nasopharyngeal carcinoma and Burkitt's lymphoma in a Canadian family. I. HLA typing, EBV antibodies and serum immunoglobulins. *Canadian Medical Association Journal* **115**: 858–60.

Jung, P.F. 1965. Familial tendency of nasopharyngeal carcinoma. *Pacific Medicine and Surgery* **73**: 242–3.

Kattwinkel, J., Lapey, A., Di Sant'Agnese, P.A. and Edwards, W.A. 1973. Hereditary pancreatitis: three new kindreds and a critical review of the literature. *Pediatrics* **51**: 55–69.

Kauppinen, R. and Mustajoki, P. 1988. Acute hepatic porphyria and hepatocellular carcinoma. *British Journal of Cancer* **57**: 117–20.

Kee, F. and Collins, B.J. 1991. How prevalent is cancer family syndrome? *Gut* **32**: 509–12.

194   T. Flanders and W. Foulkes

Kelsell, D.P., Stevens, H.P., Ratnavel, R., Bryant, S.P., Bishop, D.T., Leigh, I.M. and Spurr, N.K. 1995. Genetic linkage studies in non-epidermolytic palmoplantar keratoderma: evidence for heterogeneity. *Human Molecular Genetics* **4**: 1021–5.

Konishi, F., Wyse, N.E., Muto, T., Sawada, T., Morioka, Y., Sugimura, H. and Yamaguchi, K. 1987. Peutz-Jeghers polyposis associated with carcinoma of the digestive organs. Report of three cases and review of the literature. *Diseases of the Colon and Rectum* **30**: 790–9.

Kune, G.A., Kune, S. and Watson, L.F. 1989. The role of heredity in the etiology of large bowel cancer: data from the Melbourne Colorectal Cancer Study. *World Journal of Surgery* **13**: 124–9; discussion 129–31.

Kurahashi, H., Takami, K., Oue, T. et al. 1995. Biallelic inactivation of the APC gene in hepatoblastoma. *Cancer Research* **55**: 5007–11.

Kurtz, R.C., Sternberg, S.S., Miller, H.H. and DeCosse, J.J. 1987. Upper gastrointestinal neoplasia in familial polyposis. *Digestive Diseases and Sciences* **32**: 459–65.

La Vecchia, C., Negri, E., Franceschi, S. and Gentile, A. 1992. Family history and the risk of stomach and colorectal cancer. *Cancer* **70**: 50–5.

Laferla, G., Kaye, S.B. and Crean, G.P. 1988. Hepatocellular and gastric carcinoma associated with familial polyposis coli. *Journal of Surgical Oncology* **38**: 19–21.

Lanier, A.P., Bender, T.R., Tschopp, C.F. and Dohan, P. 1979. Nasopharyngeal carcinoma in an Alaskan Eskimo family: report of three cases. *Journal of the National Cancer Institute* **62**: 1121–4.

LeBrun, D.P., Silver, M.M., Freedman, M.H. and Phillips, M.J. 1991. Fibrolamellar carcinoma of the liver in a patient with Fanconi anemia. *Human Pathology* **22**: 396–8.

LeSher, A.R., Castronuovo, J.J., Jr. and Filippone, A.L., Jr. 1989. Hepatoblastoma in a patient with familial polyposis coli. *Surgery* **105**: 668–70.

Levine, P.H., Pocinki, A.G., Madigan, P. and Bale, S. 1992. Familial nasopharyngeal carcinoma in patients who are not Chinese. *Cancer* **70**: 1024–9.

Lewis, C.M., Neuhausen, S.L., Daley, D. et al. 1996. Genetic heterogeneity and unmapped genes for colorectal cancer. *Cancer Research* **56**: 1382–8.

Li, F.P. 1976. Familial Burkitt lymphoma and nasopharyngeal carcinoma. *Lancet* **1**: 687–8.

Li, F.P., Fraumeni, J.F., Jr., Mulvihill, J.J., Blattner, W.A., Dreyfus, M.G., Tucker, M.A. and Miller, R.W. 1988. A cancer family syndrome in twenty-four kindreds. *Cancer Research* **48**: 5358–62.

Li, J.Y. 1982. Epidemiology of esophageal cancer in China. *National Cancer Institute Monograph* **62**: 113–20.

Liaw, D., Marsh, D.J., Li, J. et al. 1997. Germline mutations of the *PTEN* gene in Cowden disease, an inherited breast and thyroid cancer syndrome. *Nature Genetics* **16**(1): 64–7.

Linares, M., Pastor, E., Gomez, A. and Grau, E. 1991. Hepatocellular carcinoma and squamous cell carcinoma in a patient with Fanconi's anemia. *Annals of Hematology* **63**: 54–5.

Lithner, F. and Wetterberg, L. 1984. Hepatocellular carcinoma in patients with acute intermittent porphyria. *Acta Medica Scandinavica* **215**: 271–4.

Liu, B., Farrington, S.M., Petersen, G.M. et al. 1995. Genetic instability occurs in the majority of young patients with colorectal cancer. *Nature Medicine* 1: 348–52.

Liu, B., Parsons, R., Papadopoulos, N. et al. 1996. Analysis of mismatch repair genes in hereditary non-polyposis colorectal cancer patients. *Nature Medicine* 2: 169–74.

Lothe, R.A., Peltomaki, P., Meling, G.I. et al. 1993. Genomic instability in colorectal cancer: relationship to clinicopathological variables and family history. *Cancer Research* 53: 5849–52.

Lovett, E. 1976. Family studies in cancer of the colon and rectum. *British Journal of Surgery* 63: 13–18.

Lowenfels, A.B., Maisonneuve, P., DiMagno, E.P., Elitsur, Y., Gates, L.K., Jr., Perrault, J. and Whitcomb, D.C. 1997. Hereditary pancreatitis and the risk of pancreatic cancer. International Hereditary Pancreatitis Study Group. *Journal of the National Cancer Institute* 6: 442–6.

Lu, J.B., Yang, W.X., Liu, J.M., Li, Y.S. and Qin, Y.M. 1985. Trends in morbidity and mortality for oesophageal cancer in Linxian County, 1959–1983. *International Journal of Cancer* 36: 643–5.

Lu, S.J., Day, N.E., Degos, L., et al. 1990. Linkage of a nasopharyngeal carcinoma susceptibility locus to the HLA region. *Nature* 346: 470–1.

Lynch, H.T., Voorhees, G.J., Lanspa, S.J., McGreevy, P.S. and Lynch, J.F. 1985. Pancreatic carcinoma and hereditary nonpolyposis colorectal cancer: a family study. *British Journal of Cancer* 52: 271–3.

Lynch, H.T., Watson, P., Kriegler, M., et al. 1988. Differential diagnosis of hereditary nonpolyposis colorectal cancer (Lynch syndrome I and Lynch syndrome II). *Disease of the Colon and Rectum* 31: 372–7.

Lynch, H.T., Fitzsimmons, M.L., Smyrk, T.C., Lanspa, S.J., Watson, P., McClellan, J. and Lynch, J.F. 1990. Familial pancreatic cancer: clinicopathologic study of 18 nuclear families. *American Journal of Gastroenterology* 85: 54–60.

Lynch, H.T., Lanspa, S., Smyrk, T., Boman, B., Watson, P. and Lynch, J. 1991a. Hereditary nonpolyposis colorectal cancer (Lynch syndromes I & II). Genetics, pathology, natural history, and cancer control, Part I. *Cancer Genetics and Cytogenetics*. 53: 143–60.

Lynch, H.T., Richardson, J.D., Amin, M., Lynch, J.F., Cavalieri, R.J., Bronson, E. and Fusaro, R.M. 1991b. Variable gastrointestinal and urologic cancers in a Lynch syndrome II kindred. *Diseases of the Colon and Rectum* 34: 891–5.

Lynch, H.T., Fusaro, L. and Lynch, J.F. 1992. Familial pancreatic cancer: a family study. *Pancreas* 7: 511–15.

Lynch, H.T., Smyrk, T.C., Watson, P. et al. 1993. Genetics, natural history, tumor spectrum, and pathology of hereditary nonpolyposis colorectal cancer: an updated review. *Gastroenterology* 104: 1535–49.

Lynch, H.T., Fusaro, L., Smyrk, T.C., Watson, P., Lanspa, S. and Lynch, J.F. 1995. Medical genetic study of eight pancreatic cancer-prone families. *Cancer Investigation* 13: 141–9.

Macklin, M.T. 1960. Inheritance of cancer of the stomach and large intestine in man. *Journal of the National Cancer Institute* 24: 551–71.

Maimon, S.N. and Zinninger, M.M. 1953. Familial gastric cancer. *Gastroenterology* 25: 139–52.

Maire, P., Morichau-Beauchant, M., Drucker, J., Barboteau, M.A., Barbier, J. and Matuchansky, C. 1984. Familial occurrence of cancer of the colon and the rectum: results of a 3-year case-control survey. *Gastroenterologie clinique et biologique* **8**: 22–7.

Mallory, S.B. 1991. Genodermatoses with malignant potential. In: *Genetic Disorders of the Skin*, ed. J.C. Alper, pp. 244–66. St. Louis: Mosby Year Book.

Marsh, D.J., Dahia, P.L.M., Zheng, Z.M., Liaw, D., Parsons, R., Gorlin, R.J. and Eng, Co. 1997. Germline mutations in *PTEN* are present in Bannayan–Zonana syndrome. *Nature Genetics* **16**(4): 333–4.

Matsukura, N., Onda, M., Tokunaga, A. et al. 1988. Simultaneous gastric cancer in monozygotic twins. *Cancer* **62**: 2430–5.

McConnell, R.B. 1966 *The Genetics of Gastrointestinal Disorders*. London: Oxford University Press

Mecklin, J.P. 1987. Frequency of hereditary colorectal carcinoma. *Gastroenterology* **93**: 1021–5.

Mecklin, J.P., Jarvinen, H.J., Hakkiluoto, A. et al. 1995. Frequency of hereditary nonpolyposis colorectal cancer. A prospective multicenter study in Finland. *Diseases of the Colon and Rectum* **38**: 588–93.

Mecklin, J.P. and Jarvinen, H.J. 1991. Tumor spectrum in cancer family syndrome (hereditary nonpolyposis colorectal cancer). *Cancer* **68**: 1109–12.

Miller, B.A., Reis, L.A.G., Hankey, B.F., Kosary, C.L. and Edwards, B.K. (Eds.).1992. *Cancer Statistics Review 1973–1989*. National Cancer Institute.

Miyanaga, O., Miyamoto, Y., Shirahama, M. and Ishibashi, H. 1989. A clinico-pathological study of hepatocellular carcinoma patients with other primary malignancies. *Gan No Rinsho – Japanese Journal of Cancer Clinics* **35**: 1729–34.

Modica, S., Roncucci, L., Benatti, P., Gafa, L., Tamassia, M.G., Dardanoni, L. and Ponz de Leon, M. 1995. Familial aggregation of tumors and detection of hereditary non-polyposis colorectal cancer in 3-year experience of 2 population-based colorectal-cancer registries. *International Journal of Cancer* **62**: 685–90.

Morita, M., Kuwano, H., Ohno, S. et al. 1994. Multiple occurrence of carcinoma in the upper aerodigestive tract associated with esophageal cancer: reference to smoking, drinking and family history. *International Journal of Cancer* **58**: 207–10.

Muir, V.M.L. 1978. Tylosis in the Orkney islands. *Journal of Biosocial Sciences* **10**: 1–6.

Muto, Y., Moriwaki, H., Ninomiya, M. et al. 1996. Prevention of second primary tumors by an acyclic retinoid, polyprenoic acid, in patients with hepatocellular carcinoma. *New England Journal of Medicine* **334**: 1561–7.

Nagase, H. and Nakamura, Y. 1993. Mutations of the APC (adenomatous polyposis coli) gene. *Human Mutation* **2**: 425–34.

Narita, T. and Takagi, K. 1984. Ataxia-telangiectasia with dysgerminoma of right ovary, papillary carcinoma of thyroid, and adenocarcinoma of pancreas. *Cancer* **54**: 1113–16.

Nelen, M.R., Padberg, G.W., Peeters, E.A.J., et al. 1996. Localization of the gene for Cowden disease to chromosome 10 q22-23. *Nature Genetics* **13**: 114–16.

Nevo, S., Meyer, W. and Altman, M. 1971. Carcinoma of nasopharynx in twins. *Cancer* **28**: 807–9.

Offerhaus, G.J., Giardiello, F.M., Krush, A.J., Booker, S.V., Tersmette, A.C., Kelley, N.C. and Hamilton, S.R. 1992. The risk of upper gastrointestinal cancer in familial adenomatous polyposis. *Gastroenterology* **102**: 1980–2.

Park, J.G., Park, K.J., Ahn, Y.O. et al. 1992. Risk of gastric cancer among Korean familial adenomatous polyposis patients. Report of three cases. *Diseases of the Colon and Rectum* **35**: 996–8.

Parkin, D.M., Laara, E. and Muir, C.S. 1988. Estimates of the worldwide frequency of sixteen major cancers in 1980. *International Journal of Cancer* **41**: 184–97.

Parkin, D.M., Pisani, P. and Ferlay, J. 1993. Estimates of the worldwide incidence of eighteen major cancers in 1985. *International Journal of Cancer* **54**: 594–606.

Phelan, C.M., Lancaster, J.M., Tonin P. et al. 1996. Mutation analysis of the BRCA2 gene in 49 site-specific breast cancer families. *Nature Genetics* **13**: 120–2.

Pickle, L.W., Greene, M.H., Ziegler, R.G., Toledo, A., Hoover, R., Lynch, H.T. and Fraumeni, J.F., Jr. 1984. Colorectal cancer in rural Nebraska. *Cancer Research* **44**: 363–9.

Pippard, E.C., Hall, A.J., Barker, D.J. and Bridges, B.A. 1988. Cancer in homozygotes and heterozygotes of ataxia-telangiectasia and xeroderma pigmentosum in Britain. *Cancer Research* **48**: 2929–32.

Pisani, P., Parkin, D.M. and Ferlay, J. 1993. Estimates of the worldwide mortality from eighteen major cancers in 1985. Implications for prevention and projections of future burden. *International Journal of Cancer* **55**: 891–903.

Pisani, P. and Parkin, D.M. 1996. Screening for gastric cancer. In: *Advances in Cancer Screening*, ed. A.B. Miller, pp. 113–20. Boston: Kluwer.

Ponz de Leon, M., Sassatelli, R., Sacchetti, C., Zanghieri, G., Scalmati, A. and Roncucci, L. 1989. Familial aggregation of tumors in the three-year experience of a population-based colorectal cancer registry. *Cancer Research* **49**: 4344–8.

Pour, P. and Ghadirian, P. 1974. Familial cancer of the esophagus in Iran. *Cancer* **33**: 1649–52.

Ranzi, T., Castagnone, D., Velio, P., Bianchi, P. and Polli, E.E. 1981. Gastric and duodenal polyps in familial polyposis coli. *Gut* **22**: 363–7.

Risk, J.M., Field, E.A., Field, J.K. et al. 1994. Tylosis oesophageal cancer mapped. *Nature Genetics* **8**: 319–21.

Ritter, S.B. and Petersen, G. 1976. Esophageal cancer, hyperkeratosis, and oral leukoplakia. Occurrence in a 25-year-old woman. *JAMA* **235**: 1723

Rozen, P. and Baratz, M. 1982. Familial juvenile colonic polyposis with associated colon cancer. *Cancer* **49**: 1500–3.

Rozen, P., Fireman, Z., Figer, A., Legum, C., Ron, E. and Lynch, H.T. 1987a. Family history of colorectal cancer as a marker of potential malignancy within a screening program. *Cancer* **60**: 248–54.

Rozen, P., Lynch, H.T., Figer, A. et al. 1987b. Familial colon cancer in the Tel-Aviv area and the influence of ethnic origin. *Cancer* **60**: 2355–9.

Russo, P. and O'Regan, S. 1990. Visceral pathology of hereditary tyrosinemia type I. *American Journal of Human Genetics* **47**: 317–24.

Sankila, R., Aaltonen, L.A., Jarvinen, H.J. and Mecklin, J.P. 1996. Better survival rates in patients with MLH1-associated hereditary colon cancer. *Gastroenterology* **110**: 682–7.

Sasajima, K., Yamanaka, Y., Inokuchi, K. et al. 1993. Multiple polyps of esophagus, stomach, colon, and rectum accompanying rectal cancer in a patient with constitutional chromosomal inversion. *Cancer* **71**: 672–6.

Seruca, R., Carneiro, F., Castedo, S., David, L., Lopes, C. and Sobrinho-Simoes, M. 1991. Familial gastric polyposis revisited. Autosomal dominant inheritance confirmed. *Cancer Genetics and Cytogenetics* **53**: 97–100.

Shine, I. and Allison, P.R. 1966. Carcinoma of the oesophagus with tylosis (keratosis palmaris et plantaris). *Lancet* **1**: 951–3.

Sholman, L. and Swift, M. 1972. Pancreatic caner and diabetes mellitus in familias of ataxia-telangietasia probands. *American Journal of Human Genetics* **24**: 48a

Simard, J., Tonin, P., Durocher, F. et al. 1994. Common origins of BRCA1 mutations in Canadian breast and ovarian cancer families. *Nature Genetics* **8**: 392–8.

Sjogren, R.W., Jr. and Johnson, L.F. 1983. Barrett's esophagus: a review. *American Journal of Medicine* **74**: 313–21.

Slattery, M.L. and Kerber, R.A. 1994. Family history of cancer and colon cancer risk: the Utah Population Database. *Journal of the National Cancer Institute* **86**: 1618–26.

Slattery, M.L., Mori, M., Gao, R. and Kerber, R.A. 1995. Impact of family history of colon cancer on development of multiple primaries after diagnosis of colon cancer. *Diseases of the Colon and Rectum* **38**: 1053–8.

Søndergaard, J.O., Bulow, S. and Lynge, E. 1991. Cancer incidence among parents of patients with colorectal cancer. *International Journal of Cancer* **47**: 202–6.

Spigelman, A.D., Murday, V. and Phillips, R.K. 1989a. Cancer and the Peutz-Jeghers syndrome. *Gut* **30**: 1588–90.

Spigelman, A.D., Williams, C.B., Talbot, I.C., Domizio, P. and Phillips, R.K. 1989b. Upper gastrointestinal cancer in patients with familial adenomatous polyposis. *Lancet* **2**: 783–5.

Spirio, L., Olschwang, S., Groden, J. et al. 1993. Alleles of the APC gene: an attenuated form of familial polyposis. *Cell* **75**: 951–7.

Spirio, L.N., Kutchera, W., Winstead, M.V. et al. 1996. Three secretory phospholipase A(2) genes that map to human chromosome 1p35-36 are not mutated in individuals with attenuated adenomatous polyposis coli. *Cancer Research* **56**: 955–8.

St.John, D.J., McDermott, F.T., Hopper, J.L., Debney, E.A., Johnson, W.R. and Hughes, E.S. 1993. Cancer risk in relatives of patients with common colorectal cancer. *Annals of Internal Medicine* **118**: 785–90.

Starink, T.M., van der Veen, J.P., Arwert, F., de Waal, L.P., de Lange, G.G., Gille, J.J. and Eriksson, A.W. 1986. The Cowden syndrome: a clinical and genetic study in 21 patients. *Clinical Genetics* **29**: 222–33.

Stephenson, B.M., Finan, P.J., Gascoyne, J., Garbett, F., Murday, V.A. and Bishop, D.T. 1991. Frequency of familial colorectal cancer. *British Journal of Surgery* **78**: 1162–6.

Stevens, H.P., Kelsell, D.P., Bryant, S.P. et al. 1996a. Palmoplantar keratoderma and malignancy (palmoplantar keratoderma ectodermal dysplasia type III) in an extensive North American pedigree is linked to the TOCG locus (17p24) and show a characteristic clinial phenotype. *Archives of Dermatology* **132**: 640–51

Stevens, H.P., Kelsell, D.P., Leigh, I.M., Ostlere, L.S., Macdermot, K.D. and Rustin, M.H.A. 1996b. Punctate pamoplantar keratodera and malignancy in a four-generation family. *British Journal of Dermatology* **134**: 720–6.

Strohmeyer, G., Niederau, C. and Stremmel, W. 1988. Survival and causes of death in hemochromatosis. Observations in 163 patients. *Annals of the New York Academy of Sciences* **526**: 245–57.

Strong, L.C., Stine, M. and Norsted, T.L. 1987. Cancer in survivors of childhood soft tissue sarcoma and their relatives. *Journal of the National Cancer Institute* **79**: 1213–20.

Swift, M., Reitnauer, P.J., Morrell, D. and Chase, C.L. 1987. Breast and other cancers in families with ataxia-telangiectasia. *New England Journal of Medicine* **316**: 1289–94.

Swift, M., Chase, C.L. and Morrell, D. 1990. Cancer predisposition of ataxia-telangiectasia heterozygotes. *Cancer Genetics and Cytogenetics* **46**: 21–7.

Thomas, H.J., Whitelaw, S.C., Cottrell, S.E. et al. 1996. Genetic mapping of the Hereditary Mixed Polyposis Syndrome to Chromosome 6q. *American Journal of Human Genetics* **58**: 770–6.

Thorlacius, S., Olafsdottir, G.H., Tryggvadottir, L. et al. 1996. A single BRCA2 mutation in male and female breast cancer families from Iceland with varied phenotypes. *Nature Genetics* **13**: 117–19.

Tonin, P., Ghadirian, P., Phelan, C. et al. 1995. A large multisite cancer family is linked to BRCA2. *Journal of Medical Genetics* **32**: 982–4.

Tonin, P., Weber, B., Offit, K. et al. 1996. Frequency of recurrent BRCA1 and BRCA2 mutations in Ashkenazi Jewish breast cancer families. *Nature Medicine* **2**: 1179–83.

Triantafillidis, J.K., Kosmidis, P. and Kottaridis, S. 1993. Familial stomach cancer. *American Journal of Gastroenterology* **93**: 1789–90.

Tsuchikame, N., Ishimaru, Y., Ohshima, S. and Takahashi, M. 1993. Three familial cases of fundic gland polyposis without polyposis coli. *Virchows Archives* **93**: 337-A.

Tulinius, H., Olafsdottir, G.H., Sigvaldason, H., Tryggvadottir, L. and Bjarnadottir, K. 1994. Neoplastic diseases in families of breast cancer patients. *Journal of Medical Genetics* **31**: 618–21.

Vasen, H.F., den Hartog Jager, F.C., Menko, F.H. and Nagengast, F.M. 1989. Screening for hereditary non-polyposis colorectal cancer: a study of 22 kindreds in The Netherlands. *American Journal of Medicine* **86**: 278–81.

Vasen, H.F., Mecklin, J.P., Khan, P.M. and Lynch, H.T. 1991. The International Collaborative Group on Hereditary Non-Polyposis Colorectal Cancer (ICG-HNPCC). *Diseases of the Colon and Rectum* **34**: 424–5.

Vasen, H.F., Wijnen, J.T., Menko, F.H. et al. 1996. Cancer risk in families with hereditary nonpolyposis colorectal cancer diagnosed by mutation analysis. *Gastroenterology* **110**: 1020–7.

Vogelstein, B., Fearon, E.R., Kern, S.E., Hamilton, S.R., Preisinger, A.C., Nakamura, Y. and White, R. 1989. Allelotype of colorectal carcinomas. *Science* **244**: 207–11.

Wang, Y.F., Chen, C.J., Harris, E.L., King, T.M., Hsu, M.M., Diehl, S.R. and Beaty, T.H. 1995. Complex segregation analysis of nasopharyngial carcinoma (NPC) in Taiwan. *American Journal of Medical Genetics* **57**: 174

Watanabe, H., Enjoji, M., Yao, T. and Ohsato, K. 1978. Gastric lesions in familial adenomatosis coli: their incidence and histologic analysis. *Human Pathology* **9**: 269–83.

Watson, P. and Lynch, H.T. 1993. Extracolonic cancer in hereditary nonpolyposis colorectal cancer. *Cancer* **71**: 677–85.

Weinberg, A.G., Mize, C.E. and Worthen, H.G. 1976. The occurrence of hepatoma in the chronic form of hereditary tyrosinemia. *Journal of Pediatrics* **88**: 434–8.

Weinberger, J.M., Cohen, Z. and Berk, T. 1981. Polyposis coli preceded by hepatocellular carcinoma: report of a case. *Diseases of the Colon and Rectum* **24**: 296–300.

Westlake, P.J., Bryant, H.E., Huchcroft, S.A. and Sutherland, L.R. 1991. Frequency of hereditary nonpolyposis colorectal cancer in southern Alberta. *Digestive Diseases and Sciences* **36**: 1441–7.

Whelan, A.J., Bartsch, D. and Goodfellow, P.J. 1995. Brief report: a familial syndrome of pancreatic cancer and melanoma with a mutation in the CDKN2 tumor-suppressor gene. *New England Journal of Medicine* **333**: 975–7.

Whitcomb, D.C., Gorry, M.C., Preston, R.A. et al. 1996. Hereditary pancreatitis is caused by a mutation in the cationic trypsinogen gene. *Nature Genetics* **14**(2): 141–5.

Williams, E.H. and de-The, G. 1974. Letter: Familial aggregation in nasopharyngeal carcinoma. *Lancet* **2**: 295–6.

Woolf, C.M. 1958. A genetic study of carcinoma of the large intestine. *American Journal of Human Genetics* **10**: 42–7.

Woolf, C.M. and Isaacson, E.A. 1961. An analysis of 5 'stomach cancer families' in the state of Utah. *Cancer* **14**: 1005–16.

Yao, T., Ida, M., Ohsato, K., Watanabe, H. and Omae, T. 1977. Duodenal lesions in familial polyposis of the colon. *Gastroenterology* **73**: 1086–92.

Yesudian, P., Premalatha, S. and Thambiah, A.S. 1980. Genetic tylosis with malignancy: a study of a South Indian pedigree. *British Journal of Dermatology* **102**: 597–600.

Yoshida, T., Haraguchi, Y., Tanaka, A. et al. 1988. A case of generalized juvenile gastrointestinal polyposis associated with gastric carcinoma. *Endoscopy* **20**: 33–5.

Zangeneh, F., Limbeck, G.A., Brown, B.I., Emch, J.R., Arcasoy, M.M., Goldenberg, V.E. and Kelley, V.C. 1969. Hepatorenal glycogenosis (type I glycogenosis) and carcinoma of the liver. *Journal of Pediatrics* **74**: 73–83.

Zanghieri, G., Di Gregorio, C., Sacchetti, C. et al. 1990. Familial occurrence of gastric cancer in the 2-year experience of a population-based registry. *Cancer* **66**: 2047–51.

Zeze, F., Ohsato, K., Mitani, H., Ohkuma, R. and Koide, O. 1983. Hepatocellular carcinoma associated with familial polyposis of the colon. Report of case. *Diseases of the Colon and Rectum* **26**: 465–8.

10

Cancers of the breast, ovary, and uterus

WILLIAM FOULKES and STEVEN NAROD

Summary

The genetic contribution to cancers that are either exclusively or mainly seen in females is considered in this review. Hereditary breast and ovarian cancers are largely attributable to mutations in *BRCA1* and *BRCA2*, whereas hereditary endometrial cancer usually occurs in the setting of a family history of colorectal cancer associated with mutations in mismatch repair genes. The similarities and differences between cancers seen in families are considered and the genes involved outlined. Finally, the practical use of this information is described.

Introduction

Breast, ovarian, and uterine cancers combined form a substantial proportion of cancers that affect women. Breast cancer is the commonest cancer in the Western world and ovarian cancer is associated with a very high mortality rate. Both endometrial and cervical cancers are less common than breast cancer but are associated with considerable morbidity. Some of the genes implicated in hereditary breast and ovarian cancers have been identified and studied in detail. Endometrial and cervical cancer are less commonly hereditary but in the case of endometrial cancer there is a clear connection with colorectal cancer and mutations in mismatch repair genes. The highly polymorphic HLA region may have an important role in determining susceptibility to cervical cancer.

Epidemiology

Descriptive epidemiology

Breast cancer is the commonest cancer in women in the developed world. In 1985, the estimated age-adjusted incidence rate of breast cancer worldwide was 32.7 per 100,000. However, this figure masks a wide variation:

in North America the rate was 84.8 per 100,000, whereas in West Africa, the corresponding rate was 11.1 Worldwide, ovarian cancer is considerably less common, (age-adjusted rate of 7.3 per 100,000). In North America the rate was 11.8 whereas in West Africa it was 6.0, thus demonstrating a much narrower international range of incidence rates for ovarian cancer compared with breast cancer. For cancer of the corpus uteri, the pattern is a somewhat similar to that seen with breast cancer, but with a much lower overall incidence rate (6.5 per 100,000 worldwide, 18.0 and 1.9 per 100,000 in North America and West Africa, respectively). For cancer of the uterine cervix, the relationship between incidence rate and geographical location is reversed. The overall age-adjusted incidence rate in 1985 was 20.0 per 100,000, but the incidence was higher (22.0) in West Africa than in North America (9.9 per 100,000). The highest rate for uterine cervix cancer was seen in Southern Africa (46.8 per 100,000) (Parkin et al., 1993). Thus rates for female cancers vary greatly in different parts of the world, with the least variation seen for ovarian cancer. This might indicate that constitutional factors are more important in cancer of the ovary than cancers of the breast and uterine corpus. This conclusion from a review of the epidemiological data is generally confirmed by genetic epidemiology studies described below.

Genetic epidemiology

Breast cancer

Early observational studies (for example, Smithers, 1948) suggested that breast cancer was more common in the relatives of women with breast cancer. Many case-control studies have confirmed and extended these early findings. However, some of the effects were rather modest, and this suggested to some observers that genetic effects were limited. Case-control studies have generally demonstrated that the relative risk of breast cancer in the first-degree relatives of breast cancer cases is greater where the proband is diagnosed at a young age (less than 45 years, about a three to fourfold increase in risk) than when the proband is diagnosed at an older age (greater than 55 years, about a 1.5 to twofold increase in risk – for a brief summary of some of these studies, see Bishop, 1992).

Cohort studies have demonstrated more modest risks in association with a family history of breast cancer. Using data from the Nurses' Health Study, Colditz et al. (1993b) monitored nearly 118,000 women to a total of 1.3 million person-years of follow-up. The overall relative risk of breast cancer associated with a maternal history of breast cancer was 1.8 (95% confidence interval –(CI): 1.5–2.0). As in the case-control studies, the risk was highest when the mother was diagnosed at a young age (less than 40 years, relative risk 2.1, 95% CI: 1.6–2.8). For the relatives of women diagnosed at 70 years or older, the risk was still elevated at 1.5 (95% CI: 1.1–2.2). This linear trend was highly significant ($p = 0.007$). In four women, both they and their mothers were diagnosed at less than 40 years of age, resulting in a relative risk of 4.1 (95% CI: 1.8–9.1). In a sub-analysis, there was little effect of years of menstruation or other potentially relevant variables on familial risk (Colditz et al., 1996). Another large cohort study (11,678 relatives of index cases) also revealed more modest risks of breast cancer associated with a family history of breast cancer. Using national statistics, Peto et al. (1996) studied the causes of cancer death in the first-degree relatives of women who were diagnosed with breast cancer at 60 years of age or less. The standardized mortality ratio (SMR) was significantly elevated at 187 (248 deaths observed and 132.7 expected, $O/E = 1.87$). Where a mother and a daughter were both affected, the risk to other sisters was significantly elevated – 13 of such women died of breast cancer, whereas only 3.28 deaths were expected ($O/E = 3.96$). This figure is substantially less than the risk associated with two first-degree relatives with ovarian cancer (see below). Other cancer deaths in excess in the first-degree relatives of breast cancer cases included endometrial cancer (SMR, 166) and laryngeal cancer (SMR, 177). The SMR for thyroid cancer was also elevated if the index case was diagnosed at under 40 years of age (SMR, 350, $p = 0.03$, but this is based on only five cases).

For a woman aged 30 with both a mother and a sister affected, the cumulative risk of breast cancer to age 70 was 17.4%. This figure is strikingly lower than the ~43% risk that would be expected if all these cases were accounted for by mutations in the breast cancer susceptibility gene, *BRCA1*, where an 87% cumulative risk to age 70 is seen (95% CI: 72% to 95%) (Ford et al., 1994). This suggests that most mother–daughter pairs are not attributable to highly penetrant genes. This is supported by the findings of the Breast Cancer Linkage Consortium and Easton et al. (1993; 1996), where only a minority of families with two or three cases of breast cancer diagnosed at age 60 or less were linked to *BRCA1*. Assuming that all the genetic effect seen in breast cancer families was due to *BRCA1*, then of 10 families with three or more cases of breast cancer, 2.4 would be predicted to be due to *BRCA1*. It is unlikely that the gene frequency or breast cancer penetrance of *BRCA2* is greater than that of *BRCA1*, and other highly-penetrant breast cancer susceptibility genes cannot be more frequent than *BRCA1*. Therefore ~40% of the excess familial breast cancer risk cannot be explained by rare, highly penetrant genes (Easton et al., 1996). However, if the affected women in a family are predominantly diagnosed when they were premenopausal, the likelihood of a *BRCA1* or *BRCA2* mutation is substantially increased.

Early evidence for a hereditary basis for breast cancer came from the observation of large families with multiple cases of breast cancer. The number of cancers in these families was too great to be explained by chance, and no known environmental factors could explain the clustering. Familial cancers tended to be of early onset and often were bilateral. This anecdotal evidence of the existence of one or more cancer susceptibility genes was later supported by segregation analysis. Using the population-based CASH (Cancer and Steroid Hormone study) registry, which contained data on families of 4370 cases of breast cancer, Claus et al. (1990) hypothesized the existence of a rare (gene frequency = 0.0033) dominant breast cancer gene with a lifetime penetrance of 92%. Other segregation analyses gave similar results (Bishop et al., 1988; Newman et al., 1988; Iselius et al., 1991). As predicted by these analyses, the risk for a woman with a mother and sister with premenopausal cancer has been reported to reach 50%, the same as for an autosomal dominant gene (Schwartz et al., 1985). The existence of such genes was proved by linkage studies (see Chapter 7). These studies led to the identification of the *BRCA1* and *BRCA2* cancer susceptibility genes in 1994 and 1995, respectively.

Ovarian cancer

The risk of ovarian cancer to age 70 is around 1% in developed countries, with higher rates seen in North America than southern Europe (Parkin et al., 1993). Population-based epidemiological studies have shown that there is an increased risk of ovarian cancer if one first-degree relative is affected by ovarian cancer – relative risk range 3–4.5 (Schildkraut and Thompson, 1988; Kerber and Slattery, 1995; Table 10.1). One hospital-based case-control study estimated a relative risk of 18.2, but the 95% confidence intervals were wide (4.8–69.0) (Hildreth et al., 1981). There is also a smaller, but still increased risk if relatives with lesser degrees of relatedness are affected (Schildkraut and Thompson, 1988; Kerber and Slattery, 1995). In a UK national study based on death certification, Easton et al. (1996) showed that the SMR for ovarian cancer associated

Table 10.1. *Risks of ovarian cancer in North America by degree of relatedness from index cases*

Affected relative	Percentage risks of ovarian cancer to age 70	Comments and references
None	1.4	From SEER statistics
One first degree	3.5–5	Most studies have given values in this range
Two first degree	33	(Easton et al., 1996)
One first degree and ≥one second degree	7	Based on three cases of cancer in Schildkraut and Thompson (1988)
One second degree	3	(Kerber and Slattery, 1995; Schildkraut and Thompson, 1988)
One third degree	2	(Kerber and Slattery, 1995; Schildkraut and Thompson, 1988)

with a diagnosis of this cancer in a first degree relative at 60 years or less was significantly elevated at 223 ($p < 0.001$, or put another way, 35 cases observed 15.72 expected, relative risk 2.23). If two first degree relatives had died from this cause, the SMR was 2415 (four cases observed, 0.17 expected, relative risk 23.5). These figures are consistent with the rarity of ovarian cancer in the population and the odds ratios estimated in case-control studies, although the point estimates of the risks from these types of studies tend to be higher than when studying cohorts. For example, from the Utah population database, a case-control study of ovarian cancer gave a relative risk of 4.31 (95% CI: 2.35–7.90) for ovarian cancer in association with a family history of a first-degree relative with this cancer (Kerber and Slattery, 1995).

There have been numerous reports of familial aggregation of ovarian cancer, beginning in 1877 (Liber, 1950). In most cases, there are also cases of breast cancer. Statistical analysis performed on a number of breast–ovary cancer families identified by Dr. Henry Lynch and his colleagues led them to conclude that the clustering of breast and ovarian cancers seen in many of these families could also be explained by the effect of a single dominant gene (Go et al., 1983). This close relationship between hereditary breast and ovarian cancer was confirmed by Narod et al.

(1991) who demonstrated linkage in breast and ovarian cancer families to the same chromosome 17 locus that had been linked to early-onset breast cancer. In fact, the presence of ovarian cancer is strongly predictive of BRCA1; families with site-specific ovarian cancer (ovarian cancer without breast cancer) are almost all due to this gene (Steichen-Gersdorf et al., 1994). Additionally, women with breast cancer are at increased risk of developing a second primary cancer of the ovary (Prior and Waterhouse, 1981); and relatives of women with breast or ovarian cancer are at roughly double the risk for either tumour (Schildkraut et al., 1989). This is interesting because the hormonal and reproductive risk factors for breast cancer tend to be inversely correlated with risk of ovarian cancer, suggesting that the genetic relationship between breast and ovarian cancers may not be dependent on hormonal and reproductive variables. From the study of Easton et al. (1996) it seems that a family history of colorectal cancer is also a risk factor for ovarian cancer. Among individuals with one relative with ovarian cancer and one with either colon or rectal cancer, there were 14 deaths from any of these three cancers, whereas only 0.23 were expected (a relative risk of 61). This strongly supports the data from family studies that show an excess of ovarian cancer in hereditary nonpolyposis colorectal cancer (HNPCC) families (Aarnio et al., 1995).

Cancer of the fallopian tube

This cancer is exceptionally rare but has been seen in several families at McGill University, Montreal, Canada with BRCA1 or BRCA2 mutations (Figures 10.1a and 10.1b). Although there have been no specific epidemiological studies of this cancer reported, it is likely that a significant proportion of cases arise in a hereditary setting.

Cancer of the uterine corpus

Epidemiological studies have demonstrated a very modest increase in relative risk for this cancer in association with a family history of endometrial cancer (Parazzini et al., 1994). Peto et al., (1996) showed a SMR of 166 for endometrial cancer in the first-degree relatives of women diagnosed with breast cancer at under 60 years of age, and a large cohort study from Sweden showed an increased risk for endometrial cancer after age 70 following a diagnosis of breast cancer (relative risk 2.4, 95% CI: 1.6–3.5) (Adami et al., 1984). This age-dependent finding was supported by a nationwide study from Finland, where the relative risk of endometrial cancer following a diagnosis of breast cancer at age 70 or more was

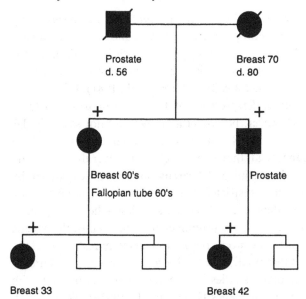

Figure 10.1(a). A breast and ovarian cancer pedigree with fallopian tube carcinoma. A *BRCA1* mutation (5382insC) has been identified in this family (Simard et al., 1994). Key: + indicated mutation carriers, the number after the site of cancer is the age at diagnosis.

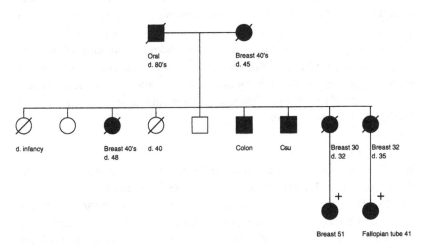

Figure 10.1(b). A breast and ovarian cancer pedigree with fallopian tube carcinoma. A *BRCA2* mutation (8764delAG) has been identified in this family (Tonin, unpublished data). Key: + indicated mutation carriers, the number after the site of cancer is the age of diagnosis; d, refers to age at death; Csu is cancer site unknown.

significantly elevated at 1.33 (Teppo et al., 1985). These results may reflect similar hormonal factors influencing breast and endometrial cancer in older women. A case-control study showed a relative risk of 3.5 for endometrial cancer in a mother or a sister if another first-degree relative had ovarian cancer (95% CI: 1.4–8.3) (Hildreth et al., 1981). It is possible that this risk could reflect the presence of HNPCC mutations in these affected individuals. However, Nelson et al. (1993) did not see a similar effect; virtually all the familial risk of endometrial cancer could be accounted for by cancers at that site in relatives. Overall, it appears that about 1% of endometrial adenocarcinoma can be explained by genetic factors. One study restricted the probands in a country-wide registry study to those diagnosed at 60 years or less – here the genetic contribution was higher, about 3% (Suomi et al., 1995). Thus, the genetic contribution to endometrial cancer appears to be largely restricted to the mismatch repair genes that predispose to HNPCC, as most of the families identified in this and other studies fit the phenotype associated with mutations in mismatch repair genes (Lynch et al., 1993a). Teppo et al. (1985) revealed the marked effect of age of diagnosis of colon cancer on subsequent endometrial cancer risk. For women diagnosed with colon cancer before age 35, there was a relative risk of 46 for a subsequent endometrial cancer. For women aged 35–49, the risk was 12, (both of these risks are significant $p < 0.001$) but for older age groups there was no significant effect. Supporting this observation is the report of an increased incidence of colorectal cancer in the first-degree relatives of women with double primary cancers of the endometrium and colorectum (Foulkes et al., 1996). The risk was largest in the first-degree relatives of women diagnosed with both endometrial and colorectal cancers at less than 55 years of age. Most of these families would fit accepted criteria for HNPCC (Vasen et al., 1991).

Cancer of the uterine cervix

By far the strongest causal factor in squamous cell carcinoma of the uterine cervix is human papilloma virus (HPV), usually subtypes 16 and 18. This virus has now been classified as a carcinogen and it is doubtful whether other important environmental causes of squamous cell carcinoma of the uterine cervix exist. There are virtually no large families reported with numerous cases of this cancer. One report has demonstrated an increased incidence of second primary cancers outside the radiation field after squamous cell carcinoma of the cervix (11 observed, 4.77 expected, relative risk 2.31, 95% CI: 1.25–4.13). Four of these 11 cancers were breast cancers (Werner-Wasik et al., 1995). From another perspective, inherited factors may be important in that the genotype may influence the likelihood of HPV infection and/or epithelial invasion. Two studies have implied that specific HLA haplotypes may be more common in those with HPV infection than in control populations, and they are described in the next section.

Genes involved in breast and ovarian cancer susceptibility

BRCA1 and *BRCA2*

Because both *BRCA1* and *BRCA2* predispose to both breast and ovarian cancer, it is more meaningful to speak of families with hereditary breast and ovarian cancers, rather than of families with hereditary breast cancer. By contrast, neither cancer of the uterine corpus nor cervix are in excess in *BRCA1* carriers (Ford et al., 1994). A conservative definition of a family with hereditary breast and ovarian cancers is one with four or more cases of breast cancer below the age of 60, or of ovarian cancer at any age. Almost all families of this type will be due to mutations in *BRCA1* or *BRCA2*.

Linkage to breast cancer was first identified in 1990 by Mary-Claire King and her colleagues (Hall et al., 1990). They found that a locus on chromosome 17 accounted for cancer susceptibility in 45% of a panel of 23 breast cancer families. The locus appeared to account for all families with a median age of breast cancer onset of 45 years or younger. This study established that familial breast cancer was genetically heterogeneous. The putative cancer susceptibility gene was named *BRCA1*.

Stratton and colleagues (1994) performed linkage analysis on a panel of 13 families with male breast cancer and found that none appeared to be linked to *BRCA1*. This unusual finding was a clue that these families might consistently be due to a second breast cancer gene. Using a panel of families with male breast cancer, as well as families that were convincingly unlinked to *BRCA1*, they found strong evidence of linkage to a second locus on chromosome 13, and called it *BRCA2* (Wooster et al., 1994). Through the examination of critical recombinants, physical mapping and the exclusion of known candidate genes, *BRCA1* and *BRCA2* were identified in 1994 and 1995, respectively (Miki et al., 1994; Wooster et al., 1995). In a study of 145 breast–ovarian cancer families, approximately 80% were due to *BRCA1* and the remainder appeared linked to *BRCA2* (Narod et al., 1995a,b). There was no convincing example in this data set of a family unlinked to both loci. Most families with breast cancer alone appear to be due to *BRCA2*, and the greater the number of breast cancers, the greater is the probability of linkage to *BRCA2*. This is because the penetrance of ovarian cancer in *BRCA1* carriers is roughly 50% and it is therefore unlikely that families with many (e.g. six or more) breast cancers will not include a case of ovarian cancer as well. In Canada, there has been only a single site-specific breast cancer family with a *BRCA1* mutation identified to date (Simard et al., 1994; Durocher et al., 1996), all others contain cases of ovarian cancer as well. Among families with male breast cancer, 80% are linked to *BRCA2* and 20% are linked to *BRCA1* (examples of *BRCA1* families with male breast cancer are described in Hogervorst et al., 1995; Struewing et al., 1995; Serova et al., 1996).

Roughly one in 70 women will be diagnosed with ovarian cancer in Canada by the age of 70, and approximately 4% of these (1 in 1750 women overall) are members of families with hereditary breast and ovarian cancers (Narod et al., 1994a). Assuming that 50% of women with *BRCA1* mutations will develop ovarian cancer by the age of 70, this implies a frequency of *BRCA1* mutations of 1 in 875 in the Canadian population. Easton et al. (1995) estimate the carrier frequency of *BRCA1* mutant alleles in the UK to be 1 in 833, based on 44 breast cancer deaths occurring among the relatives of 1203 cases of ovarian cancer (31.8 expected). From these two estimates, it is probable that between one in 500 and one in 1000 women are carriers of *BRCA1* mutations.

The relative risk for breast cancer among *BRCA1* carriers varies from 100 at age 30 to 1.6 at age 75 (Easton et al. 1993). Easton et al. (1995) estimate the proportion of breast cancers due to *BRCA1* in the population to be 5.3% below age 40 and less than 1% over age 70.

In a study of the Breast Cancer Linkage Consortium, 76 cancers other than breast or ovary were observed among 33 *BRCA1*-linked families (62 expected) (Ford et al., 1993). Prostate cancer accounted for a portion of the excess (relative risk 2.0), but it is unlikely that more than 10% of familial prostate cancer can be explained by *BRCA1* mutations (Eeles, unpub. data). The other site found to be significantly over-represented in the *BRCA1*-linked families was cancer of the colon (relative risk 2.8). However, in a study of 220 Ashkenazi Jewish families with breast and ovarian cancers, only pancreatic cancer was significantly over-represented in those families with *BRCA1* or *BRCA2* mutations compared with all families (relative risk 3.73, $p < 0.05$) (Tonin et al., 1996b). An unusual family with a striking susceptibility to both early-onset breast and early-onset colon cancer has been described (Miller et al., 1992), and the risks of breast cancer in the female relatives of women with double primary cancers of both the breast and colorectum are greater than the familial risks associated with a proband with breast cancer alone (Foulkes et al., 1996). There are few data available on the range of cancers in *BRCA2* families. However, it appears from early reports that *BRCA2* is a multi-site cancer gene (Berman et al., 1996a; Tonin et al., 1996a).

TP53 *mutations and Li–Fraumeni syndrome*

The Li–Fraumeni syndrome is the association of early-onset breast cancer and childhood cancers, including soft tissue sarcomas, osteosarcomas, adrenocortical cancers, and leukaemia (Li and Fraumeni, 1969). The paediatric aspects of this syndrome are discussed in Chapter 19. Of relevance here is that the diagnosis should be considered when a woman with early-onset breast cancer is found to have a relative with childhood cancer. In a follow-up study of 24 families, breast cancer accounted for 15 of 52 new cases of cancer (Garber et al., 1991). The relative risk for breast cancer among relatives under age 45 was 17.9, much greater than the relative risk of 1.8 observed for women over age 45. In 1990, mutations of the *TP53* gene were reported in families with the Li–Fraumeni syndrome (Malkin et al., 1990). Constitutional *TP53* mutations are infrequent in women with breast cancer; only three *TP53* mutations were found in a total of 463 women with breast cancer (Børresen et al., 1992; Sidransky et al., 1992). *TP53* mutations are also very uncommon in hereditary breast and ovarian cancers. In one reported family with a splice-site mutation in *TP53* (Jolly et al., 1994), the only person affected by ovarian cancer developed this cancer at age 21, and later was diagnosed with colon cancer at age 31. The proband had a choroid plexus carcinoma, seen in Li–Fraumeni families, but not in hereditary breast–ovarian cancer families. Ovarian cancer is very rarely diagnosed in the third decade in gene carriers in hereditary breast and ovarian cancer families (W.F and S.N, unpub. obs).

Cowden disease

This is another rare syndrome associated with an increased risk of breast cancer. The cardinal clinical features of this autosomal dominant disor-

212 — W. Foulkes and S. Narod

Table 10.2. *Commonly reported clinical findings in Cowden disease**

Clinical features	Frequency (%)
Mucocutaneous lesions (trichilemmomas, papillomas)	75–90
Thyroid disease (benign and malignant neoplasms)	7–70
Breast disease (benign and maligant neoplasms)	18–75
Reproductive organ neoplasms (uterine and ovarian)	40
Gastrointestinal polyps (< 10% associated with cancer)	40
Macrocephaly	35
Mental retardation	10

Note: *Adapted from Starink, 1984; Mallory, 1991; Hansen and Fryns, 1995.

der are shown in Table 10.2. The gene for Cowden disease has been localized to chromsome 10q by linkage (Nelen et al., 1996), and mutations in the previously-identified gene, PTEN (Li et al., 1997) have been discovered in families with Cowden disease (Liaw et al., 1997). The gene is thought to be a protein tyrosine phosphatase, and is mutated somatically in several different cancers, notably breast, prostate and brain cancers (Li et al., 1997). Some commentators have speculated that it is much more common than is generally believed, as bilateral fibrocystic breast disease and wart-like skin lesions are not uncommon in the general population. However, we believe this to be unlikely. The gastrointestinal features of Cowden disease have been discussed in Chapter 9.

Ataxia-telangiectasia and breast cancer

Another gene that has attracted interest as a candidate breast cancer gene is the gene for ataxia-telangiectasia (A-T). The homozygote frequency of this recessive disease is 1 in 100,000 (Pippard et al., 1988). This prevalence is equivalent to a gene frequency of 0.006 (i.e. 1.2% of the population are heterozygote carriers). The gene (*ATM*) and the clinical features of those with mutations in this gene are discussed in Chapter 18. There may be a risk of breast cancer associated with heterozygous carriage of *ATM* alleles associated with the syndrome. Swift et al. (1991) found 23 cases of breast cancer in relatives of cases of ataxia-telangiectasia. This rate was 5.1 times higher than expected, based on the observation of three cases of breast cancer in a spouse control group. However, from North American tumour registry data there were 4.0 cases expected in this control group, so the true relative risk is likely to be smaller (e.g. 3.8). Indeed, recent studies of A-T families suggest that the risk of breast cancer for *ATM* heterozygotes is elevated 3.8-fold compared to non-carriers (Athma et al., 1976). Easton (1993) estimated the proportion of breast cancer due to A-T heterozygotes to be 7%. Swift et al. (1991) also reported a greater use of diagnostic and therapeutic X-rays in the cases of breast cancer than among healthy controls. Markers from the A-T region were typed on 16 breast cancer families, including 10 which appeared to be unlinked to *BRCA1*, but there was no evidence that *ATM* accounted for the cancer susceptibility in these families (Wooster et al., 1993). Because of the large size of this gene, and because most mutations are unique, it will be difficult to determine the frequency of *ATM* mutations among women with breast cancer. Nevertheless, the *ATM* gene was completely screened in 38 women with breast cancers and no germline variants were found that were not also present in the general population (Vorechovsky et al., 1996). Following this, FitzGerald et al. (1997) searched for germline mutations in 401 women with breast cancer diagnosed at 40 years or younger. They found only two heterozygotes, and this was a lower frequency than observed in the control group. Although the sample size precluded identifying a small relative risk, it does now seem unlikely that mutations in *ATM* are responsible for a significant proportion of early-onset breast cancer. It is likely that studying sporadic breast cancers from populations where founder mutations have been located (Telatar et al., 1996) will be the most efficient way to determine the role of *ATM* in breast cancer.

Modifying genes and breast cancer risk

It is possible that polymorphic variants of genes exist which are associated with a small or moderate increased risk of breast cancer. A gene associated with risk ratio of two to five would rarely lead to a large family cluster of cancer, but could be responsible for a significant proportion of breast cancer in the population. One candidate gene is *RASH*, (formerly known as *HRAS*). The presence of one of the 'rare alleles' of a minisatellite polymorphism located near to the *RASH* proto-oncogene was found in a meta-analysis to be associated with a 1.93-fold increased risk of breast cancer (Krontiris et al., 1993). However, among carriers of *BRCA1* mutations, rare alleles of the *RASH* locus do not appear to increase the risk of breast cancer (Phelan et al., 1996).

Genes involved in uterine cancer susceptibility

Uterine corpus

As stated above, it appears that most, if not all of the genetic risk of endometrial cancer at a young age is borne by the mismatch repair genes which are mutated in HNPCC (see Chapter 9). The cumulative risk of endometrial cancer to age 80 in HNPCC gene carriers is about 43%, at least 10 times the expected figure (Aarnio et al., 1995). The peak incidence of the disease occurs at least 15 years earlier in gene carriers than in the general population (Watson et al., 1994). Whether there are genes that predispose to breast and/or endometrial cancer at an older age is not known, but it possible that polymorphisms in genes such as those encoding the oestrogen or progesterone receptor might influence risk of these two cancers.

Uterine cervix

The critical involvement of HPV16 and 18 in squamous cell carcinoma of the uterine cervix is now established. Recent studies have suggested that there may be an association between particular HLA haplotypes and cancer risk (Wank and Thomssen, 1991; Apple et al., 1994, 1995) but this remains controversial as other groups have found no such correlation (Glew et al., 1993; Vandenvelde et al., 1993). Wank and Thomssen (1991) noted an association between serologically-defined DQw3 and increased risk of cervical cancer. Subsequently, using PCR-based technology, Apple et al. (1994) showed that certain HLA class II haplotypes were associated with cervical carcinoma, whereas DR13 haplotypes were protective. In a study of Hispanic women from New Mexico, the same group found that DRB1*1501-DQB1*0602 was seen in 13 out of 53 HPV16+ invasive cancer cases and in 14 out of 220 ethnically-matched Pap smear-negative controls, giving an odds ratio of 4.78, $p = 0.00007$). A similar odds ratio was seen for severe dysplasia, but this and other haplotypes were not over-represented in slight-to-moderate dysplasia cases. It should be noted that this haplotype is common in many ethnic groups. DR13 was again protective; odds ratio 0.26, $p = 0.009$ for HPV16+ invasive cancers (Apple et al., 1995). DR13 was not protective in HPV16− cancers.

   Adenoma malignum is a rare form of cervical cancer which probably does not share a viral aetiology with squamous cell carcinoma. It has been reported in individuals with Peutz–Jeghers syndrome (see Chapter 9,

Table 9.4) (Spigelman et al., 1995). The gene responsible for Peutz–Jeghers syndrome has been localised to chromosome 19p by comparative genomic hybridization of a polyp and subsequent linkage (Hemminki et al., 1997).

Risk modifiers for breast and ovarian cancer

Genetic modifiers

Not all women with *BRCA1* mutations develop cancer; some develop breast but not ovarian cancer, and vice versa, and the ages of onset are highly variable. It is not yet clear if the variation is due largely to chance, or if there are factors which are predictive of cancer. When *BRCA1* was identified, it became possible to study whether different mutations were associated with different risks. The great majority of *BRCA1* mutations lead to a truncated (and presumably non-functional) protein, and there is no obvious reason why the effects of inactivating mutations should differ. Gayther et al. (1995) studied 32 families with *BRCA1* mutations and found that mutations in the 3' end of the gene were associated with significantly fewer cases of ovarian cancer than mutations in the 5' end. There are many families that are exceptions to this. In a study of Ashkenazi Jewish families with *BRCA1* mutations, there was no significant difference in the average number of cases of ovarian cancer in families with 5' 185delAG mutations (1.25 cases) compared with families with 5382insC mutations at the 3' end of the gene (1.00 cases) (Tonin et al., 1996b).

It is equally possible that the variation is due to modifying genes. If the modifier gene were on chromosome 17q, near *BRCA1*, then the variation within a family would be less than the variation between families. If the modifier were on another chromosome then there would be great variation within families, and there might be systematic differences between ethnic groups, depending on the frequency of the polymorphic alleles of the modifier genes in the populations studied. The presence of a rare allele of the *RASH* polymorphism on chromosome 11 increased the risk of ovarian cancer, but not of breast cancer, among *BRCA1* carriers (Phelan et al., 1996). Rebbeck et al. (1995) found that the mean age of diagnosis of familial breast cancer was younger in women carrying a null allele of the glutathione *S*-transferase polymorphism. It would make sense to study groups such as the Ashkenazim where relatively few mutations have been reported and other risk factors may differ less than within other less genetically and culturally homogenous groups.

Reproductive factors

Multiparity is associated with a reduced risk of breast cancer in the general population (Kelsey, 1979) and in *BRCA1* carriers (Narod et al., 1995c). Sellers and colleagues (1992) studied a cohort of 37,105 women, of whom 493 developed breast cancer. They found that the risks associated with low parity were greater among women with one or more first-degree relatives affected with breast cancer. This was not seen in the Nurses' Health Study Research Group report (Colditz et al., 1996), where no protection was offered by multiple birth or early first birth in women with a family history of breast cancer. By contrast, in a historical cohort study of *BRCA1* carriers, Narod and colleagues (1995c) found the risk of breast cancer decreased by 15% for each additional birth.

In the Sellers study, a first pregnancy after age 30 was associated with a 5.8-fold increase in risk of breast cancer in the familial subgroup. Similarly, Dupont and Page (1987) reported an eightfold risk of breast cancer associated with first birth over the age of 30 (versus below age 20) among women with a positive family history of the disease. In these two epidemiology studies it is expected that only a minority of cases would be among *BRCA1* carriers. In a study of 333 known *BRCA1* carriers an early age of first birth was not found to be protective, after adjusting for parity (Narod et al., 1995c), in agreement with the findings of the Nurses' Health Study Group (Colditz et al., 1996).

Hereditary breast cancer appears to be more frequent in recent generations (Narod et al., 1995c). The risk of breast cancer was 2.75 times greater for women born after 1930 than for those born before 1930. The factors that influence the increasing trend are unknown, but they do not seem to be limited to reproductive variables.

For *BRCA1* carriers, parity appears to be predictive of ovarian cancer risk, even when taking into account the protective effect of the oral contraceptive pill. Interestingly, a late birth was protective (Narod et al., 1995c). This finding was supported in a case-control study of French-Canadian women with ovarian cancer – those with a strong family history were most protected by a late first birth (Godard et al., 1998).

Nothing is known about reproductive risk factors and risk of endometrial cancer in mismatch repair gene carriers.

Predictive testing, diagnosis and management issues in hereditary breast, ovary, and uterine cancer

Breast and ovarian cancers

Overview

The clinical cancer geneticist must estimate the probability that a particular case of breast cancer is hereditary. This probability is used to estimate the risk of recurrence in the patient and to estimate the risk of cancer occurrence in other family members. Factors to be considered include the number and sites of cancer in the woman's family, her past history of cancer, and the age-of-onset, laterality, and histology of her tumour. It is important to note that if a woman has few female relatives, if she is adopted or if the family history is not known, a woman with hereditary cancer may report no relatives with the disease. As discussed above, the risk of breast cancer among relatives increases with early age-of-onset in the index case. Also, the risk of breast cancer is greater for relatives of bilateral cases than for unilateral cases.

Histopathological features

There is no convincing evidence for the existence of a characteristic pre-neoplastic state in the hereditary breast cancer families. However, among women undergoing breast biopsy, atypical hyperplasia is associated with a fourfold risk of developing breast cancer (Dupont and Page, 1987). There appears to be a positive association between atypical hyperplasia and a family history of breast cancer. Carter et al. (1988) documented that 20% of women with atypical hyperplasia had a first-degree relative with breast cancer, but only 11.9% of controls had an affected relative ($p < 0.01$). Dupont and Page (1985) found the risk of breast cancer to be increased 11 times if a woman had both atypical hyperplasia and a family history of breast cancer. To date there is no evidence that atypical hyperplasia or carcinoma-in-situ are frequent features of breast cancer associated with *BRCA1* mutations (Sun et al., 1996). It appears that *in situ* carcinoma may be a feature of *BRCA2* families. All types of breast cancer may appear in *BRCA1* and *BRCA2* families, and there is no concordance of cancer types within a family. Malignant cells from *BRCA1*-associated cancers are notable for their high proliferation rates and mean S-phase fraction (Marcus et al., 1996). They also appear to be more often of medullary or 'atypical medullary' histology than expected. Tubulolobular cancers are over-represented in *BRCA2*-associated cancers (Marcus et al., 1996).

It has been reported that there is an association between mutation position in *BRCA1* and proliferation – in one study, mutations at the conserved 5' and 3' extremes of the gene (including the recurrent Askenazi mutations 185delAG and 5282insC) were more likely to result in highly-proliferating breast cancers than mutations elsewhere in the gene (Sobol et al., 1996). This finding is supported in part by data from 149 breast cancers in Ashkenazi Jewish patients, where those with the two common recurrent mutations were significantly more likely to have a high nuclear grade and to be poorly differentiated than those without mutations (Karp et al., 1997). *BRCA1*-positive breast cancers were also significantly more likely to be oestrogen receptor-negative.

Ovarian cancer in a hereditary setting is commonly of the serous papillary type, with mucinous carcinoma significantly under-represented (Bewtra et al., 1992a; Piver et al., 1993a). In families where linkage to *BRCA1* has been demonstrated, a woman with a mucinous ovarian cancer is most likely not to be a gene carrier (Narod et al., 1994b). Borderline ovarian tumours are also under-represented in *BRCA1*-linked families (Bewtra et al., 1992).

Identifying mutation carriers

Carriers of mutations in *BRCA1* and *BRCA2* can be identified either by linkage analysis or by direct mutation detection. Mutation detection techniques are discussed in Chapter 8. Linkage analysis is an indirect method and does not provide proof of the presence of a mutation in the family or in the individual. However, linkage analysis can be used to establish if a family is linked to *BRCA1* or to *BRCA2* before more extensive mutation analyses are undertaken. Linkage analysis is discussed in Chapter 7.

BRCA1 and *BRCA2* are both large genes (Table 10.3). As such, it is helpful if linkage analysis can eliminate one or both genes from further consideration. The techniques of linkage analysis are simple, but the interpretation of linkage data may be problematic. In contrast, direct mutation analysis requires a greater investment of resources, but the data generated are relatively easy to interpret. Ideally, a screening programme should incorporate both techniques. However, when there is only a single affected female in a family available for testing, linkage analysis is generally not possible. In the absence of strong evidence of linkage, a negative mutation test is not generally useful – i.e., it is not possible to reassure individuals that they are not at elevated risk, because of the possibility that a mutation may have been missed, and because of

Table 10.3. *Comparative features of* BRCA1 *and* BRCA2

Gene	Chromosomal position	Size of open reading frame (amino acids)	Size of messenger RNA	Cancers commonly seen in gene carriers	Other cancers in excess in families
BRCA1	17q12-21	1863aa	7.8 kb	Breast (rarely male), ovary	Fallopian tube, ?pancreas, ?colorectal, ?prostate
BRCA2	13q12-13	3418aa	11-12 kb	Breast (female and male), ovary, (?depending on mutation site)	Pancreas, ?lymphoma, ?larynx ?fallopian tube

genetic heterogeneity. This may be less of a problem in ethnic groups where very few mutations have been reported, e.g. the Ashkenazim (Tonin et al., 1996b).

Not all *BRCA1* mutations are in the coding region of the gene. In some cases, examination of lymphocyte RNA permits the identification of mutations that are not present in the DNA (Serova et al., 1996). The protein truncation test is a rapid screening test for *BRCA1* mutations (Hogervorst et al., 1995). Although this technique is not sensitive to missense mutations, less than 10% of all *BRCA1* mutations are missense mutations (see Chapter 8). Single strand conformation analysis (SSCA) is another method of screening for mutations in the coding region prior to sequencing. Over 80% of *BRCA1* mutations in families identified to date are due to insertions or deletions of small stretches of DNA (Shattuck-Eidens et al., 1995).

It is also important to know the ethnic origin of the individual tested because this may provide some information about the most likely mutations. For example, the majority of families of Ashkenazi Jewish descent with hereditary breast and ovarian cancers carry a mutation of either the 185delAG- or the 5382insC-type (Tonin et al., 1996b). The 185delAG mutations is almost specific for Jews, but the 5382insC mutation is seen in several groups from Eastern Europe. It is prudent to screen first for these two mutations in Jewish women before a more exhaustive search. In both cases a particular genetic haplotype is carried on the copy of chromosome 17q that is associated with these mutations. By first typing the individuals in a family with *BRCA1* markers, it may be possible to predict the presence of a particular mutation. Other mutations seen in the Ashkenazim include 188del11 in *BRCA1* and 6174delT in BRCA2, but it is not certain that these mutations are restricted to the Ashkenazim (Berman et al., 1996a,b).

The risk of breast and ovarian cancers to relatives of women diagnosed with these forms of cancer has been established and there are several papers published that present empiric risks which can be used in most counselling situations (Schwartz et al., 1985; Ottman et al., 1986; Gail et al., 1989). It is now possible, using several methods, to identify with a high degree of probability, women in predisposed families who carry *BRCA1* or *BRCA2* mutations before the onset of clinical cancer. The use of genetic linkage and mutation analysis in counselling women from high-risk breast cancer families is now established in several centres.

Prevention: breast cancer

Current strategies for breast cancer prevention in high risk women are inadequate. Because of the limitations of screening mammography, and because the benefit of tamoxifen or other chemopreventive agents in preventing breast cancer is unproven, some women at very high risk opt for prophylactic surgical removal of breasts. In the Breast Cancer Linkage consortium study (Ford et al., 1993), 23 contralateral breast cancers were observed more than three years after the initial diagnosis of breast cancer. The cumulative risk for contralateral cancer among affected carriers was 85% to age 70. Because of the high risk of recurrent cancer in *BRCA1* carriers, some authors recommend that contralateral mastectomy be considered at the time of the initial surgery (Lynch et al., 1993b).

Mammographic screening is routinely recommended for high risk women in most family cancer clinics. Mammography has not been proven to reduce mortality from breast cancer in young women (Miller et al., 1992), but the subgroup of women with a strong family history has not been studied.

Early menopause, whether natural or surgically induced, offers some protection against breast cancer (Kelsey, 1979). It has not yet been determined to what extent oophorectomy diminishes the risk of hereditary breast cancer, if at all. Surgical menopause is also associated with increased risks of cardiovascular disease and of osteoporosis. These risks may be diminished by oestrogen replacement, but the safety of post-menopausal oestrogen replacement in women who are at high risk for cancer is under debate. There is probably a modest increase in breast cancer risk for women taking prolonged hormone replacement (Colditz et al., 1993a, 1995), but this is offset by a reduction in cardiovascular disease incidence and mortality. In a meta-analysis of hormone replacement therapy and breast cancer risk, it was concluded that women with a positive family history of breast cancer had a 3.4-fold increase in breast cancer risk if they had ever used hormone replacement therapy ($p < 0.05$) (Steinberg et al., 1991). The size of the effect was smaller for those women without a family history of breast cancer. From the Nurses' Health Study, Colditz et al. (1993b) did not find family history to modify the risk of oestrogen use, which they estimate as 1.23 for greater than 10 years of oestrogen use.

The ideal drug to give under these circumstances would diminish the risks of breast cancer and cardiovascular disease and osteoporosis. It may be that tamoxifen will become a useful drug in this setting; McDonald et al. (1995) showed a decreased risk of cardiovascular disease in women following treatment with tamoxifen. A large trial evaluating the use of tamoxifen in preventing breast cancer in high risk women is now underway.

A meta-analysis of oral contraceptive use and breast cancer risk showed a slight elevation in risk which diminished once the contraceptive was discontinued (Calle et al., 1996). Currently, a family history of breast cancer is not considered to be a contraindication for oral contraceptive use. In the Nurses' Health Study Research Group report (Colditz et al., 1996), there was no additional effect on risk of past use of oral contraception in those with a positive family history compared to those with no family history. It will be important to note the effect of oral contraception on ovarian cancer risk in *BRCA1* and *BRCA2* carriers.

Prevention: reproductive, hormonal and other risk factors in ovarian cancer

Oral contraceptive use, tubal ligation and previous hysterectomy all protect against ovarian cancer. In contrast, low parity is a risk factor for ovarian cancer, and among those who do have children, those who have children and complete their families at a young age are at a higher risk than those who have a late age of first birth (Adami et al., 1994). Thus from this study, when controlling for parity, it is age of first birth that is most predictive of ovarian cancer risk. The oral contraceptive pill has been shown to be highly protective – a meta-analysis of 20 studies from 1970–91 gave a relative risk for ovarian cancer of 0.64 (95% CI: 0.57–0.73) in association with use of oral contraception (Hankinson et al., 1992). However, protection from ovarian cancer may cease after six years of use (Whittemore et al., 1992). Early menopause does not appear to be protective (Whittemore et al., 1992), so neither these findings nor those of Adami and colleagues fit into either of the two main hypotheses of ovarian carcinogenesis – incessant ovulation and excessive gonadotrophic ovarian stimulation. It is interesting that a recent case-control study of ovarian cancer among French-Canadians showed that oral contraceptive use was most protective in those who last used the oral contraceptive pill at age 35–43 (adjusted relative risk of ovarian cancer: 0.2, 95% CI: 0.09–0.47; compared with no use). In those who last used the oral contraceptive pill at age 17–25 the adjusted relative risk was 1.0 (Godard et al., 1998). Thus the timing of hormonal intervention may be very important in ovarian cancer prevention.

Whether or not these risk factors will translate to hereditary forms of ovarian cancer is uncertain – Narod and colleagues showed that increasing parity was a risk factor for hereditary ovarian cancer, a finding at variance with results from case-control studies in unselected cases (Narod et al., 1995c). In Godard's study there was a suggestion that familial cases were afforded more protection by tubal ligation and late age of last use of oral contraceptives than non-familial cases, but the numbers were too small for definitive conclusions. Large studies of *BRCA1* and *BRCA2* mutation carriers will be required to answer these important questions. These answers will aid management decisions such as the role of oral contraceptives, tubal ligation and prophylactic oophorectomy in those predisposed to ovarian cancer as result of mutations in highly penetrant dominant cancer associated genes.

Early detection of ovarian cancer

In the general population, clinical examination, transabdominal (Campbell et al., 1989), transvaginal (Kurjak and Zalud, 1992) ultrasound (with or without colour-flow Doppler), and serum CA-125 screening tests (Cuckle and Wald, 1990) either alone or in combination (Jacobs et al., 1993) have all been assessed as potential screening tests in various settings. However, no single test has yet proved to be practical for population screening. Women at increased risk of ovarian cancer as a result of their family history and/or *BRCA1* test are a subgroup that are likely to be more suitable for screening. Using transvaginal ultrasound, and colour-flow Doppler monitoring, 61 abnormal lesions were detected in 1601 self-referred women with family history of ovarian, breast, and other cancers. These 61 women were referred for surgical investigation and six were found to have cancers, five of which were early stage, but only one woman had a family history of ovarian cancer only (Bourne et al., 1993). Using transvaginal ultrasound with colour flow imaging, Weiner et al. (1993) found ovarian cancer in 4 of 600 women with a past history of breast cancer (this group is at roughly double the risk of ovarian cancer as is the general public). Muto et al. (1993) screened 386 women with a family history of ovarian cancer using transvaginal sonography, colour flow Doppler and CA-125. The ultrasound examination was abnormal in 23% of the women, but no malignant ovarian lesion was detected. Thus even in high, or moderately high risk groups, the yield is low. It will be easier to assess the role of ultrasound now that specific groups with different risks can be differentitated on the basis of mutation analysis.

Screening with multiple serum markers has been proposed in an attempt to improve detection of early ovarian cancers. At least one of three markers (M-CSF, OVX1 and CA-125) were elevated in the serum of 45 out of 46 women with stage 1 ovarian carcinomas. Unfortunately 51% of women with benign pelvic masses also had elevated levels of one or more markers (Woolas et al., 1993). Using these multiple markers in conjunction with other screening tests may be useful in high-risk women.

Prophylactic oophorectomy is another possible way of preventing ovarian cancer. Because of the high lifetime risk of ovarian cancer associated with *BRCA1*, and because the sensitivity and effectiveness of the current methods of screening are uncertain, several groups currently recommend prophylactic removal of the ovaries of *BRCA1* mutation carriers around the time of menopause (Kerlikowske et al., 1992; Lynch et al., 1995). Unfortunately, about 5% of these women will later develop peritoneal cancer (Tobacman et al., 1982; Piver et al., 1993b). The hormonal conseqences of prophylactic oophorectomy in young women should also be considered (Speroff et al., 1991). Oophorectomy in the woman at average risk of breast cancer should probably be followed by hormone replacement therapy, as the beneficial effects of hormone replacement therapy on the cardiovascular system and on bone mineral density probably outweigh the increased risk of breast cancer (Nayfield et al., 1991). However, the use of hormone replacement therapy in the high-risk woman is worrisome, because this therapy probably increases the risk of breast cancer, particularly in those who have used hormones for more than five years (Adami and Persson, 1995; Davidson, 1995). A possible alternative might be tamoxifen, particularly if the woman has not had a prophylactic mastectomy. The role for tamoxifen in the management of the high risk women deserves attention, and may become clearer when results from the NSABP tamoxifen breast cancer prevention trial become available.

Cancer of the uterine corpus

Established risk factors for endometrial adenocarcinoma include use of hormone replacement therapy (especially but not exclusively unopposed oestrogen therapy), nulliparity and/or multigravidity, early age at menarche, late age of natural menopause, total length of ovulation span and medical conditions such as obesity, diabetes mellitus and possibly hypertension (Nason and Nelson, 1994; Grady et al., 1995;

Mcpherson et al., 1996). Infertility may be a risk factor and oral contraceptive use appears to be protective (Stanford et al., 1993). Hereditary endometrial cancer is rather infrequently encountered in clinical practice, and for this reason, it has been difficult to study risk factors that might influence the occurrence of this cancer in its hereditary setting. Collaborative studies that address these issues are now underway.

Prevention: endometrial cancer
Preventive hysterectomy has been recommended by some authors for HNPCC-associated gene carriers as the lifetime risk of endometrial adenocarcinoma in these women approaches 50% (Aarnio et al., 1995). However, no formal recommendations have been made.

Conclusions

The genetic contribution to cancers that are solely or mainly seen in women appears to be largest for ovarian cancer, where between 5 and 10% of ovarian carcinoma can be explained by hereditary factors. In families where *BRCA1* is mutated, gene carriers have a risk to age 70 of ovarian cancer of about 50%. For breast cancer, genetic effects are far more marked in the relatives of women diagnosed with breast cancer at a young age than in those diagnosed older, the cut-off point being around the menopause. In large *BRCA1* families, the risk of breast cancer to age 70 in gene carriers is about 85%. Only about 1% of endometrial cancer is explained by inheritance of highly penetrant genes, but again, effects are more marked in those diagnosed at a younger age. For HNPCC-associated gene carriers, the risk of endometrial cancer is about 45% to age 80. Squamous cell carcinoma of the uterine cervix is rarely if ever hereditary, and HPV infection is by far the most important risk factor. A rare form of cervical cancer has been reported in Peutz–Jeghers syndrome. For breast, ovary, and endometrial cancer, the simple enquiry as to the presence of a family history of cancer (at all sites) in first- and second-degree relatives may be all that is required to detect those at highest risk of primary or second primary cancer. Suitable interventions can then be initiated.

Acknowledgements

We thank Dr. Patricia Tonin for Figures 10.1a and 10.1b and for comments on the text.

226   *W. Foulkes and S. Narod*

References

Aarnio, M., Mecklin, J.P., Aaltonen, L.A., Nystromlahti, M. and Jarvinen, H.J. 1995. Life-time risk of different cancers in hereditary non-polyposis colorectal cancer (HNPCC) syndrome. *International Journal of Cancer* **64**: 430–3.

Adami, H.O., Bergkvist, L., Krusemo, U. and Persson, I. 1984. Breast cancer as a risk factor for other primary malignant diseases. A nationwide cohort study. *Journal of the National Cancer Institute* **73**: 1049–55.

Adami, H.O., Hsieh, C.C., Lambe, M. et al. 1994. Parity, age at first childbirth, and risk of ovarian cancer. *Lancet* **344**: 1250–4.

Adami, H.O. and Persson, I. 1995. Hormone replacement and breast cancer. A remaining controversy? *JAMA* **274**: 178–9.

Apple, R.J., Erlich, H.A., Klitz, W., Manos, M.M., Becker, T.M. and Wheeler, C.M. 1994. HLA DR-DQ associations with cervical carcinoma show papillomavirus-type specificity. *Nature Genetics* **6**: 157–62.

Apple, R.J., Becker, T.M., Wheeler, C.M. and Erlich, H.A. 1995. Comparison of human leukocyte antigen DR-DQ disease associations found with cervical dysplasia and invasive cervical carcinoma. *Journal of the National Cancer Institute* **87**: 427–36.

Athma, P., Rappaport, R. and Swift, M. 1996. Molecular genotyping shows that ataxia-telangiectasia heteroxygotes are predisposed to breast cancer. *Cancer Genetics and Cytogenetics* **92**(2): 130–4.

Berman, D.B., Costalas, J., Schultz, D.C., Grana, G., Daly, M. and Godwin, A.K. 1996a. A common mutation in *BRCA2* that predisposes to a variety of cancers is found in both Jewish Ashkenazi and non-Jewish individuals. *Cancer Research* **56**: 3409–14.

Berman, D.B., Wagner-Costalas, J., Schultz, D.C., Lynch, H.T., Daly, M. and Godwin, A.K. 1996b. Two distinct origins of a common *BRCA1* mutation in breast-ovarian cancer families – a genetic study of 15 185delAG-mutation kindreds. *American Journal of Human Genetics* **58**: 1166–76.

Bewtra, C., Watson, P., Conway, T., Read-Hippee, C. and Lynch, H.T. 1992. Hereditary ovarian cancer: a clinicopathological study. *International Journal of Gynecological Pathology* **11**: 180–7.

Bishop, D.T. 1992. Family history of breast cancer: how important is it? *Journal of Medical Genetics* **29**: 152–3.

Bishop, D.T., Cannon-Albright, L., McLellan, T., Gardner, E.J. and Skolnick, M.H. 1988. Segregation and linkage analysis of nine Utah breast cancer pedigrees. *Genetic Epidemiology* **5**: 151–69.

Børresen, A.L., Andersen, T.I., Garber, J. et al. 1992. Screening for germ line TP53 mutations in breast cancer patients. *Cancer Research* **52**: 3234–6.

Bourne, T.H., Campbell, S., Reynolds, K.M. et al. 1993. Screening for early familial ovarian cancer with transvaginal ultrasonography and colour blood flow imaging. *British Medical Journal* **306**: 1025–9.

Calle, EE., Heath, C.W., Miracle-McMahill H.L. et al. 1996. Breast cancer and hormonal contraceptives–collaborative re-analyis of individual data on 53,297 women with breast cancer and 100,239 women without breast cancer from 54 epidemiological studies. *Lancet* **347**:1713–27.

Campbell, S., Bhan, V., Royston, P., Whitehead, M.I. and Collins, W.P. 1989. Transabdominal ultrasound screening for early ovarian cancer. *British Medical Journal.* **299**: 1363–7.

Carter, C.L., Corle, D.K., Micozzi, M.S., Schatzkin, A. and Taylor, P.R. 1988. A prospective study of the development of breast cancer in 16, 692 women with benign breast disease. *American Journal of Epidemiology* **128**: 467–77.

Claus, E.B., Risch, N.J. and Thompson, W.D. 1990. Age at onset as an indicator of familial risk of breast cancer. *American Journal of Epidemiology* **131**: 961–72.

Colditz, G.A., Egan, K.M. and Stampfer, M.J. 1993a. Hormone replacement therapy and risk of breast cancer: results from epidemiologic studies. *American Journal of Obstetrics and Gynecology* **168**: 1473–80.

Colditz, G.A., Willett, W.C., Hunter, D.J., Stampfer, M.J., Manson, J.E., Hennekens, C.H. and Rosner, B.A. 1993b. Family history, age, and risk of breast cancer. Prospective data from the Nurses' Health Study. *JAMA* **270**: 338–43.

Colditz, G.A., Hankinson, S.E., Hunter, D.J. et al. 1995. The use of estrogens and progestins and the risk of breast cancer in postmenopausal women. *New England Journal of Medicine* **332**: 1589–93.

Colditz, G.A., Rosner, B.A. and Speizer, F.E. 1996. Risk factors for breast cancer according to family history of breast cancer. *Journal of the National Cancer Institute* **88**: 365–71.

Cuckle, H.S. and Wald, N.J. 1990. The evaluation of screening tests for ovarian cancer. In *Ovarian Cancer: Biological and Therapeutic Challenges*, ed. F. Sharp, P. Mason and R.E. Leake, pp. 229–39. London: Chapman and Hall.

Davidson, N.E. 1995. Hormone-replacement therapy–breast versus heart versus bone. *New England Journal of Medicine* **332**: 1638–9.

Dupont, W.D. and Page, D.L. 1985. Risk factors for breast cancer in women with proliferative breast disease. *New England Journal of Medicine* **312**: 146–51.

Dupont, W.D. and Page, D.L. 1987. Breast cancer risk associated with proliferative disease, age at first birth, and a family history of breast cancer. *American Journal of Epidemiology* **125**: 769–79.

Durocher, F., Tonin, P., Shattuck-Eidens, D., Skolnick, M., Narod, S.A. and Simard, J.S. 1996. Mutation analysis of the BRCA1 gene in 24 families with cases of cancer in the breast, ovary, and multiple other sites. *Journal of Medical Genetics* **33**: 819–24.

Easton, D., Ford, D. and Peto, J. 1993. Inherited susceptibility to breast cancer. *Cancer Surveys* **18**: 95–113.

Easton, D.F., Bishop, D.T., Ford, D. and Crockford, G.P. 1993. Genetic linkage analysis in familial breast and ovarian cancer: results from 214 families. The Breast Cancer Linkage Consortium. *American Journal of Human Genetics* **52**: 678–701.

Easton, D.F., Ford, D. and Bishop, D.T. 1995. Breast and ovarian cancer incidence in *BRCA1*-mutation carriers. Breast Cancer Linkage Consortium. *American Journal of Human Genetics* **56**: 265–71.

Easton, D.F., Matthews, F.E., Ford, D., Swerdlow, A.J. and Peto, J. 1996. Cancer mortality in relatives of women with ovarian cancer – the OPCS study. *International Journal of Cancer* **65**: 284–94.

FitzGerald, M.G., Bean, J.M., Hedge, S.R. et al. 1997. Heterozygous ATM mutations do not contribute to early onset of breast cancer. *Nature Genetics* **15**(3): 307–10.

Ford, D., Easton, D. and Bishop, D.T. 1993. The risks of cancer in BRCA1 mutation carriers. *American Journal of Human Genetics* **53S**: A298

Ford, D., Easton, D.F., Bishop, D.T., Narod, S.A. and Goldgar, D.E. 1994. Risks of cancer in *BRCA1*-mutation carriers. Breast Cancer Linkage Consortium. *Lancet* **343**: 692–5.

Foulkes, W., Flanders, T., Lambert, D. and Narod, S. 1996. Increased incidence of cancer in the first-degree relatives of women with double primary cancers of the colon and endometrium: a registry-based study. *American Journal of Human Genetics* **59S**: A67, p. 347.

Foulkes, W.D., Bolduc, N., Lambert, D. et al. 1996. Increased incidence of cancer in first degree relatives of women with double primary carcinomas of the breast and colon. *Journal of Medical Genetics* **33**: 534–9.

Gail, M.H., Brinton, L.A., Byar, D.P., Corle, D.K., Green, S.B., Schairer, C. and Mulvihill, J.J. 1989. Projecting individualized probabilities of developing breast cancer for white females who are being examined annually. *Journal of the National Cancer Institute* **81**: 1879–86.

Garber, J.E., Goldstein, A.M., Kantor, A.F., Dreyfus, M.G., Fraumeni, J.F., Jr. and Li, F.P. 1991. Follow-up study of twenty-four families with Li–Fraumeni syndrome. *Cancer Research* **51**: 6094–7.

Gayther, S.A., Warren, W., Mazoyer, S. et al. 1995. Germline mutations of the *BRCA1* gene in breast and ovarian cancer families provide evidence for a genotype-phenotype correlation. *Nature Genetics* **11**: 428–33.

Glew, S.S., Duggan-Keen, M., Ghosh, A.K. et al. 1993. Lack of association of HLA polymorphisms with human papillomavirus-related cervical cancer. *Human Immunology* **37**: 157–64.

Go, R.C., King, M.C., Bailey-Wilson, J., Elston, R.C. and Lynch, H.T. 1983. Genetic epidemiology of breast cancer and associated cancers in high-risk families. I. Segregation analysis. *Journal of the National Cancer Institute* **71**: 455–61.

Godard, B., Foulkes, W.D., Provencher, D. et al. 1998. Risk factors for familial and sporadic ovarian cancer among French-Canadians: a case-control study. *American Journal of Obstetrics and Gynecology*. (In press.)

Grady, D., Gebretsadik, T., Kerlikowske, K., Ernster, V. and Petitti, D. 1995. Hormone replacement therapy and endometrial cancer risk: a meta-analysis. *Obstetrics Gynecology* **85**: 304–13.

Hall, J.M., Lee, M.K., Newman, B., Morrow, J.E., Anderson, L.A., Huey, B. and King, M.C. 1990. Linkage of early-onset familial breast cancer to chromosome 17q21. *Science* **250**: 1684–9.

Hankinson, S.E., Colditz, G.A., Hunter, D.J., Spencer, T.L., Rosner, B. and Stampfer, M.J. 1992. A quantitative assessment of oral contraceptive use and risk of ovarian cancer. *Obstetrics Gynecology* **80**: 708–14.

Hanssen, A.M. and Fryns, J.P. 1995. Cowden syndrome. *Journal of Medical Genetics* **32**(2): 117–19.

Hemminki, A., Tomlinson, I., Markie, D. et al. 1997. Localization of a susceptibility locus for Peutz-Jeghers syndrome to 19p using comparative genomic hybridization and targeted linkage analysis. *Nature Genetics* **15**: 87–90.

Hildreth, N.G., Kelsey, J.L., LiVolsi, V.A. et al. 1981. An epidemiologic study of epithelial carcinoma of the ovary. *American Journal of Epidemiology* **114**: 398–405.

Hogervorst, F.B., Cornelis, R.S., Bout, M. et al. 1995. Rapid detection of *BRCA1* mutations by the protein truncation test. *Nature Genetics* **10**: 208–12.

Iselius, L., Slack, J., Littler, M. and Morton, N.E. 1991. Genetic epidemiology of breast cancer in Britain. *Annals of Human Genetics* **55**: 151–9.

Jacobs, I., Davies, A.P., Bridges, J. et al. 1993. Prevalence screening for ovarian cancer in postmenopausal women by CA 125 measurement and ultrasonography. *British Medical Journal.* **306**: 1030–4.

Jolly, K.W., Malkin, D., Douglass, E.C., Brown, T.F., Sinclair, A.E. and Look, A.T. 1994. Splice-site mutation of the p53 gene in a family with hereditary breast–ovarian cancer. *Oncogene* **9**: 97–102.

Karp, S., Tonin, P.N., Bégin, L.R., Martinez J.J., Zhang J.C., Pollak, M.N. and Foulkes, W.D. 1997. Influence of *BRCA1* mutations on nuclear grade and estrogen receptor status on breast carcinoma in Ashkenazi Jewish women. *Cancer* **80**: 435–41.

Kelsey, J.L. 1979. A review of the epidemiology of human breast cancer. *Epidemiological Reviews* **1**: 74–109.

Kerber, R.A. and Slattery, M.L. 1995. The impact of family history on ovarian cancer risk. The Utah Population Database. *Archives International Medicine* **155**: 905–12.

Kerlikowske, K., Brown, J.S. and Grady, D.G. 1992. Should women with familial ovarian cancer undergo prophylactic oophorectomy? *Obstetrics and Gynecology* **80**: 700–7.

Krontiris, T.G., Devlin, B., Karp, D.D., Robert, N.J. and Risch, N. 1993. An association between the risk of cancer and mutations in the HRAS1 minisatellite locus. *New England Journal of Medicine* **329**(8): 517–23.

Kurjak, A. and Zalud, I. 1992. Transvaginal colour flow Doppler in the differentiation of benign and malignant ovarian masses. In *Ovarian Cancer 2*, ed. F. Sharp, P. Mason and W. Creasman, pp. 249–64. London: Chapman and Hall.

Liaw, D., Marsh, D.J., Li, J. et al. 1997. Germline mutations of the PTEN gene in Cowden disease, an inherited breast and thyroid cancer syndrome. *Nature Genetics* **16**(1): 64–7.

Li, F.P. and Fraumeni, J.F. 1969. Soft-tissue sarcomas, breast cancer, and other neoplasms. A familial syndrome? *Annals of Internal Medicine* **71**: 747–52.

Li, J., Yen, C., Liaw, D. et al. 1997. PTEN, a putative protein tyrosine phosphatase gene mutated in human brain, breast, and prostate cancer. *Science* **275**(5308): 1943–47.

Liber, A.F. 1950. Ovarian cancer in a mother and five daughters. *Archives of Pathology* **49**: 280–90.

Lynch, H.T., Smyrk, T.C., Watson, P. et al. 1993a. Genetics, natural history, tumor spectrum, and pathology of hereditary nonpolyposis colorectal cancer: an updated review. *Gastroenterology* **104**: 1535–49.

Lynch, H.T., Watson, P., Conway, T.A. et al. 1993b. DNA screening for breast/ovarian cancer susceptibility based on linked markers. A family study. *Archives of Internal Medicine* **153**: 1979–87.

Lynch, H.T., Severin, M.J., Mooney, M.J. and Lynch, J. 1995. Insurance adjudication favoring prophylactic surgery in hereditary breast-ovarian cancer syndrome. *Gynecology Oncology* **57**: 23–6.

Malkin, D., Li, F.P., Strong, L.C. et al. 1990. Germ line p53 mutations in a familial syndrome of breast cancer, sarcomas, and other neoplasms. *Science* **250**: 1233–8.

Mallory, S.B. 1991. Genodermatoses with malignant potential. In *Genetic Disorders of the Skin*, ed. J.C. Alper, pp. 244–66. St. Louis: Mosby Year Book.

Marcus, J.N., Watson, P., Page, D.L. et al. 1996. Hereditary breast cancer: pathobiology, prognosis, and BRCA1 and BRCA2 gene linkage. *Cancer* **77**: 697–709.

McDonald, C.C., Alexander, F.E., Whyte, B.W., Forrest, A.P. and Stewart, H.J. 1995. Cardiac and vascular morbidity in women receiving adjuvant tamoxifen for breast cancer in a randomised trial. The Scottish Cancer Trials Breast Group. *British Medical Journal* **311**: 977–80.

Mcpherson, C.P., Sellers, T.A., Potter, J.D., Bostick, R.M. and Folsom, A.R. 1996. Reproductive factors and risk of endometrial cancer - the Iowa Women's Health Study. *American Journal of Epidemiology* **143**: 1195–202.

Miki, Y., Swensen, J., Shattuck-Eidens, D. et al. 1994. A strong candidate for the breast and ovarian cancer susceptibility gene BRCA1. *Science* **266**: 66–71.

Miller, A.B., Baines, C.J., To, T. and Wall, C. 1992. Canadian National Breast Screening Study: 1. Breast cancer detection and death rates among women aged 40 to 49 years. *Canadian Medical Association Journal* **147**: 1459–76.

Miller, S., Jothy, S., Shibata, H., Parboosingh, J. and Narod, S.A. 1992. Early onset breast and colon cancer in a large sibship. *American Journal of Human Genetics* **51S**: A66

Muto, M.G., Cramer, D.W., Brown, D.L. et al. 1993. Screening for ovarian cancer: the preliminary experience of a familial ovarian cancer center. *Gynecology Oncology* **51**: 12–20.

Narod, S.A., Feunteun, J., Lynch, H.T., Watson, P., Conway, T., Lynch, J. and Lenoir, G.M. 1991. Familial breast-ovarian cancer locus on chromosome 17q12-q23. *Lancet* **338**: 82–3.

Narod, S.A., Madlensky, L., Bradley, L., Cole, D., Tonin, P., Rosen, B. and Risch, H.A. 1994a. Hereditary and familial ovarian cancer in southern Ontario. *Cancer* **74**: 2341–6.

Narod, S.A., Tonin, P., Lynch, H., Watson, P., Feunteun, J. and Lenoir, G. 1994b. Histology of BRCA1-associated ovarian tumours. *Lancet* **343**: 236

Narod, S.A., Ford, D., Devilee, P. et al. 1995a. Genetic heterogeneity of breast-ovarian cancer revisited. Breast Cancer Linkage Consortium. *American Journal of Human Genetics* **57**: 957–8.

Narod, S.A., Ford, D., Devilee, P. et al. 1995b. An evaluation of genetic heterogeneity in 145 breast-ovarian cancer families. Breast Cancer Linkage Consortium. *American Journal of Human Genetics* **56**: 254–64.

Narod, S.A., Goldgar, D., Cannon-Albright, L. et al. 1995c. Risk modifiers in carriers of BRCA1 mutations. *International Journal of Cancer* **64**: 394–8.

Nason, F.G. and Nelson, B.E. 1994. Estrogen and progesterone in breast and gynecologic cancers. Etiology, therapeutic role, and hormone replacement. *Obstetrics and Gynecology Clinics of North America* **21**: 245–70.

Nayfield, S.G., Karp, J.E., Ford, L.G., Dorr, F.A. and Kramer, B.S. 1991. Potential role of tamoxifen in prevention of breast cancer. *Journal of the National Cancer Institute* **83**: 1450–9.

Nelen, M.R., Padberg, G.W., Peeters, E.A.J., et al. 1996. Localization of the gene for Cowden disease to chromosome 10 q22-23. *Nature Genetics* **13**: 114–16.

Nelson, C.L., Sellers, T.A., Rich, S.S., Potter, J.D., McGovern, P.G. and Kushi, L.H. 1993. Familial clustering of colon, breast, uterine, and ovarian cancers as assessed by family history. *Genetic Epidemiology* **10**: 235–44.

Newman, B., Austin, M.A., Lee, M. and King, M.C. 1988. Inheritance of human breast cancer: evidence for autosomal dominant transmission in high-risk families. *Proceedings of the National Academy of Sciences USA* **85**: 3044–8.

Ottman, R., Pike, M.C., King, M.C., Casagrande, J.T. and Henderson, B.E. 1986. Familial breast cancer in a population-based series. *American Journal of Epidemiology* 123: 15–21.

Parazzini, F., La Vecchia, C., Moroni, S., Chatenoud, L. and Ricci, E. 1994. Family history and the risk of endometrial cancer. *International Journal of Cancer* 59: 460–2.

Parkin, D.M., Pisani, P. and Ferlay, J. 1993. Estimates of the worldwide incidence of eighteen major cancers in 1985. *International Journal of Cancer* 54: 594–606.

Peto, J., Easton, D.F., Matthews, F.E., Ford, D. and Swerdlow, A.J. 1996. Cancer mortality in relatives of women with breast cancer: the OPCS study. *International Journal of Cancer* 65: 275–83.

Phelan, C.M., Rebbeck, T.R., Weber, B.L. et al. 1996. Ovarian cancer risk in BRCA1 carriers is modified by the HRAS1 variable number of tandem repeat (VNTR) locus. *Nature Genetics* 12: 309–11.

Pippard, E.C., Hall, A.J., Barker, D.J. and Bridges, B.A. 1988. Cancer in homozygotes and heterozygotes of ataxia-telangiectasia and xeroderma pigmentosum in Britain. *Cancer Research* 48: 2929–32.

Piver, M.S., Baker, T.R., Jishi, M.F. et al. 1993a. Familial ovarian cancer. A report of 658 families from the Gilda Radner Familial Ovarian Cancer Registry 1981–1991. *Cancer* 71: 582–8.

Piver, M.S., Jishi, M.F., Tsukada, Y. and Nava, G. 1993b. Primary peritoneal carcinoma after prophylactic oophorectomy in women with a family history of ovarian cancer. A report of the Gilda Radner Familial Ovarian Cancer Registry. *Cancer* 71: 2751–5.

Prior, P. and Waterhouse, J.A. 1981. Multiple primary cancers of the breast and ovary. *British Journal of Cancer* 44: 628–36.

Rebbeck, T.R., Walker, A. and Hoskins, K. 1995. Modification of familial breast cancer penetrance by glutathione-S-transferase genotypes. *American Journal of Human Genetics* 11: 428–33.

Schildkraut, J.M., Risch, N. and Thompson, W.D. 1989. Evaluating genetic association among ovarian, breast, and endometrial cancer: evidence for a breast/ovarian cancer relationship. *American Journal of Human Genetics* 45: 521–9.

Schildkraut, J.M. and Thompson, W.D. 1988. Familial ovarian cancer: a population-based case-control study. *American Journal of Epidemiology* 128: 456–66.

Schwartz, A.G., King, M.C., Belle, S.H., Satariano, W.A. and Swanson, G.M. 1985. Risk of breast cancer to relatives of young breast cancer patients. *Journal of the National Cancer Institute* 75: 665–8.

Sellers, T.A., Kushi, L.H., Potter, J.D., Kaye, S.A., Nelson, C.L., McGovern, P.G. and Folsom, A.R. 1992. Effect of family history, body-fat distribution, and reproductive factors on the risk of postmenopausal breast cancer. *New England Journal of Medicine* 326: 1323–9.

Serova, O., Montagna, M., Torchard, D. et al. 1996. A high incidence of BRCA1 mutations in 20 breast-ovarian cancer families. *American Journal of Human Genetics* 58: 42–51.

Shattuck-Eidens, D., McClure, M., Simard, J. et al. 1995. A collaborative survey of 80 mutations in the BRCA1 breast and ovarian cancer susceptibility gene. Implications for presymptomatic testing and screening. *JAMA* 273: 535–41.

Sidransky, D., Tokino, T., Helzlsouer, K. et al. 1992. Inherited p53 gene mutations in breast cancer. *Cancer Research* 52: 2984–6.

Simard, J., Tonin, P., Durocher, F. et al. 1994. Common origins of BRCA1 mutations in Canadian breast and ovarian cancer families. *Nature Genetics* 8: 392–8.

Smithers, D.W. 1948. Family history of 459 patients with cancer of the breast. *British Journal of Cancer* 2: 163–7.

Sobol, A., Stoppa-Lyonnet, D., Bressac-de Paillerets, B. et al. 1996. Truncation at conserved terminal regions of BRCA1 protein is associated with highly proliferative hereditary breast cancers. *Cancer Research* 56: 3216–19.

Speroff, T., Dawson, N.V., Speroff, L. and Haber, R.J. 1991. A risk-benefit analysis of elective bilateral oophorectomy: effect of changes in compliance with estrogen therapy on outcome. *American Journal of Obstetrics and Gynecology* 164: 165–74.

Spigelman, A.D., Arese, P. and Phillips, R.K. 1995. Polyposis: the Peutz-Jeghers syndrome. *British Journal of Surgery* 82: 1311–14.

Stanford, J.L., Brinton, L.A., Berman, M.L., Mortel, R., Twiggs, L.B., Barrett, R.J., Wilbanks, G.D. and Hoover, R.N. 1993. Oral contraceptives and endometrial cancer: do other risk factors modify the association? *International Journal of Cancer* 54: 243–8.

Starink, T.M. 1984. Cowden's disease: analysis of fourteen new cases. *Journal of the American Academy of Dermatology* 11(6): 1127–41.

Steichen-Gersdorf, E., Gallion, H.H., Ford, D. et al. 1994. Familial site-specific ovarian cancer is linked to BRCA1 on 17q12-21. *American Journal of Human Genetics* 55: 870–5.

Steinberg, K.K., Thacker, S.B., Smith, S.J., Stroup, D.F., Zack, M.M., Flanders, W.D. and Berkelman, R.L. 1991. A meta-analysis of the effect of estrogen replacement therapy on the risk of breast cancer. *JAMA* 265: 1985–90.

Stratton, M.R., Ford, D., Neuhasen, S. et al. 1994. Familial male breast cancer is not linked to the BRCA1 locus on chromosome 17q. *Nature Genetics* 7: 103–7.

Struewing, J.P., Brody, L.C., Erdos, M.R. et al. 1995. Detection of eight BRCA1 mutations in 10 breast/ovarian cancer families, including 1 family with male breast cancer. *American Journal of Human Genetics* 57: 1–7.

Sun, C.C., Lenoir, G., Lynch, H. and Narod, S.A. 1996. In situ breast cancer and BRCA1. *Lancet* 348: 408

Suomi, R., Hakala-Ala-Pietila, T., Leminen, A., Mecklin, J.P. and Lehtovirta, P. 1995. Hereditary aspects of endometrial adenocarcinoma. *International Journal of Cancer* 62: 132–7.

Swift, M., Morrell, D., Massey, R.B. and Chase, C.L. 1991. Incidence of cancer in 161 families affected by ataxia-telangiectasia. *New England Journal of Medicine* 325: 1831–6.

Telatar, M., Wang, Z., Udar, N et al. 1996. Ataxia-telangiectasia: mutations in ATM cDNA detected by protein-truncation screening. *American Journal of Human Genetics* 59: 40–4.

Teppo, L., Pukkala, E. and Saxen, E. 1985. Multiple cancer – an epidemiologic exercise in Finland. *Journal of the National Cancer Institute* 75: 207–17.

Tobacman, J.K., Greene, M.H., Tucker, M.A., Costa, J., Kase, R. and Fraumeni, J.F., Jr. 1982. Intra-abdominal carcinomatosis after prophylactic oophorectomy in ovarian-cancer-prone families. *Lancet* 2: 795–7.

Tonin, P., Ghadirian, P, Phelan, C.M. et al. 1996a. Case report: large multisite cancer family is linked to BRCA2. *Journal of Medical Genetics* 32: 982–4.

Tonin, P., Weber, B., Offit, K. et al. 1996b. Frequency of recurrent BRCA1 and BRCA2 mutations in Ashkenazi Jewish breast cancer families. *Nature Medicine* **2**: 1179–83

Vandenvelde, C., De Foor, M. and van Beers, D. 1993. HLA-DOB1*03 and cervical intraepithelial neoplasia grades I-III. *Lancet* **341**: 442

Vasen, H.F., Mecklin, J.P., Khan, P.M. and Lynch, H.T. 1991. The International Collaborative Group on Hereditary Non-Polyposis Colorectal Cancer (ICG-HNPCC). *Diseases of the Colon and Rectum* **34**: 424–5.

Vorechovsky, I., Rasio, D., Luo, L.P. et al. 1996. The ATM gene and susceptibility to breast cancer – analysis of 38 breast tumors reveals no evidence for mutation. *Cancer Research* **56**(1): 2726–32.

Wank, R. and Thomssen, C. 1991. High risk of squamous cell carcinoma of the cervix for women with HLA-DQw3. *Nature* **352**: 723–5.

Watson, P., Vasen, H.F., Mecklin, J.P., Jarvinen, H. and Lynch, H.T. 1994. The risk of endometrial cancer in hereditary nonpolyposis colorectal cancer. *American Journal of Medicine* **96**: 516–20.

Weiner, Z., Beck, D., Shteiner, M., Borovik, R., Ben-Shachar, M., Robinzon, E. and Brandes, J.M. 1993. Screening for ovarian cancer in women with breast cancer with transvaginal sonography and color flow imaging. *Journal of Ultrasound Medicine* **12**: 387–93.

Werner-Wasik, M., Schmid, C.H., Bornstein, L.E. and Madoc-Jones, H. 1995. Increased risk of second malignant neoplasms outside radiation fields in patients with cervical carcinoma. *Cancer* **75**: 2281–5.

Whittemore, A.S., Harris, R. and Itnyre, J. 1992. Characteristics relating to ovarian cancer risk: collaborative analysis of 12 US case-control studies. II. Invasive epithelial ovarian cancers in white women. Collaborative Ovarian Cancer Group. *American Journal of Epidemiology* **136**: 1184–203.

Woolas, R.P., Xu, F.J., Jacobs, I.J. et al. 1993. Elevation of multiple serum markers in patients with stage I ovarian cancer. *Journal of the National Cancer Institute* **85**: 1748–51.

Wooster, R., Ford, D., Mangion, J., Ponder, B.A., Peto, J., Easton, D.F. and Stratton, M.R. 1993. Absence of linkage to the ataxia telangiectasia locus in familial breast cancer. *Human Genetics* **92**: 91–4.

Wooster, R., Neuhausen, S.L., Mangion, J. et al. 1994. Localization of a breast cancer susceptibility gene, BRCA2, to chromosome 13q12-13. *Science* **265**: 2088–90.

Wooster, R., Bignell, G., Lancaster, J. et al. 1995. Identification of the breast cancer susceptibility gene BRCA2. *Nature* **378**: 789–92.

11
Cancers of the kidney and urothelium
EAMONN MAHER

Summary

Only a small proportion of renal cell and urothelial cancers are attributable to an inherited predispostion, but the rare conditions which are
associated with an increased risk of these cancers have provided an
insight into mechanisms of carcinogenesis in the more common sporadic
cancers. Thus this chapter provides a detailed clinical and molecular
analysis of von Hippel–Lindau disease, which is a rare disorder in itself,
but mutations in the causative gene, *VHL*, are very common in sporadic
renal cell cancer. Other types of familial clear and non-clear cell renal
cancer are also discussed. Urothelial cancer is associated with other
inherited syndromes such as hereditary non-polyposis colorectal cancer,
but more relevant in most cases is the population variation in the physiological response to carcinogens, operating via enzymes such as *N*-
acetyl transferase.

Renal cell carcinoma

This is the most common adult renal neoplasm and each year at least
25,000 cases are diagnosed in the US alone. Smoking is the main risk
factor and only a small fraction of cases are familial (~2%), however, as
with other familial cancer syndromes, investigations of rare familial disorders predisposing to renal cell carcinoma (RCC) have provided important clues to the genetic basis of non-familial RCC.

von Hippel–Lindau (VHL) disease

This disorder is the most frequent cause of inherited susceptibility to
RCC. Although only about 10% of VHL patients present with RCC,

this is the most common cause of death and the risk of RCC exceeds 70% by age 60 years (Maher et al., 1990a). Furthermore at least 50% of patients with RCC have bilateral or multicentric tumours and the mean age at onset of RCC is in the fourth decade, at least 15 years before that of sporadic cases (Maher et al., 1990b). Early detection of small asymptomatic RCC improves the prognosis of VHL patients and regular renal imaging from age 15 years is now recognized to be an important requirement for the optimal management of VHL disease families (Maher, 1994; Choyke et al., 1995). Renal cysts are frequent in VHL disease and although annual ultrasonography is the primary method of renal surveillance in many centres, CT scanning is more sensitive and may be preferred in the presence of severe cystic disease. MRI scanning may be a useful adjunct to CT scanning and ultrasonography (Choyke et al., 1995). The identification of small (< 2 cm) solid lesions does not necessitate immediate removal and some lesions may enlarge slowly (Choyke et al., 1992). However, tumours > 3 cm are usually excised because of the risk of metastatic disease. A conservative nephron-sparing approach to surgical management is now undertaken in most centres (Walther et al., 1995). Although many patients subsequently develop further primary tumours, the conservative approach does seem to be associated with only a small risk of metastatic spread and the need for dialysis or transplantation may be delayed for many years with this pproach (Steinbach et al.,1995).

The other major complications of VHL disease are retinal, cerebellar and spinal haemangioblastomas, phaeochromocytoma (adrenal and extra-adrenal) and renal, pancreatic and epididymal cysts. Although visceral cysts are common in VHL, symptomatic disease is infrequent (Thompson et al., 1989). Rarer complications of VHL disease include pancreatic tumours (usually islet cell) which are often malignant and endolymphatic sac tumours (Binkovitz et al., 1990; Choyke et al., 1995). Early detection of VHL tumours may reduce morbidity and mortality, and affected patients and at risk relatives should be offered regular screening (see Table 11.1).

VHL disease displays age-dependent penetrance (86% and 97% at 40 and 60 years respectively) and variable expression, and the diagnosis is often delayed, particularly in isolated cases (Maher et al., 1990a). The standard clinical diagnostic criteria require only a single manifestation (haemangioblastoma or visceral lesion) in the presence of a family history of retinal or cerebellar haemangioblastoma, but either two haemangioblastomas or a single hamangioblastoma and a visceral lesion are

Table 11.1. *Example of a screening protocol for von Hippel–Lindau disease in affected patients and at risk relatives*

Affected Patient
1. Annual physical examination and urine testing.
2. Annual direct and indirect ophthalmoscopy
3. MRI (or CT) brain scan every three years to age 50 and every five years thereafter.
4. Annual abdominal (renal/pancreas/adrenal) ultrasound scan, with CT scan every three years
5. Annual 24-hour urine collection for VMAs and normetadrenaline.

At Risk Relative*
1. Annual physical examination and urine testing.
2. Annual direct and indirect ophthalmoscopy from age 5. Annual fluoroscein angioscopy or angiography from age 10 (see text) until age 60.
3. MRI (or CT) brain scan every three years to from age 15 to 40 years and then every five years until age 60 years.
4. Annual abdominal (renal/pancreas/adrenal) ultrasound scan, with abdominal CT scan every three years from age 16 to 65 years.
5. Annual 24-hour urine collection for VMAs and normetadrenaline.

Note: Adapted from Maher et al. (1990).
*Screening can be relaxed or discontinued in individuals shown to be at low risk or negligible risk by DNA analysis.
MRI: magnetic resonance imaging; CT: computed tomography; VMA: vanillyl-mandelic acid (3-methyoxy-4-hydroxy mandelic acid).

required if there is no clear family history (Melmon and Rosen, 1964). The first degree relatives of all isolated cases should be carefully investigated for subclinical manifestations of VHL, but after careful investigation, most isolated cases appear to represent de novo mutations (Richards et al., 1995). Although the presence of renal, pancreatic, or epididymal cysts in an at risk relative satisfies the standard diagnostic criteria, these lesions can occur in normal individuals and do not provide unequivocal evidence of carrier status. The variability of expression of VHL disease requires that all unusual or new symptoms should be promptly investigated, but in addition, regular surveillance of heterozygotes and at risk relatives allows complications to be detected early and reduces morbidity and mortality. A typical surveillance protocol is detailed in Table 11.1.

The gene for VHL disease was isolated by a positional cloning approach in 1993, five years after the initial mapping to chromosome 3p25 by linkage studies (Seizinger et al., 1988; Latif et al., 1993). The

VHL coding sequence is represented in three exons and germline *VHL* gene mutations may be identified in ~75% of VHL patients and in some patients with familial phaeochromocytoma (Crossey et al., 1994a; Richards et al., 1994; Chen et al., 1995a; Crossey et al., 1995; Neumann et al., 1995; Maher et al., 1996). Up to 20% of patients have large deletions detected by Southern analysis or pulsed field gel electrophoresis, and a further 55% small intragenic mutations. DNA based predictive testing (by direct mutation analysis or linked DNA markers) is possible in the majority of families, and enables annual screening to be discontinued in relatives who are shown not to be gene carriers. The characterization of *VHL* germline mutations has enabled correlations between genotype and phenotype to be established (Crossey et al., 1994a; Richards et al., 1994; Chen et al., 1995b; Maher et al., 1996). The most striking association is with predisposition to phaeochromocytoma, the incidence of which varies widely between families. Most VHL families without phaeochromocytoma have deletions or mutations predicted to cause a truncated pVHL, while predisposition to phaeochromocytoma is strongly associated with the presence of missense mutations. Specific missense mutations may have differing phenotypes. Substitution of an arginine at codon 167 causes a high incidence of phaeochromocytoma and of RCC and other VHL complications. In contrast, Tyr98His also produces a high risk of phaeochromocytoma and haemangioblastomas, but a low risk of RCC (Brauch et al., 1995). Some missense mutations may predispose to phaeochromocytoma only (Crossey et al., 1995; Neumann et al., 1995). These findings suggest that pVHL has tissue specific functions (Maher et al., 1996). Intragenic *VHL* gene mutations are not distributed randomly through the coding sequence. Many mutations appear to interfere with the function of the elongin binding domain (codons 157 to 189) (see below), but no mutations have been described in the first 54 codons. This 5' region is poorly conserved between the human and rodent *VHL* genes (Duan et al., 1995a; Gao et al., 1995).

VHL gene product binds to the B and C subunits of the elongin heterotrimer and so prevents assembly of the complete elongin complex (Duan et al., 1995b; Kibel et al., 1995). The elongin complex (S3 transcription factor) upregulates transcription of target genes by reducing RNA polymerase II pausing, thereby increasing the rate of transcriptional elongation. pVHL inhibits transcriptional elongation in vitro and has been demonstrated to downregulate expression of vascular endothelial growth factor, which is known to be overexpressed in haemangioblastomas and sporadic RCC (Brown et al., 1993; Wizigmann-

Voos et al., 1995; Siemeister et al., 1996). It has been proposed that the localization of pVHL within the cell is dependent on cell density such that it is predominantly cytoplasmic in confluent cultures and nuclear in sparse cultures (Lee et al., 1996).

VHL tumours characteristically demonstrate loss or inactivation of the wild-type *VHL* allele irrespective of the tumour type or nature of the germline mutation (Crossey et al., 1994b; unpub. obs.), so that the *VHL* gene appears to function as a classic tumour suppressor gene. RCC in VHL patients has a clear cell appearance, as do almost 80% of sporadic RCC. Chromosome 3p allele loss is the most frequent genetic event in clear cell RCC and appears to occur early in tumourigenesis. Although detailed analysis of the pattern of chromosome 3p allele loss in sporadic RCC provided evidence for at least three distinct critical regions (at 3p14, 3p21 and 3p25) (van der Hout et al., 1991; Yamakawa et al., 1991; Foster et al., 1994a), recent studies have shown that the *VHL* gene is inactivated in the majority of sporadic clear cell RCC (Foster et al., 1994b; Gnarra et al., 1994; Shuin et al., 1994). In addition to somatic mutations, the *VHL* gene may also be inactivated by de novo methylation which silences *VHL* expression (Herman et al., 1994). Both 3p allele loss and *VHL* gene mutations appear to be infrequent in non-clear cell (papillary) RCC. Introduction of wild-type VHL protein into a VHL deficient RCC cell line has been reported to suppress tumourigenicity in a nude mice assay, but the effects on in vitro growth have been inconsistent (Chen et al., 1995a; Iliopoulos et al., 1995).

Familial clear cell RCC without evidence of VHL disease

Isolated, familial clear cell RCC occurs rarely, and large families are uncommon. Although *VHL* gene mutations have been identified in some cases of familial phaeochromocytoma (Crossey et al., 1995; Neumann et al., 1995), so far, germline *VHL* gene mutations have not been reported in familial clear cell RCC kindreds. However, in a few cases, susceptibility to clear cell RCC has been associated with constitutional rearrangements of chromosome 3p. In these cases the translocation breakpoint are distant from the *VHL* gene in chromosome 3p14. In the best studied case, a t(3;8) was associated with a high risk of RCC in a large North American kindred (Cohen et al., 1979). The translocation breakpoint was cloned and two candidate tumour suppressor genes, *HRCA1* and *FHIT*, were isolated from the peritranslocation region (Boldog et al., 1993; Ohta et al., 1996). Although *HRCA1* has not been implicated in the pathogenesis of sporadic RCC, deletions of *FHIT* are frequent in a variety of cancers and inactivation of this gene may be relevant. However, analysis of renal cancers from the t(3;8) family has revealed that the derivative chromosome 8 (containing 3p14-p26) has been lost from the tumour and somatic *VHL* mutations occur on the retained chromosome 3 (Gnarra et al., 1994; Schmidt et al., 1995). These results would appear to suggest that the translocation associated RCC susceptibility may not result from disruption of a tumour suppressor gene at the translocation site, but rather that the translocated chromosome is unstable and easily lost from cells in which a somatic *VHL* gene mutation has occurred.

Non-clear cell renal cancer

The infrequency of both chromosome 3p allele loss and *VHL* gene mutations in sporadic non-clear cell RCC suggests genetic heterogeneity in sporadic RCC, and similar findings have been reported in familial RCC. Thus Zbar et al. (1994, 1995), described 10 kindreds with familial papillary non-clear cell RCC. Inheritance was compatible with an age-dependent autosomal dominant predisposition with incomplete penetrance. Screening of at risk relatives often revealed asymptomatic multiple tumours. Linkage to the *VHL* gene was excluded in those families suitable for linkage analysis (Zbar et al., 1995). The most frequent cytogenetic abnormality in non-clear cell RCC is trisomy 7 (van den Berg et al., 1993) and a specific chromosomal translocation between chromosomes X and 1 (t(X;1)(p11;q21)) has been described for a subgroup of human papillary RCC (Meloni et al., 1993). Molecular genetic analysis of sporadic RCC has indicated that, compared to clear cell tumours, deletions of the long arms of chromosome 11 and 21 are common in papillary RCC (Thrash-Bingham et al., 1995). It seems reasonable to expect that clues to the location of susceptibility genes might be obtained from animal models of renal cancer. The gene mutated in the Eker rat model of familial papillary renal cancer has been isolated and is the rat homologue of the human tuberous sclerosis (TSC2) gene (The European Chromosome 16 Tuberous Sclerosis Consortium 1993; Yeung et al., 1994; Kobayashi et al., 1995). Although an increased incidence of RCC has been reported in tuberous sclerosis, the absolute risk of RCC appears to be small (~2%) and the most frequent renal complications of tuberous sclerosis are angiomyolopipomas (49%) and renal cysts (32%) (Cook et al., 1996). Eker rat tumours show loss of the wild type *tsc2* allele, but somatic *TSC2* mutations or allele loss have not yet been reported in sporadic non-clear cell human RCC.

Renal pelvis cancer

Carcinoma of the renal pelvis, may be a feature of hereditary nonpolyposis colorectal cancer (HNPCC) syndrome (Chapter 9), but somatic mutations DNA-mismatch repair genes such as *MSH2* and *MLH1* do not appear to have a major role in the pathogenesis of sporadic RCC (Thrash-Bingham et al., 1995).

Urothelial cancer

Although cancers of the ureter and bladder may be seen in HNPCC (Chapter 9) and there may be an increased risk of bladder cancer in patients with germline *RB-1* mutations, familial bladder cancer is rare and the most important contribution of genetic factors to bladder cancer risk is probably in determining individual susceptibility to environmental carcinogens such as tobacco or occupational exposure to aromatic amine compounds. As many chemical carcinogenes become hazardous as a result of host metabolism, interindividual variations in the activity of metabolic enzymes might influence individual susceptibility. Hence many studies have attempted to associate various cancers with genetic polymorphisms in metabolic enzymes. Initial studies have often relied on phenotyping assays. However, such studies are difficult to perform and may be influenced by host factors such as concomitant drug therapy, coexisting disease, smoking status and renal function, and often initial associations have not been confirmed. Definition of the molecular basis for variations in metabolic phenotypes allows direct genotyping to be performed. Some of these studies relevant to tobacco-related cancers are discussed in detail in Chapter 17. Genotype studies are likely to be more robust, but the selection of suitable controls remains an important problem (Wolf et al., 1994). Phenotypic variations at the cytochrome P450 *CYP2D6* gene had been associated with susceptibility to bladder cancer. Daly et al., (1993) reported a higher frequency of homozygotes for the *GSTM1* null allele in bladder tumour patients than controls. However, although the GSTM1 pathway is thought to be involved in the metabolism of tobacco carcinogens, there was no difference in the *GSTM1* genotypes of smokers and non-smokers with bladder cancer and the findings were not confirmed by Zhong et al. (1993). *N*-acetyltransferase (NAT) activity has been implicated in the metabolism of arylamines which, in addition to their role in occupational bladder cancer, are also found in cigarette smoke. Using molecular genetic methods to define NAT2 status, Risch et al. (1995) confirmed previous phenotyping studies which had associated slow acetylators with occupational bladder cancer. In addition, Risch et al. (1995) also demonstrated an association between slow-acetylators and bladder cancer in cigarette smokers. The determination of the genetic basis for additional variations in metabolic phenotypes will allow the more precise genotype association studies to be performed and enable the possible effects of interactions between polymorphic variants in different genes to be studied in relevant patient groups. This should provide a clearer picture of the relevance of inherited factors in susceptibility to environmental carcinogens in the pathogenesis of bladder cancer.

Bladder tumours are frequently synchronous or metachronous. However, while these features are classical indicators of genetic susceptibility, molecular studies have suggested that multicentricity does not reflect a high incidence of multiple primary tumours, but rather that a single primary transformation event may seed other tumours by spread across the urothelium. Under this model, inactivation of a chromosome 9 tumour suppressor gene occurs early in tumourigenesis and precedes the spread of malignant cells along the urothelium. Later mutational events including loss of tumour suppressor genes on chromosomes 13 (retinoblastoma gene), 17 (*TP53*) and 18 may determine cancer invasiveness (Sidransky et al., 1992; Habuchi et al., 1993).

Conclusion

Renal cell cancers are increasing in incidence in the western world. Although cigarette smoking is an important factor, there have been very few clues to the aetiology of these cancers, so the identification of genes that predispose to renal clear cell cancers has been particularly welcome. Thus identifying *VHL*, the gene responsible for the rare von Hippel–Lindau syndrome has proved to be a crucial step in the understanding of the molecular events that lead to sporadic renal cell cancer. Other rarer types of renal cancer are less well investigated, but a number of attractive candidate genes remain to be studied in detail. Urothelial cancers are also smoking-related, but do not feature in von Hippel–Lindau disease. They have been noted in HNPCC families and bladder cancer is seen in association with mutations in *RB-1*. The role of metabolic enzyme polymorphisms in determining risk is as yet uncertain, but N-acetyl transferase in particular is worthy of further study.

References

Binkovitz, L.A., Johnson, C.D. and Stephens, D.H. 1990. Islet cell tumors in von Hippel-Lindau disease: increased prevalence and relationship to the multiple endocrine neoplasias. *American Journal of Roentgenology* **155**: 501–5.

Boldog. F.L., Gemmill, R.M., Wilkie, C.M. et al. 1993. Positional cloning of the hereditary renal carcinoma 3;8 chromosome translocation breakpoint. *Proceedings of the National Academy of Sciences, USA* **90**: 8509–13.

Brauch, H., Kishida, T., Glavac, D. et al. 1995. Von Hippel–Lindau (VHL) disease with pheochromocytoma in the Black Forest region of Germany: evidence for a founder effect. *Human Genetics* **95**: 551–6.

Brown L, Berse B, Jackman R, Tognazzi K, Manseau E, Dvorak H, Senger D. 1993. Increased expression of vascular permeability factor (vascular endothelial growth factor) and its receptors in kidney and bladder carcinomas. *American Journal of Pathology* **143**: 1255-1262.

Chen, F., Kishida, T., Duh, F.M., Renbaum, P., Orcutt, M.L., Schmidt, L., Zbar, B. 1995a. Suppression of growth of renal carcinoma cells by the von Hippel–Lindau tumor suppressor gene. *Cancer Research* **55**: 4804–7.

Chen, F., Kishida, T., Yao, M. et al. 1995b. Germline mutations in the von Hippel-Lindau disease tumor suppressor gene: correlations with phenotype. *Human Mutation* **5**: 66–75.

Choyke, P.L., Glenn, G.M., Walther, M.M. et al. 1992. The natural history of renal lesions in von Hippel–Lindau disease: a serial CT study in 28 patients. *American Journal of Roentgenology* **159**: 1229–34.

Choyke, P.L., Glenn, G.M., Walther, M.M., Patronas, N.J., Linehan, W.M. and Zbar, B. 1995. von Hippel–Lindau disease: genetic, clinical, and imaging features. *Radiology* **194**: 629–42.

Cohen, A.J., Li, F.P., Berg, S. et al. 1979. Hereditary renal cell carcinoma associated with a chromosomal translocation. *New England Journal of Medicine* **301**: 592–5.

Cook, J.A., Oliver, K., Meuller, R.F. and Sampson, J. 1996. A cross sectional study of renal involvement in tuberous sclerosis. *Journal of Medical Genetics* **33**: 480–4.

Crossey, P.A., Eng, C., Ginalska-Malinowska, M., Lennard, T.W.J., Wheeler, D.C., Ponder, B.A.J. and Maher, E.R. 1995. Molecular genetic diagnosis of von Hippel–Lindau disease in familial phaeochromocytoma. *Journal of Medical Genetics* **32**: 885–6.

Crossey, P.A., Foster, K., Richards, F.M. et al. 1994a. Molecular genetic investigations of the mechanism of tumourigenesis in von Hippel–Lindau disease: analysis of allele loss in VHL tumours. *Human Genetics* **93**: 53–8.

Crossey, P.A., Richards, F.M., Foster, K. et al. 1994b. Identification of intragenic mutations in the von Hippel–Lindau disease tumour suppressor gene and correlation with disease phenotype. *Human Molecular Genetics* **3**: 1303–8.

Daly, A.K., Thomas, D.J., Cooper, J., Pearson, W.R., Neal, D. E. and Idle, J.R. 1993. Homozygous deletion of the gene for glutathione S-transferase M1 in bladder cancer. *British Medical Journal* **307**: 481–2.

Duan, D.R., Humphrey, J.S., Chen, D.Y. et al. 1995a Characterization of the VHL tumor suppressor gene product: localization, complex formation, and the effect of natural inactivating mutations. *Proceedings of the National Academy of Sciences, USA* **92**: 6459–63

Duan, D.R., Pause, A., Burgess, W.H. et al. 1995b. Inhibition of transcription elongation by the VHL tumor suppressor protein. *Science* **269**: 1402–6.

Foster, K, Crossey, P.A., Cairns, P. et al. 1994a. Molecular genetic investigation of sporadic renal cell carcinoma: analysis of allele loss on chromosomes 3p, 5q, 11p, 17 and 22. *British Journal of Cancer* **69**: 230–4.

Foster, K., Prowse, A., van den Berg, A. et al. 1994b. Somatic mutations of the von Hippel–Lindau disease tumour suppressor gene in non-familial clear cell renal carcinoma. *Human Molecular Genetics* **3**: 2169–73.

Gao, J., Naglich, J.G., Laidlaw, J., Whaley, J.M., Seizinger, B.R. and Kley, N. 1995. Cloning and characterization of a mouse gene with homology to the human von Hippel–Lindau disease tumor suppressor gene: implications for the potential organization of the human von Hippel–Lindau disease gene. *Cancer Research* **55**: 743–7.

Gnarra, J.R., Tory, K., Weng, Y. et al. 1994. Mutations of the VHL tumour suppressor gene in renal carcinoma. *Nature Genetics* **7**: 85–90.

Habuchi, T., Ogawa, O., Kakehi, Y. et al. 1993. Accumulated allelic losses in the development of invasive urothelial cancer. *International Journal of Cancer* **53**: 579–84.

Herman, J.G., Latif, F., Weng, Y. et al. 1994. Silencing of the VHL tumor-suppressor gene by DNA methylation in renal carcinoma. *Proceedings of the National Academy of Sciences USA* **91**: 9700–4.

Iliopoulos, O., Kibel, A., Gray, S. and Kaelin, W., Jr. 1995. Tumour suppression by the human von Hippel–Lindau gene product. *Nature Medicine* **1**: 822–6.

Kibel, A., Iliopoulos, O., DeCaprio, J.A. and Kaelin, W., Jr. 1995. Binding of the von Hippel–Lindau tumor suppressor protein to Elongin B and C. *Science* **269**: 1444–6.

Kobayashi, T., Hirayama, Y., Kobayashi, E., Kubo, Y. and Hino, O. 1995. A germline insertion in the tuberous sclerosis (Tsc2) gene gives rise to the Eker rat model of dominantly inherited cancer. *Nature Genetics* **9**: 70–4.

Latif, F., Tory, K., Gnarra, J. et al. 1993. Identification of the von Hippel–Lindau disease tumor suppressor gene. *Science* **260**: 1317–20.

Lee, S., Chen, D.Y.T., Humphrey, J.S., Gnarra, J.R., Linehan, W.M. and Klausner, R.D. 1996. *Proceedings of the National Academy of Sciences USA* **93**: 1770–5.

Maher, E.R. 1994. Von Hippel–Lindau disease. *European Journal of Cancer* **30A**: 1987–90.

Maher E.R., Webster, A.R., Richards, F.M., Green, J.S., Crossey, P.A., Payne, S.J. and Moore, A.T. 1996. Phenotypic expression in von Hippel–Lindau disease: correlations with germline VHL gene mutations. *Journal of Medical Genetics* **33**: 328–32.

Maher, E.R., Yates, J.R.W. and Ferguson-Smith, M.A. 1990b. Statistical analysis of the two stage mutation model in von Hippel–Lindau disease and in sporadic cerebellar haemangioblastoma and renal cell carcinoma. *Journal of Medical Genetics* **27**: 311–14.

Maher, E.R., Yates, J.R.W., Harries, R., Benjamin, C., Harris, R. and Ferguson-Smith, M.A. 1990a. Clinical features and natural history of von Hippel–Lindau disease. *Quarterly Journal of Medicine* **77**: 1151–63.

Melmon, K.L. and Rosen, S.W. 1964. Lindau's disease. *American Journal of Medicine* **36**: 595–617.

Meloni, A.M., Dobbs, R.M., Pontes, J.E. and Sandberg, A.A. 1993. Translocation (X;1) in papillary renal cell carcinoma. A new cytogenetic subtype. *Cancer Genetics and Cytogenetics* **65**: 1–6.

Neumann, H.P.H., Eng, C., Mulligan, L., Glavac, D. et al. 1995. Consequences of direct genetic testing for germline mutations in the clinical management of families with multiple endocrine neoplasia type 2. *JAMA* **274**: 1149–51.

Ohta, M., Inoue, H., Cotticelli, M. et al. 1996. The FHIT gene, spanning the chromosome 3p14.2 fragile site andd renal carcinoma-associated t(3;8) breakpoint, is abnormal in digestive tract cancers. *Cell* **84**: 587–97.

Richards, F.M., Crossey, P.A., Phipps, M.E. et al. 1994. Detailed mapping of germline deletions of the von Hippel–Lindau disease tumour suppressor gene. *Human Molecular Genetics* **3**: 595–8.

Richards, F.M., Payne, S.J., Zbar, B., Affara, N.A., Ferguson-Smith, M.A. and Maher, E.R. 1995. Molecular analysis of de novo germline mutations in the Von Hippel–Lindau disease gene. *Human Molecular Genetics* **4**: 2139–43.

Risch, A., Wallace, D. M., Bathers, S. and Sim, E.. 1995. Slow N-acetylation genotype is a susceptibility factor in occupational and smoking related bladder cancer. *Human Molecular Genetics* **4**(2): 231–6.

Schmidt, L., Li, F., Bron, R.S. et al. 1995. Mechanism of tumorigenesis of renal carcinomas associated with the constitutional 3;8 translocation. *Cancer Journal from Scientific American* **1**: 191–5.

Seizinger, B.R., Rouleau, G.A., Ozelius, L.J. et al. 1988. Von Hippel–Lindau disease maps to the region of chromosome 3 associated with renal cell carcinoma. *Nature* **332**: 268–9.

Shuin, T., Kondo, K., Torigoe, S. et al. 1994. Frequent somatic mutations and loss of heterozygosity of the von Hippel–Lindau tumor suppressor gene in primary human renal cell carcinomas. *Cancer Research* **54**: 2852–5.

Sidransky, D., Frost, P., von Eschenbach, A., Oyasu, R., Preisinger, A.C. and Vogelstein, B. 1992. Clonal origin bladder cancer. *New England Journal of Medicine* **326**: 737–40.

Siemeister, G., Weindel, K., Mohrs, K., Barleon, B., Martiny-Brown, G. and Marme, D. 1996. Reversion of deregulated expression of vascular endothelial growth factor in human renal carcinoma cells by von Hippel–Lindau tumor suppressor protein. *Cancer Research* **56**: 2299–301.

Steinbach, F., Novick, A.C., Zincke, H. et al., Treatment of renal cell carcinoma in von Hippel–Lindau disease: a multicenter study. *Journal of Urology* **153**: 1812–6.

The European Chromosome 16 Tuberous Sclerosis Consortium. 1993. Identification and characterization of the tuberous sclerosis gene on chromosome 16. *Cell* **751**: 305–15.

Thompson, R.K., Peters, J.I., Sirinek, K. R. and Levine, B.A. 1989. von Hippel–Lindau syndrome presenting as pancreatic endocrine insufficiency: a case report. *Surgery* **105**: 598–604.

Thrash-Bingham, C.A., Salazar, H., Freed, J.J., Grenberg, R.E. and Tartof, K.D. 1995. Genomic alterations and instabilities in renal cell carcinomas and their relationship to tumor pathology. *Cancer Research* **55**: 6189–95.

Van den Berg, E., Van der Hout, A.H., Oosterhuis, J. et al. 1993. Cytogenetic analysis of epithelial renal-cell tumors: relationship with a new histopathological classification. *International Journal of Cancer* **55**: 223–7.

van der Hout, A.H., van der Vlies, P., Wijmenga, C., Li, F.P., Oosterhuis, J.W. and Buys, C.H. 1991. The region of common allelic losses in sporadic renal cell carcinoma is bordered by the loci D3S2 and THRB. *Genomics* **11**: 537–42.

Walther, M.M., Choyke, P.L., Weiss, G. et al. 1995. Parenchymal sparing surgery in patients with hereditary renal cell carcinoma. *Journal of Urology* **153**: 913–6.

Wizigmann-Voos, S., Breier, G., Risau, W. and Plate, K.H. 1995. Up-regulation of vascular endothelial growth factor and its receptors in von Hippel–Lindau disease-associated and sporadic hemangioblastomas. *Cancer Research* **55**: 1358–64.

Wolf, C.R., Smith, C.A.D. and Forman, D. 1994. Metabolic polymorphisms in carcinogen metabolising enzymes and cancer susceptibility. *British Medical Bulletin* **50**: 718–31.

Yamakawa, K., Morita, R., Takahashi, E., Hori, T., Ishikawa, J. and Nakamura, Y. 1991. A detailed deletion mapping of the short arm of chromosome 3 in sporadic renal cell carcinoma. *Cancer Research* **51**: 4707–11.

Yeung, R. S., Xiao, G.H., Jin, F., Lee, W.C., Testa, J.R. and Knudson, A.G. 1994. Predisposition to renal carcinoma in the Eker rat is determined by germ-line mutation of the tuberous sclerosis 2 (TSC2) gene. *Proceedings of the National Academy of Sciences, USA* **91**: 11413-16.

Zbar, B., Glenn, G., Lubensky, I. et al. 1995. Hereditary papillary renal cell carcinoma: clinical studies in 10 families. *Journal of Urology* **153**: 907–12.

Zbar, B., Tory, K., Merino, M. et al. 1994. Hereditary papillary renal cell carcinoma. *Journal of Urology* **151**: 561–6.

Zhong, S., Wyllie, A.H., Barnes, D., Wolf, C.R. and Spurr, N.K. 1993. Relationship between the GSTM1 genetic polymorphism and susceptibility to bladder, breast and colon cancer. *Carcinogenesis* **14**: 1821–4.

12

Cancers of the prostate and testes

STEVEN NAROD, BONNIE KING and DAVID HOGG

Summary

Two cancers that are restricted to males, but are otherwise rather different – prostate cancer, which affects mainly older men, and testicular cancer, which affects a much younger age group – are reviewed in this chapter. While linkage to chromosome 1q has been reported for some prostate cancer families, the genetic basis of testicular cancer is not established. Linkage studies in prostate cancer are discussed, focusing on the exciting development of linkage to a chromosome 1 locus. The strong evidence for genetic heterogeneity is commented on, and the possible role of candidate genes is examined. Finally, the topic of the use of a family history to discriminate those at higher risk (who might be suitable candidates for screening) is introduced. Little is known about the genetics of testicular cancer, although linkage studies have been performed. This section of the chapter reviews these data and also discusses the mouse model for testicular cancer, probably the strongest evidence that susceptibility genes exist in humans. The chapter concludes with a brief review of somatic changes in testicular cancer that may provide clues to the location of susceptibility genes.

Genetic predisposition to prostate cancer – introduction

Prostate cancer is caused by a combination of genetic and environmental factors. It is known that genetic factors are important because of the wide variation in prostate cancer rates between different ethnic groups, and because a family history of prostate cancer is a risk factor for the development of this cancer. A gene for prostate cancer susceptiblity has been mapped to chromosome 1. The identification of this gene location confirms our belief that prostate cancer aggregation in families may be due to inherited susceptibility. Genetic variation may influence the rate at which prostate cancer develops, or the rate at which this cancer progresses or is metastasized. The family history is also important for interpreting a screening test as an increased level of prostate specific antigen (PSA) in the blood is more likely to lead to the diagnosis of prostate cancer if there is a family history of the disease. It is hoped that by increasing our knowledge of genetic factors in prostate cancer, we will be able to individualize risk assessment and screening protocols. This knowledge will also be central to our understanding of the development of the disease.

Linkage studies in prostate cancer

The first chromosomal localization of a gene for prostate cancer was reported in *Science* in November, 1996 (Smith et al., 1996). Isaacs and his colleagues identified a cluster of linked markers on chromosome 1, which contains the locus of a prostate cancer susceptibility gene. This gene, named *HPC1*, accounted for roughly 34% of families in a panel of 66 North American pedigrees with three or more men affected with prostate cancer. These findings provide the best evidence to date that in some cases prostate cancer can appear as a dominant genetic trait, and their report catalysed the worldwide search for the prostate cancer susceptibility gene. There was no evidence that men with prostate cancer in families linked to chromosome 1q were diagnosed earlier than men from unlinked families, or that *HPC1* was associated with an increased risk for cancer at other sites. Based on the estimates that 1 in 170 men might carry a prostate cancer predisposing mutation, and that 34% of such mutations may be of the *HPC1* gene, the authors estimated that up to 1 in 500 men may carry a mutation in *HPC1*.

As was pointed out by Isaacs and his colleagues, it is very difficult to study the genetic basis of prostate cancer by linkage analysis (Smith et al., 1996). Prostate cancer typically occurs at a late age, and it is rare to have DNA available from living affected men in more than one generation. It is difficult to define clearly the age-of-onset of prostate cancer for an individual or to standardize ages between studies. This is because the diagnosis is only rarely made on men with symptoms due to cancer. More commonly the diagnosis is made when a man undergoes a prostatectomy for symptoms of benign hyperplasia and malignant cells are found in the examined pathology specimen. A second common scenario is that an elevated PSA is found during a routine screening examination, and that this prompts a clinical investigation, which leads to the diagnosis of prostate cancer. For these reasons it is difficult to speak of the age of cancer onset in an unequivocal way, or to ask if ages of onset are systematically different between familial and non-familial cases.

Prostate cancer families are usually small and rarely include more than four living affected men. It is difficult to determine whether a particular family is linked to *HPC1* and all such judgements are probabilistic. With the rare exception of very large families, it is always possible that the *HPC1* markers could co-segregate with the cancer phenotype by chance. In order for a family to provide sufficient independent evidence of linkage to chromosome 1, it is typically necessary to have six or more informative meiotic events to examine (an informative meiosis is one where there is an opportunity for recombination – two siblings provide less information than two first cousins). Similarly, it cannot be said with certainty if a given case of prostate cancer in a linked family is hereditary or is due to chance. For these reasons it will be difficult to identify critical recombinants in a prostate cancer family – i.e., it will not be possible to exclude completely the alternative possibilities of a non-linkage family or of sporadic cases. Because of the inherent difficulties with linkage analysis, several other approaches to prostate cancer genetics have been taken.

Redefining the phenotype in hereditary prostate cancer – are other cancers in excess?

It is not yet clear if a family history of prostate cancer is associated with an increased risk of cancer at other sites – the results to date have been contradictory. Several studies have reported that a family history of prostate cancer increases the risk of breast cancer (Theissen, 1974; Cannon et al., 1982; Tulinius et al., 1992; Anderson and Badzioch, 1993, Sellers et al., 1994) but there have been negative studies as well (Isaacs et al., 1995). It is not yet clear to what extent the clustering in families of breast and prostate cancer is due to the *BRCA1* or *BRCA2* genes. Prostate cancer has been reported in excess in families with mutations of both types (Ford et al., 1994; Tonin et al., 1995; Thorlacius et al., 1996). Langston et al. (1996) screened for *BRCA1* mutations in a set of 49 men with either very early onset prostate cancer (< 53 years of age at diagnosis) or with prostate cancer and a family history of premenopausal breast cancer or of prostate cancer. Only one clear example of a *BRCA1* mutation (185delAG) was found; however, the 185delAG mutation is present in up to 1% of Jewish individuals (Struewing et al., 1995) and this may have been a chance finding. From the Gilda Radner Familial Ovarian Cancer Registry, Jishi et al. (1995) found an excess of prostate cancer in families with three or more cases of ovarian cancer. It is assumed that for the majority of these families the prostate cancer was due to mutations in *BRCA1* or *BRCA2*.

Isaacs et al. (1995) did not find an excess of breast cancer in prostate cancer families but found an excess risk of tumours of the central nervous system. Slattery and Kerber (1994) reported a familial association between colon cancer and prostate cancer in the Utah Population Database. In Norway, a significant deficit of prostate cancer was reported in the fathers of patients with testicular cancer (Heimdal et al., 1996).

Patterns of transmission – evidence for genetic heterogeneity

Twin studies provide strong evidence for a genetic component to prostate cancer. From a registry of 4840 male twin pairs in Sweden, 458 cases of prostate cancers were identified. There were 16 concordant pairs among 1649 monozygotic twins, but only six concordant pairs among 2983 dizygotic twin pairs (Grönberg et al., 1994). The average age in the concordant monozygous pairs was younger (72.6 years) than that of the dizygous pairs (75.1 years).

Twin studies cannot be used to infer the genetic mode of transmission and results from family studies of prostate cancer have not lead to a consistently favoured genetic model. Most studies have suggested that prostate cancer susceptibility is best modelled as a dominant trait. In a large case-control study (691 cases) a relative risk (RR) for prostate cancer of 3.0 was found for brothers, 2.0 for fathers, 1.9 for grandfathers, and 1.7 for uncles of men with prostate cancer (Steinberg et al. 1990). A segregation analysis performed on this set of families led these investigators to conclude that prostate cancer inheritance best fits an autosomal dominant model, where a rare susceptibility gene with a high lifetime penetrance was transmitted (Carter et al., 1992). The principal weakness of this and other case-control genetic studies of prostate cancer is that the history of prostate cancer in family members is based on the recollection of the index patient and is not confirmed by pathology reports. Reported histories of prostate cancer in second-degree relatives tend to be inaccurate. Prostate cancer patients may be more likely to be aware of the diagnosis in relatives, may be more diligent in their search for additional cases, or may be more likely to misinterpret benign disease as cancer, than are healthy controls. The effect of this recall bias will be to increase

the magnitude of the relative risks associated with a family history, especially for second-degree relatives, where the information is less certain.
For example, the odds ratio for a first-degree relative in the Steinberg
study (Steinberg et al., 1990) was 2.1, and was not significantly different
from the odds ratio for a second-degree relative (1.8). For both dominant
and recessive genetic diseases, the attenuation of relative risk between
first and second-degree relatives is expected to be greater than this.
Furthermore, the frequency of prostate cancer was reported to be 7.5%
in the fathers of unaffected controls but only 2.7% in uncles of controls.
The difference in these two estimates is most likely due to recall bias.
Ideally, the family history of prostate cancer should be taken before the
diagnosis is made – e.g., in the interval between the report of an eleveted
PSA and the diagnostic biopsy.

Not all studies of prostate cancer have concluded that the data best fit
a dominant model. In several studies the risk for brothers was found to be
significantly greater than the risk for sons or fathers of cases. This is
consistent with a recessive or X-linked component to prostate cancer
inheritance. In 1960, Woolf studied familial risks of prostate cancer in
Utah (Woolf, 1960). Deaths from prostate cancer among 228 cases and
their relatives were identified by review of Utah state vital statistics
records, thereby eliminating the possibility of recall bias. The observed
numbers of deaths were compared to the expected number based on rates
from the Utah State Bureau of Vital Statistics and to deaths in a control
group. There were 12 deaths from prostate cancer among brothers of
prostate cancer cases, compared to 4.3 expected (RR = 2.81;
$p = 0.002$), and three deaths in fathers compared to 2.4 expected
(RR = 1.25; not significant). An X-linked susceptibility gene is possible,
but a deficit of allele sharing among siblings with prostate cancer suggest
that the androgen receptor, on the X chromosome, is not the responsible
gene (Sun et al., 1995).

Narod and colleagues (1995) recorded prostate cancer family histories
from 6390 men attending a screening clinic in Quebec City. Family histories were taken prior to screening, and recall bias was not possible.
Prostate cancer was found in 10.2% of subjects who reported a brother
affected; this number was 2.6 times higher than that for men with no
reported affected relative. The corresponding relative risk for men with
an affected father was only 1.2. Monroe and colleagues (1995) studied a
population-based cohort of blacks, whites, Japanese and Hispanics and
found that the relative risk for prostate cancer was approximately twofold larger if the brother was affected than if the father was affected. This

was true for all four ethnic populations. Greater relative risks for brothers were also found by Whittemore et al. (1995) and by Hayes et al. (1995).

In summary, there is likely to be a great deal of genetic heterogeneity in familial prostate cancer. The study by Smith et al. (1996) confirms the existence of at least one highly penetrant dominant susceptibility gene, and there are probably others. However, it is likely that additional susceptibility genes with X-linked, or autosomal recessive, modes of activity will also be found.

There is no clear benign precursor for hereditary prostate cancer, and familial cancers do not appear to be systematically different from sporadic ones (Bastacky et al., 1995). Narod et al. (1995) observed an increase in the frequency of abnormal rectal examinations in relatives of prostate cancer patients. The exact nature of these lesions is unclear, but a proportion of these were likely to be cases of benign prostatic hyperplasia. A second study reported that a family history of prostate disease (cancer or hyperplasia) was more frequent in relatives of men with benign hyperplasia (20%) than in relatives of men with prostate cancer (12.8%) or healthy controls (5.1%) (Schuman et al., 1977). These results suggest that common genetic mechanisms may predispose to benign and malignant prostate disease.

Ethnic studies

Rates of prostate cancer vary markedly between different ethnic groups. This variation is probably due to a combination of genetic and environmental factors, although the relative contribution of each is not yet known. Differences in diet appear to explain only a small proportion of observed ethnic variation. African-American men have the highest incidence and mortality rate of any population studied. The rates in Asian men may be fiftyfold less. Although prostate cancer is more frequent among African-American men, it is not known if the fraction attributable to genetic factors is higher in this group. In the study by Whittemore et al. (1995) a report of two or more affected first-degree relatives with prostate cancer was associated with a higher relative risk in blacks (RR = 9.7) than it was in whites (RR = 3.9) or in Asians (RR = 1.6). However, no differences were seen in the magnitudes of the familial relative risks between blacks and whites in the study by Hayes et al. (1995).

Association studies

Because of the inherent difficulties in the linkage approach to prostate cancer, several investigators have taken the candidate gene approach. An association study is one strategy for assessing the importance of candidate genes. As a first step, polymorphic genetic variation is sought within the candidate gene, or in a nearby region. In some cases the polymorphic alleles may differ in the amino acid sequence of the protein. These coding polymorphisms are given priority for study because it is felt that the different forms of the protein may have different functional activities. A second class of polymorphisms of interest are those which are present in the untranslated region of the RNA. These polymorphic variants are believed to influence transcript stability. The most common class of polymorphisms are in the non-coding region of the DNA.

Candidate genes are often chosen either because they code for enzymes or for receptors of hormones which are known to be involved in prostate gland growth and differentiation, or because they are involved in carcinogenesis at other sites. Cancer genes of interest may be active in cell cycle control, DNA stability or repair, or mutagen sensitivity.

Androgen receptor studies

Testosterone is the principal steroid hormone involved in prostate growth. Dihydrotestosterone is the most active metabolite. It exerts its effect on cell growth through binding to the androgen receptor in the cytoplasm and then passing into the nucleus. There is a well studied polymorphic CAG tract in exon 1 of the androgen receptor which has been used for several prostate cancer association studies. The frequency of short alleles of the androgen receptor (those with fewer than 20 repeat units) is higher in blacks than in whites (Coetzee and Ross, 1994). It has been proposed that this distributional difference may account to some degree for the higher cancer incidence in blacks. In a case-control study, Ingles et al. (1997) found that prostate cancer cases with short CAG repeat lengths (fewer than 20 repeat units) had an increased risk of prostate cancer in their relatives. In summary, there are limited data that suggest that germline variation in the androgen receptor is involved in susceptibility to prostate cancer. There is also evidence that somatic mutations of the androgen receptor may influence prostate cancer growth and androgen independence (Taplin et al., 1995).

The vitamin D receptor

There are several polymorphisms of the vitamin D receptor which have been studied. Taylor et al. (1996) studied a TaqI RFLP at codon 352. The allele with the restriction site present is referred to as allele t. Only 8% of 108 cases were homozygous tt, as opposed to 22% of white controls ($p < 0.01$) A second polymorphism is found in the non-coding 3' untranslated region of the Vitamin D receptor. The polymorphism is based on variation in the length of a poly A tract in the 3' untranslated region of the gene. Ingles and colleagues found that the presence of a long allele of this vitamin D receptor polymorphism (i.e., greater than 17 repeat units) was associated with a fourfold increase in risk (Ingles et al., 1997). However, 95% of the control population carried at least one copy of the susceptibility allele. Only a small subgroup of 5% of the population has two short alleles and could be considered at low risk. Because the high risk allele is the common allele, this polymorphism is not expected to account for the clustering of prostate cancer in extended families. Doll et al. (1996) reported an association between a specific allele of the poly (ADP ribose) polymerase gene (*PADPRP*) and prostate cancer in black Americans, but their sample size was small and their observations have not yet been replicated.

The importance of genetic factors in the progresion of prostate cancer

Theoretically, genetic factors might influence any of the stages of prostate carcinogenesis, and may affect either the cancer incidence rate or the rate of progression. For example, the observation that an increased incidence of prostate cancer is associated with a particular allele might be because the allele increases susceptibility to prostate cancer or, that once established, the allele is associated with an increased rate of tumour growth or a tendency to metastasize. For this reason, it is possible that different genetic patterns may be observed or that different susceptibility genes described, depending on how the cancer phenotype is defined. For example, studies based on the occurrence of prostate cancer at autopsy may give different results from studies of men who are known to have died from prostate cancer. Similarly, a study of men with metastatic disease may give results that differ from a study based on a series of men with prostate cancer detected through an elevated PSA at age 50.

Screening – can family history help?

One of the main goals of identifying genetic markers for prostate cancer is that these markers will allow clinicians to identify men at high risk of cancer for preventive strategies. Because little is known about environmental causes of prostate cancer, current preventive strategies focus on early detection through screening. Family history is probably the most important known factor which can be used to identify men at high risk. The serum test for PSA is proposed to be a sensitive and specific means of detecting asymptomatic prostate cancer prior to metastatic spread. It is hoped that population-based screening programmes using PSA will be successful in reducing mortality from the disease. The positive predictive value of a screening test will increase with the prevalence of the condition in the screened population. Narod and colleagues (1995) found that the positive predictive value of a PSA test above 3.0 µg/l was higher for men with a postive family history of prostate cancer. For example, among men with a normal rectal examination and a PSA greater than 3.0 µg/l per liter, 12% were found to have cancer if the family history was negative, but 27% were found to have cancer if there was an affected first degree relative. It is currently recommended in many centres that PSA screening be offered to men with a family history of prostate cancer, but there is no consensus yet as to the appropriate age at which screening should begin. McWhorter et al. (1992) screened 34 healthy men from high risk prostate cancer families. Each family contained two brothers affected with prostate cancer. Screening was performed using both PSA and random four quadrant needle biopsies. Prostate cancer was found in eight (24%) of the men. The PSA level was elevated in only three of the men with cancer. This study suggests that enhanced surveillance is warranted in high risk men based on family history and that such surveillance should include a random biopsy, although controlled trials would be welcome.

Familial testicular cancer – introduction

Testicular teratoma is one of the commonest cancers in young men. Advances in treatment of teratoma have resulted in substantial improvements in survival. Testicular tumours are rarely seen in the same family, but the relative risks associated with a first degree relative with testicular cancer can be substantial, rather like Hodgkin's disease, which is also rarely seen in close relatives of affected cases. Linkage studies are hampered by this fact, and also by the absence of any clear pattern of transmission. Non-parametric studies may be more informative. Mouse models suggest that susceptibility genes do exist, but there are significant differences between the murine and human disease. Somatic mutation studies may point towards the location of genes that are mutated in the germline, but up until now, this has not been a useful avenue for the identification of inherited cancer genes. Triplet expansions have not been associated with human cancer, but early results in testicular cancer families suggest they may play a role in susceptibility to this cancer.

Pathology

Testicular germ cell tumours may be classified by the age of presentation into those affecting infants, those affecting adolescents and young adults, and those affecting older men (De Jong et al., 1990). Adult germ cell tumours are divided into seminomas and non-seminomas in roughly equal numbers. Non-seminomas include embryonal carcinomas, teratocarcinomas and choriocarcinomas, and mixed tumours, including mixed seminomas/non-seminomas and mixed non-seminomas. The malignant cells likely arise from gonocytes, the immature precursors of spermatogonia (Bailey et al., 1986). During the development of germ cell tumours, cells pass through an intermediate stage of carcinoma in situ in the seminiferous tubules (Haillot et al., 1992). Tumours in infants are commonly yolk sac tumours, whereas tumours in older men are commonly spermatocytic seminoma. Yolk cell tumours are not discussed further in this review.

Evidence for inherited susceptibility to testicular cancer

The lifetime risk for developing testicular cancer is estimated to be 1 in 286 Caucasian males. The risk is much higher in patients with a previous history of testicular cancer and in patients with a family history of the disease (Nicholson and Harland, 1995). Familial predisposition to testicular cancer (as measured by relative risks for the first degree relatives of affected cases) may be as great as, or greater than, that for cancer of the breast, colon, or skin. The risk for germ cell tumours differs greatly between populations – the incidence is about four times greater in the white population than in the black population (Daniels et al., 1981). This ethnic variation may be due in part to different genetic susceptibility but the specific genes and environmental factors involved have not been identified. Within the limits of current demographic studies, these differences seem to be related to genetic background, as incidence rates do not appear to vary with migration (Daniels et al., 1981). Children with cryptorchidism are at an increased risk of testicular cancer. The risk persists after relocation of the testicle to the scrotum, suggesting an underlying predisposition to both conditions. Patients with a history of testis cancer have a relative risk for a second germ cell tumour in the contralateral testis up to 35 times higher than that of the general population (Van Leeuwen et al., 1993). Cannon-Albright et al. (1994) correlated genealogical records in Utah with the State Cancer Registry and found that a number of malignancies clustered in families. The tumour sites demonstrating the greatest tendency towards familial clustering included the testes, small intestine, lip, and thyroid (Cannon-Albright et al., 1994). This observation fits well with studies of familial testicular cancer that have reported a relative risk to brothers of between 6 and 10 (Nicholson and Harland, 1995). It also fits with the clinical observation that large pedigrees with mutliply affected members are rarely, if ever, seen for any of these four cancers. Because several studies have oberved that the risk of developing testicular cancer appears to have doubled over the past 25 years, environmental factors may also play a role in accelerating the development of this malignancy (Hoff Wanderas et al., 1995; Bergstrom et al., 1996).

Nicholas and Harland (1995) reviewed the published reports of families with multiple cases of testicular cancer. The age of presentation of the familial cases was found to be slightly younger (mean of 29 years) than non-familial controls (mean of 36 years). The risk of bilateral disease was also higher in the familial cases (15% vs. 5%). Interestingly, the age at first tumour presentation of bilateral cases in the general population is similar to that of familial cases, suggesting that bilateral cases may represent unrecognized familial cases. Based on the assumption that most, if not all, bilateral cases are hereditary, this ratio yields a hereditary fraction of testicular cancer of 33%. However, it is not clear that this assumption is correct. Certainly for other early-onset tumours without a strong familial component, such as Wilms', there is no clear evidence that bilateral tumours are more likely to be hereditary than unilateral tumours (see Chapter 19). Affected sibling-pairs were more commonly reported than affected father–son pairs. Even allowing for reduced fertility rates in fathers, these observations might be explained by a recessive testicular cancer gene with a frequency of the susceptibility allele of 5%. Alternate explanations for the predominance of sibling-pairs include an X-linked component or strong environmental factors.

Mouse models for germ cell tumours

The mouse strain SV-129/ter is susceptible to testicular teratomas (Noguchi and Noguchi, 1985). Genetic analyses have demonstrated that four to five loci appear to contribute to the cancer susceptibility phenotype (J. Nadeau, 1996, pers. comm.). One of these loci, designated ter, appears to be particularly important. Homozygous ter/ter animals are germ cell deficient and most develop teratomas, 75% of which are bilateral. Heterozygous ter/+ mice are not germ cell deficient and 17% develop teratomas, most of which are unilateral. Interestingly, mice that are ter/ter do not develop testicular cancer when moved to a genetic background other than the SV-129 strain (Noguchi and Noguchi, 1985). This observation suggests the presence of modifier genes that act in an epistatic fashion to strongly influence the phenotypic effect of the ter gene. The ter gene is located on mouse chromosome 18 in a region which is syntenic to human chromosome 5q31 (Asada et al., 1994; Sakurai et al., 1994). No specific sequences mapping to these loci have been associated with testicular cancers mouse or humans, respectively. The genetic similarity of the murine to human disease is striking, although heterozygous mice do develop tumours, while most humans presumably do not.

Linkage studies in human testicular cancer

Two linkage studies of testicular cancer have been reported to date. An initial study from the Imperial Cancer Research Fund group in 1995 was based on the analysis of 35 sibling pairs types for 220 markers throughout the genome yielded six regions with LOD (logarithm of odds) scores in excess of 1.0 (Leahy et al., 1995). One region on chromosome 4 gave a LOD score of 2.6. A follow-up study by the International Testis Cancer Linkage Consortium (1996) was unable to verify the chromosome 4 linkage but did identify another locus on chromosme 12q at a LOD score of 2.0. LOD scores of this magnitude are often due to chance. Linkage was not found to 5q31, the region syntenic to the mouse ter loucs.

Cytogenetic and molecular genetic changes in testicular cancer

Some clues as to the location of putative testicular cancer susceptibility genes may be obtained from the examination of somatic mutations or rearrangements in tumours. While chromosomal changes in germ cell tumours are marked by a high incidence of numerical and structural chromosomal abnormalities, a consistent cytogenetic finding is that of an isochromosome 12p, i(12p), which is found in over 85% of germ cell tumours (Chaganti et al., 1993). The i(12p) marker is more common in seminomas than in non-seminomas, and its copy number increases with the stage of the disease, being especially common in metastatic lesions. The significance of the i(12p) is currently a subject of investigation, but may parallel the expression of the cyclin D2 gene on 12p (Sicinski et al., 1996) There have been no reports to date of constitutional involvement of chromosome 12p, (or of any other chromosome region) in familial testicular cancers.

A number of studies of sporadic testicular cancers have examined loss of heterozygosity (LOH) at various loci (Mathew et al., 1994; Murty et al., 1994; Lothe et al., 1995; Peng et al., 1995; Smith and Rukstalis, 1995). These studies have been hampered by the considerable chromosomal aneuploidy observed in these neoplasms, which render interpretation of LOH difficult due to non-specific chromosomal loss. Whether any of the regions identified by various laboratories, such as 18q LOH, do contain genes that predispose to testicular cancer is as yet unproven. *TP53* has been extensively studied in germ cell tumours. Despite the presence of increased amounts of immunostainable material in testicular tumours and in carcinoma in situ (Bartkova et al., 1991) there is a lack of *TP53* mutations in sporadic testicular tumours (Peng et al., 1993) and in germline DNA from individuals with familial testicular cancer (Heimdal et al. 1993). This latter finding is not surprising as testicular cancer is rarely featured in Li–Fraumeni syndrome (see Chapters 10 and 19). A recent study has demonstrated that the p53 protein in murine teratocarcinoma cells is present in increased amounts and while physically normal is functionally inactive, being unable to transactivate the mdm-2 and p21 genes (Lutzker and Levine, 1996). Interestingly, treatment of cells with etoposide appears to functionally activate p53, leading to transcription of target genes and apoptosis of the cells. This response may explain the exquisite sensitivity of testicular cancers to DNA-damaging agents and the ability to cure many patients with radiation and chemotherapy.

Triplet expansion in testicular cancer

Microsatellite instability has been observed in a variety of tumours, particularly in those arising in patients with hereditary non-polyposis colorectal cancer (HNPCC). This instablity has been linked, in some instances, to a defect in DNA repair associated with constitutional or acquired mutations in repair genes (Eshleman et al., 1996; see Chapters 9 and 18). Such dinucleotide repeat instability has not been observed in testicular tumours, with the possible exception of a localized replication error-type genomic instability at 1q42-43 in human male germ cell tumours (Murty et al., 1994b). In contrast, Huddart et al. (1995) observed instablity of trincucleotide and tetranucleotide repeats in testicular cancers.

The intergenerational expansion of triplet repeat microsatellite sequences underlies the transmission of a number of heritable neurological disorders but has not been previously observed in association with malignant disease (Ashley and Warren, 1995). King et al. (1997) used the repeat expansion technique (RED) technique to determine whether (CAG) triplet repeat expansions were present in DNA from malignant cells and observed expanded (CAG) tracts in 5/11 testicular tumour cell lines with concordance between germline and tumour (CAG) tract size. Furthermore, estimation of germline DNA from kindreds predisposed to testicular cancer revealed in increase in (CAG) tract size in five of five families and was particularly striking in one large pedigree where expansions were observed in three of four affected brothers. It is thus possible that a single expanded (CAG) tract may define a locus that resides within or near a gene important to testicular tumorigenesis. Alternatively, a form of genomic instability affecting triplet repeats may be associated with this malignancy.

Conclusion

The age-standardized rates of prostate cancer are increasing in most western countries, particularly for those countries where PSA screening has been introduced. Along with the late age of onset of the disease, this has hampered linkage and gene identification studies. A location for a putative prostate cancer susceptibility gene has nevertheless been identified on chromosome 1, but requires confirmation. The problem with identifying susceptibility genes in testicular cancer is different – very few large pedigrees exist. It may require a candidate gene mutation screen approach, or the use of association studies. It would not be surprising if genes that determine susceptibility to testicular cancer have a role in development of the testes.

References

Anderson, D.E. and Badzioch, M.D. 1993. Familial breast cancer risks. *Cancer* **72**: 114–19.

Asada, Y., Varnum, D.S., Frankel, W.N. and Nadeau, J.H. 1994. A mutation in the Ter gene causing increased susceptibility to testicular teratomas maps to mouse chromosome 18. *Nature Genetics* **6**: 363–8.

Ashley, C.T. and Warren ST. 1995. Trinucleotide repeat expansion and human disease. *Annual Review of Genetics* **29**: 703–28.

Bailey, D., Baumal, R., Law, J. et al. 1986. Production of a monoclonal antibody specific for seminomas and dysgerminomas. *Proceedings of the National Academy of Sciences, USA* **83**: 5291–5.

Bartkova, J., Bartek, J., Lukas, J. et al. 1991. p53 protein alterations in human testicular cancer including pre-invasive intratubular germ-cell neoplasia. *International Journal of Cancer* **49**: 129–202.

Bastacky, S.I., Wojno, K.J., Walsh, P.C., Carmichael, M.J. and Epstein, J.I. 1995. Pathological features of hereditary prostate cancer. *Journal of Urology* **153**: 987–92.

Bergstrom, R., Adami, H.O., Mohner, M. et al. 1996. Increase in testicular cancer incidence in six European countries: a birth cohort phenomenon. *Journal of the National Cancer Institute* **88**: 727–33.

Cannon-Albright, L.A., Thomas, A., Goldgar, D.E. et al. 1994. Familiality of cancer in Utah. *Cancer Research* **54**: 2378–85.

Cannon L, Bishop DT, Skolnick M, Hunt S, Lyon JL, Smart CR. 1982 Genetic epidemiology of prostate cancer in the Utah Mormon genealogy. *Cancer Surveys* **1**: 47-69.

Carter, B.S., Beaty, T.H., Steinberg, G.D., Childs, B. and Walsh, P.C. 1992. Mendelian inheritance of familial prostate cancer. *Proceedings of the National Academy of Sciences USA* **89**: 3367–71.

Chaganti, R.S., Rodriguez, E. and Bosl, G.J. 1993. Cytogenetics of male germ cell tumours. *Urology Clinics of North America* **20**: 55–6.

Coetzee, G.A. and Ross, R.K. 1994. Prostate cancer and the androgen receptor. *Journal of the National Cancer Institute* **86**: 871–2.

Daniels, J.L., Stutzman, R.E. and McLeod, D.G. 1981. A comparison of testicular tumours in black and white patients. *Journal of Urology* **125**: 341–2.

De Jong, B., Oosterhuis, J.W., Castedo, S.M., Vos, A. and te Meerman, G.J. 1990. Pathogenesis of adult testicular germ cell tumours. A cytogenetic model. *Cancer Genetics and Cytogenetics* **48**: 143–67.

Doll, J.A., Suarez, B.K. and Donis-Keller, H. Association between prostate cancer in black Americans and an allele of the PADPRP pseudogene on chromosome 13. *American Journal of Human Genetics* **58**: 425–8.

Eshleman, J.R. and Markowitz, S.D. 1996 Mismatch repair defects in human carcinogenesis. *Human Molecular Genetics* **5**: 1489–94.

Ford, D., Easton, D.F., Bishop, Dt., Narod, S.A., Goldgar, D.E. and the Breast Cancer Linkage Consortium. 1994. Risks of cancer in BRCA1-muation carriers. *Lancet* **343**: 692–5.

Grönberg, H., Damber, L. and Damber, J-E. 1994. Studies of genetic factors in prostate cancer in a twin population. *Journal of Urology* **152**: 1484–9.

Haillot, O., Fetissof, F., Janin, P. and Lanson, Y. 1992. Carcinoma in situ of the testis. *Progress in Urology* **2**: 680–8.

Hayes, R.B., Liff, J.M., Pottern, L.M. et al. 1995. Prostate cancer risk in U.S. blacks and whites with a family history of cancer. *International Journal of Cancer* 60: 361–4.

Heimdal K., Lothe, R.A., Lystad, S. et al. 1993. No germline TP53 mutations detected in familial and bilateral testicular cancer. *Genes Chromosomes and Cancer* 6: 92–7.

Heimdal, K., Olsson, H., Tretli, S., Flodgren, P., Børresen, A.L. and Fossa, S.D. 1996. Risk of cancer in relatives of testicular cancer patients. *British Journal of Cancer* 73: 970–3.

Hoff Wanderas, E., Tretli, S. and Fossa, S.D. 1995. Trends in incidence of testicular cancer in Norway 1955–1992. *European Journal of Cancer* 31A: 2044–8.

Huddart, R.A., Wooster, R., Horwich, E. and Cooper, C.S. 1995. Microsatellite instability in human germ cell tumours. *British Journal of Cancer* 72: 642–5.

IARC. 1992. *Cancer Incidence in Five Continents*, vol. VI, ed. D.M. Parkin, C.S. Muir, S.L. Whelan, Y.T. Gao, J. Ferlay and J. Poull. Lyon, France: IARC.

Ingles, S.A., Ross, R.K., Yu, H.C., Irvine, R.A., La Pera, G., Haile, R.W. and Coetzee, G.A. 1977. Association of prostate cancer risk with genetic polymorphisms in vitamin D receptor and androgen receptor. *Journal of the National Cancer Institute* 89(2): 166–70.

International Testis Cancer Linkage Consortium. 1996. Evidence for a testicular cancer susceptibility locus (TECA1) on 12q. Presented at the American Association of Cancer Research conference, Washington DC.

Isaacs, S.D., Kiemeny, L.A.L.M., Baffoe-Bonnie, A., Beaty, T.H. and Walsh, P.C. 1995. Risk of cancer in relatives of prostate cancer probands. *Journal of the National Cancer Institute* 87: 991–6.

Jishi, M.F., Intrye, J.H., Oakley-Girvan, I.A., Piver, M.S. and Whittemore, A.S. 1995. Risks of cancer among members of families in the Gilda Radner Familial Ovarian Cancer Registry. *Cancer* 76: 1416–21.

King, B.L., Peng, H.Q., Goss, P. et al. 1997. Repeat Expansion Detection analysis of (CAG)n tracts in tumor cell lines, testicular tumours and testicular cancer families. *Cancer Research* 57: 209–14.

Langston, A.A., Stanford, J.L., Wicklund, K.G. et al. 1996. Germ-line BRCA1 mutations in selected men with prostate cancer. *American Journal of Human Genetics* 58: 881–5.

Leahy, M.G., Tonks, S., Moses, J.H. et al. 1995. Candidate regions for a testicular cancer susceptibility gene. *Human Molecular Genetics* 4: 1551–5.

Lothe, R.A., Pelotmaki, P., Tommerup, D. et al. 1995. Molecular genetic changes in human male germ cell tumours. *Laboratory Investigation* 73: 606–14.

Lutzker, S.G. and Levine, A.J. 1996. A functionally inactive p53 protein in teratocarcinoma cells is activated by either DNA damage or cellular differentiation. *Nature Medicine* 2: 804–10.

Mathew, S., Murty, V.V., Bosl, G.J. and Chaganti, R.S. 1994. Loss of heterozygosity identifies multiple sites of allelic deletions on chromosome 1 in human male germ cell tumours. *Cancer Research* 54: 6265–9.

McWhorter, W.P., Hernadez, A.D., Meikle, A.W. et al. 1992. A screening study of prostate cancer in high risk families. *Journal of Urology* 148: 826–8.

Monroe, K.R., Yu, M.C., Kolonel, L.N. et al. 1995. Evidence of an X-linked or recessive genetic component to prostate cancer risk. *Nature Medicine* 1: 827–32.

262   S. Narod, B. King and D. Hogg

Murty, V.V., Li, R.G., Houldsworth, J. et al. 1994a. Frequent allelic deletions and loss of expression characterize the DCC gene in male germ cell tumours. *Oncogene* **9**: 3227–31.

Murty, V.V., Li, R.G., Mathew, S. et al. 1994b. Replication error-type genetic instability at 1q42-43 in human male germ cell tumours. *Cancer Research* **54**: 3983–5.

Narod, S.A., Dupont, A., Cusan, L., Diamond, P., Gomez, J.-L., Suburu, R. and Labrie, F. 1995. The impact of family history on early detection of prostate cancer. *Nature Medicine* **1**: 99–101.

Nicholson, P.W. and Harland, S.J. 1995. Inheritance and testicular cancer. *British Journal of Cancer* **71**: 421–6.

Noguchi, T. and Noguchi, M. 1985. A recessive mutation (ter) causing germ cell deficiency and a high incidence of congenital testicular teratomas in 129/Sv ter mice. *Journal of the National Cancer Institute* **75**: 385–92.

Peng, H.Q., Bailey, D., Bronson, D., Goss, P.E. and Hogg, D. 1995. Loss of heterozygosity of tumor suppressor genes in testis cancer. *Cancer Research* **55**: 2871–5.

Peng, H.Q., Hogg, D., Malkin, D. et al. 1993. Mutations of the p53 gene do not occur in testis cancer. *Cancer Research* **53**: 3574–8.

Sakurai, T., Katoh, H., Moriwaki, K., Noguchi, I. and Noguchi, M. 1994. The ter primordial germ cell deficiency mutation maps near Grl-1 on mouse chromosome 18. *Mammalian Genome* **5**: 333–6.

Schuman, L., Mandel, M., Blackard, C., Bauer, H., Scarlett, J. and McHugh, R. 1997. Epidemiologic study of prostatic cancer; a preliminary report. *Cancer Treatment Report* **61**: 181–6.

Sellers, T.A., Potter, J.D., Rich, S.S. et al. 1994. Familial clustering of breast and prostate cancers and risk of postmenopausal breast cancer. *Journal of the National Cancer Institute* **86**: 1860–5.

Sicinksi, P., Donaher, J.L., Geng, Y. et al. 1996. Cyclin D2 is an FSH responsive gene involved in gonadal cell proliferation and oncogenesis. *Nature* **384**: 470–4.

Slattery, M.L. and Kerber, R.A. 1994. Family history of cancer and colon cancer risk; the Utah Population Database. *Journal of the National Cancer Institute* **86**: 1618–26.

Smith, J.R., Freije, D., Carpten, J.D. et al. 1996. Major susceptibility locus for prostate cancer on chromosome 1 suggested by a genome-wide search. *Science* **274**: 1371–4.

Smith, R.C. and Rukstalis, D.B. 1995. Frequent loss of heterozygosity at 11p loci in testicular cancer. *Journal of Urology* **153**: 1684–7.

Steinberg, G.D., Carter, B.S., Beaty, T.H., Childs, B. and Walsh, P.C. 1990. Family history and the risk of prostate cancer. *Prostate* **17**: 337–47.

Struewing, J.P., Abeliovich, D., Peretz, T., Avishai, N., Kaback, M.M., Collins, F.S. and Brody, L.C. 1995. The carrier frequency of the BRCA1 185delAG mutation is approximately 1 percent in Ashkenazi Jewish individuals. *Nature Genetics* **11**: 198–200.

Sun, S., Narod, S.A., Aprikian, A., Ghadirian, P. and Labrie, F. 1995. Androgen receptor and familial prostate cancer. *Nature Medicine* **1**: 848–9.

Taplin, M.E., Bubley, G.J., Shuster, T.D. et al. 1995. Mutant androgen receptor detected in metastatic androgen-independent prostate cancer. *New England Journal of Medicine* **332**: 1393–8.

Taylor, J., Hirvonen, A., Watson, M., Pittman, G., Mohler, J.L. and Bell, D.A. 1996. Association of prostate cancer with vitamin D receptor gene polymorphism. *Cancer Research* **56**: 4108–10.

Theissen, E.U. 1974. Concerning a familial association between breast cancer and both prostatic and uterine malignancies. *Cancer* **34**: 1102–7.

Thorlacius, S., Olafsdottier, G., Tryggvadottir, L. et al. 1996. A single BRCA2 mutation in male and female breast cancer families from Iceland with varied cancer phenotypes. *Nature Genetics* **13**: 117–19.

Tonin, P., Ghadirian, P., Phelan, C. et al. 1995. A large multisite cancer family is linked to BRCA2. *Journal of Medical Genetics* **32**: 982–4.

Tulinius, H., Egilsson, V., Olafsdottir, G.H. and Sigvaldason, H. 1992. Risk of prostate ovarian and endometrial cancer among relatives of breast cancer patients. *British Medical Journal* **305**: 855–7.

Van Leeuwen, F.E., Stigglebout, A.M., Van den Belt-Dusebout, A.W. et al. 1993. Second cancer risk following testicular cancer: a follow-up study of 1,909 patients. *Journal of Clinical Oncology* **11**: 415–24.

Whittemore, A.S., Wu, A.H., Kolonel, L.N. et al. 1995. Family history and prostate cancer risk in black, white and Asian men in the United States and Canada. *American Journal of Epidemiology* **141**: 732–40.

Woolf, C.M. 1960. An investigation of the familial aspects of carcinoma of the prostate. *Cancer* **13**: 739–44.

13
The neurofibromatoses and other neuro-oncological syndromes

MARTIN RUTTLEDGE and GUY ROULEAU

Summary

Primary solid tumours of the central and peripheral nervous system account for only a small proportion of all human neoplasms. However, the high rate of morbidity and mortality associated with these nervous system tumours makes them important not only to patients and their families, but to a wide variety of medical specialists who are involved in their treatment and management. A number of well documented hereditary syndromes predispose individuals to a variety of specific nervous system tumours. These diseases are interesting in that they enable researchers to identify specific genes that are involved in the genesis of these familial tumours and their sporadic counterparts. This chapter focuses mainly on the neurofibromatoses, NF1 and NF2, including a detailed discussion of the genetic basis of these conditions, mutation studies of the genes involved and phenotype/genotype correlations. Some variants of these diseases are also discussed.

Introduction

In adults, primary central nervous system (CNS) tumours constitute approximately 2–3% of all surgically treated cancer cases. The gliomas, which arise from neuroglial cells and are predominantly sporadic in origin, account for 30–40% of all primary intracranial tumours (Russel and Rubenstein, 1989). There are some inherited diseases where there is a predisposition to these glial tumours. For example, symptomatic optic nerve gliomas are found in approximately 2% of neurofibromatosis type 1 (NF1) patients (Riccardi and Eichner, 1986; Huson et al., 1988); astrocytomas and other brain tumours are often found in the Li–Fraumeni syndrome, which is predominantly characterized by bone and soft tissue tumours (sarcomas) and early onset breast cancer, combined with a number of other malignancies (Li and Fraumeni, 1969, 1982; Li et al., 1988). Gliomas may also be encountered in the context of the rare Turcot syndrome, where they are found together with familial adenomatous polyposis (FAP). Meningiomas (tumours arising from the meninges) and schwannomas (arising from Schwann cells surrounding nerve axons and dendrites) together account for another 25–30% of all primary adult CNS tumours (Kepes, 1982; Zulch, 1986; Russell and Rubinstein, 1989). The majority of these lesions (greater than 95%) occur as sporadic, solitary lesions and are generally identified in patients over 50 years of age. In some instances, however, both schwannomas and meningiomas are found in much younger individuals, predominantly in the context of the inherited syndrome, neurofibromatosis type 2 (NF2). Families in which meningiomas are the only CNS tumours have also been reported, but these are quite rare (Memon, 1980; McDowell, 1990). Interestingly, one such family has been shown to be unlinked to the NF2 locus on chromosome 22, suggesting that a separate gene is involved in these cases (Pulst et al., 1993). Ependymomas (tumours arising from ependymal cells lining the ventricles) are also found at an increased incidence in NF2, albeit in a small percentage of patients.

In children, approximately one-fifth of all cancers involve the CNS (Robbins et al., 1981; Silverberg and Lubera, 1986; Friedman et al., 1991). The most common of these are the astrocytomas (26–28%), followed by the medulloblastomas or primitive neuroectodermal tumours (18–25%), other types of gliomas and a number of other, rarer neoplasms. There are several important syndromes which predispose children to develop these cancers. Medulloblastomas, for example, are found in Gorlin syndrome, an inherited disease with a prevalence of approximately 1 per 55,000 (Gorlin and Goltz, 1960; Evans et al., 1991). Childhood gliomas and other CNS tumours are found in 5% of Li–Fraumeni cases and, as stated above, optic gliomas are found at an increased incidence in NF1 patients.

Neurofibromatosis type 1

NF1, also known as von Recklinghausen's disease or peripheral neurofibromatosis, is one of the most common, autosomal dominantly inherited disorders in humans (Riccardi, 1981). It affects approximately 1 in 3000 people, appears to be race-independent and displays marked clinical variability (Crowe et al., 1956; Riccardi, 1981; Riccardi & Eichner, 1986; Huson et al., 1989). The penetrance of the gene is close to 100%, but some cases show only minor features of the disease (i.e. variable expressivity is common; Sergeyev, 1975; Riccardi and Eichner, 1986; Riccardi and Lewis, 1988) Primarily, tissues of neural crest origin appear to be involved. Characteristic manifestations of NF1 include *café au lait* macules, Lisch nodules of the iris, neurofibromas (of cutaneous nerves), axillary freckling, learning difficulties and other congenital abnormalities (Riccardi, 1992). Affected individuals are usually identified in infancy or early childhood. However, the initial presenting signs may range from multiple congenital abnormalities in a newborn to a solitary mass in an older individual. Greater than 90% of affected cases have more than six *café au lait* spots (diameter greater than 1.5 cm) and one or more skin neurofibromas. The majority of patients may only have one or two clearly visible signs of the disease. However, there are some who develop large numbers of skin lesions (there are a number of reports of patients with more than 1000 neurofibromas). Given this extreme variability, it may be difficult to make a diagnosis in the absence of further detailed examination.

Approximately half of all NF1 patients have no family history and are thus believed to be the result of new mutations in the NF1 gene (see below). These cases of de novo NF1 probably arise as a result of a mutation during gametogenesis, most frequently spermatogenesis. Thus, their offspring are at 50% risk of inheriting the mutated copy of the NF1 gene and developing the disorder. Alternatively, patients with no family history may be the result of somatic mosaiscism, whereby only certain tissues harbour the mutant gene. This situation arises when the mutation occurs early in embryogenesis, generally within a week of fertilization.

Neurofibromatosis type 2

NF2, also previously called central neurofibromatosis or bilateral acoustic neurofibromatosis (BANF), is a syndrome characterized by multiple intracranial and intraspinal tumors, predominantly vestibular schwannomas (arising from the vestibular branch of the eighth cranial nerve), meningiomas and to a lesser extent ependymomas (Eldridge, 1981; Martuza and Eldridge, 1988; Evans et al. 1992a). Posterior capsular lens opacities are also found in a substantial proportion of NF2 cases (Pearson-Webb et al., 1986; Kaiser-Kupfer et al., 1989). The hallmark of the disease is classically bilateral vestibular schwannomas (approximately 85% of patients), but schwannomas of other cranial nerves and the spinal cord are also common. Approximately half of all patients with NF2 develop meningiomas. These tumours are usually multiple and are often the cause of mortality, especially if they become malignant or if they are located close to sensitive intracranial structures. In approximately 5% of cases ependymomas are also present. The investigation of choice for identifying small intracranial and intraspinal tumours in NF2 is gadolinium enhanced MRI (Pastores et al., 1991).

NF2 is transmitted in an autosomal dominant fashion and has an incidence of about 1 in 40,000 individuals (Narod et al., 1992; Evans et al., 1992b). Penetrance of the predisposing gene is similiar to NF1, being close to 100% (Kanter et al., 1980; Evans et al., 1992a). However, there is often not the extreme intrafamilial clinical variability observed in NF1, suggesting that other secondary genes may not play such a significant role in the phenotypic expression of NF2. Lack of family history in approximately 50% of all NF2 patients suggests that these cases arose as the result of a new mutation in the predisposing gene. This relatively high new mutation rate is similar to that observed for NF1 (Crowe et al., 1956).

Clinically, it is now generally accepted that there are at least two forms of NF2; a severe (Wishart) subtype and a mild (Gardner) subtype (Eldridge et al., 1991; Evans et al., 1992b). Although there are presently no formal criteria used to distinguish these two forms of the disease, most investigators agree that severe NF2 presents before 20–25 years of age, and is characterized by multiple (more than three) tumours requiring repeated surgical intervention. By contrast, mild NF2 patients are not usually symptomatic until after 25 years of age and often the only tumours present are bilateral vestibular schwannomas. Average survival for patients with the severe form of the disease is approximately 15 years after diagnosis, whereas in mild NF2 life expectancy may not vary significantly from the general population. Some affected individuals do not clearly fall into either one of these two clinical groups as they may have numerous tumours presenting after 25 years of age or they develop symptoms of only bilateral vestibular schwannomas at an early age. These patients can be classified clinically as of unknown severity, or as having moderate NF2.

Identification of the *NF1* and *NF2* genes

Although various forms of neurofibromatosis have been described clinically for more than 100 years, it was not until 1987 with the advent of modern genetic linkage analysis (using polymorphic DNA markers in families with clinically defined features) that the genes for both NF1 and NF2 were localized to separate chromosomes (Seizinger et al., 1987a; Barker et al., 1987; Rouleau et al., 1987).

The search for the NF1 gene on chromosome 17 ended in 1990 when two groups simultaneously identified chromosomal translocations and mutations in a candidate cDNA (Cawthon et al., 1990a; Viskochil et al., 1990; Wallace et al., 1990). The NF1 gene comprises approximately 300 kb of genomic DNA and is divided up into 59 exons. Interestingly, three smaller genes are embedded in the first intron of *NF1* (Cawthon et al., 1990b; O'Connell et al., 1990; Xu et al., 1990; Viskochil et al., 1991; Cawthon et al., 1991). However, the biological significance of this finding is not yet understood. The NF1 gene encodes a protein, neurofibromin, which has a GTPase activating protein (GAP) like domain (Buchberg et al., 1990; Xu et al., 1990). Neurofibromin is believed to act as a negative regulator of cell growth by accelerating the conversion of active GTP-bound RAS to the inactive GDP-bound state. If neurofibromin function is diminished or is absent, as in tumours from NF1 patients, elevated levels of active GTP-bound RAS will predominate. This increase in cellular RAS-GTP promotes cell growth and thereby contributes to the tumourigenic phenotype. This hypothesis is supported by the fact that approximately 25% of all human cancers show mutations in the *RAS* gene which result in an inhibition of the intrinsic GTPase of the RAS proteins.

The NF2 gene was mapped to the long arm of human chromosome 22 by genetic linkage analysis in 1987 (Rouleau et al., 1987). Its location was refined several times in the following five years using flanking DNA markers (Rouleau et al., 1990; Ruttledge et al., 1993), but it was not until 1993 that the gene was finally cloned (Rouleau et al., 1993; Trofatter et al., 1993). A number of interstitial germline deletions were essential in pinpointing the NF2 gene from a panel of candidate cDNA clones. After direct sequencing of patient and tumour DNA, a host of inactivating mutations were identified thus confirming its identity as the NF2 gene. The gene spans approximately 120 kb of genomic DNA and encodes 17 exons. Its protein product, alternatively named schwannomin (SCH) or Merlin, is a member of the ERM family of proteins which include merosin, ezrin and radixin. Based on its homology to these proteins, it is believed that SCH plays a role in maintaining a communication between the cytoskeleton and the plasma membrane (Rouleau et al., 1993; Trofatter et al., 1993; Takeshima et al., 1995). However, it is still not clear whether the tumour suppressor activity of SCH is related to this function; that is, whether this activity is encoded by the region of homology to the other members of the ERM family of proteins. Investigators have localized SCH to the cytoplasmic side of the plasma membrane, but its precise interaction with other cytoskeletal proteins is still not completely clear. Immunostaining using polyclonal and monoclonal antibodies against SCH have shown that it co-localizes with F-actin and other elements of the cytoskeleton. There is predominant staining in the motile areas of cells such as in the leading or ruffling edges.

Mutation screening in *NF1* and *NF2*

To date, more than 160 different disease causing mutations have been identified in the NF1 gene (Cawthon et al., 1990a; Viskochil et al., 1990; Wallace et al., 1990; B. Korf, 1996, pers. comm.) . The majority of these alterations are germline and are predicted to result in a truncated NF1 protein (over 80% result in premature translation termination and a truncated protein) or a protein with reduced activity in the Gap Related Domain (GRD). Approximately one-quarter of all the changes identified thus far involve deletion of all or part of the NF1 gene. Many of the mutations that have been identified are in the GRD, which is encoded by exons 20-27, but this predominance may represent an ascertainment bias due to the fact that many investigators originally concentrated on this part of the gene. Some reports have shown up to 30% missense mutations in the *NF1-GRD*. These changes are more likely to be pathogenic as this region is highly conserved.

Identification of mutations in the NF2 gene has proceeded far more rapidly than for NF1. This is due to the smaller size of the NF2 gene and the fact that the *NF2* exons are particularly suitable for rapid mutation screening by such techniques as single strand conformation analysis (SSCA) and denaturing gradient gel electrophoresis (DGGE). There are, to date, several hundred different mutations reported in the NF2 gene in NF2 individuals and sporadic tumours associated with NF2 (MacCollin et al., 1993, 1994; Rouleau et al., 1993; Sainz et al., 1993; Sanson et al., 1993; Trofatter et al., 1993; Bianchi et al., 1994; Bourn et al., 1994a,4b; Irving et al., 1994; Jacoby et al., 1994; Lekanne Deprez et al., 1994; Ruttledge et al., 1994; Twist et al., 1994; Merel et al., 1995; Wellenreuther et al., 1995). More than 95% of these alterations are predicted to result in the production of a truncated NF2 protein. These include nonsense mutations, small deletions and insertions which result in a frameshift and the introduction of a premature stop codon, and splice site alterations. In approximately 5% of cases, constitutional missense mutations have been found in the NF2 gene. It is believed that these missense changes will be helpful in identifying functionally important regions of SCH, which in turn may lead to a better understanding of the role of SCH in normal tissues and why its absence or dysfunction in NF2 patients contributes to tumorigenesis. Ultimately, the goal is to identify the cellular components that interact with SCH and to try and devise a treatment regime which compensates for this loss of function in tumour cells. However, unfortunately this idealistic vision may be a long way off for such multi-tumour syndromes as NF2.

From the NF2 mutation studies performed by many different laboratories, it appears that there are no significant hot spots. Although some sequence variants have been identified in several presumably unrelated individuals and sporadic meningiomas and schwannomas, these cases make up a relatively small percentage of the total. However, it is possible that an as yet unidentified hot-spot region may be uncovered, as up to 40% of NF2 patients so far do not show any causative mutation despite a thorough investigation of the entire coding region of the NF2 gene. Furthermore, mutations may also be identified in the regulatory portions of the gene which have not yet been studied.

Phenotype–genotype correlations in *NF1* and *NF2*

As discussed previously, there is often marked clinical variability within NF1 families (Carey et al., 1979; Riccardi et al., 1979; Huson et al., 1989) suggesting that, in addition to the NF1 gene, other secondary genes play a role in the phenotypic expression of the disease. This hypothesis is supported by the fact that monozygotic twins often show strong correlation with respect to clinical expression, whereas distant relatives may show marked variability in severity of disease (Easton et al., 1993). It has not been possible (with some notable exceptions) to find any significant correlation between mutations that affect the NF1 gene and clinical outcome. This may be due to the fact that only a relatively small number of NF1 kindreds have been studied in detail clinically where mutations have been characterized. Alternatively, it may reflect the fact that there is little or no correlation between the type and location of mutation within the NF1 gene and clinical severity. In order to answer this question, a large number of carefully studied patients with characterized mutations need to be investigated. Given the large size of the NF1 gene, this type of study probably needs several hundred affected individuals with a limited number of pathogenic mutations in order to be statistically significant.

There is, however, one group of NF1 patients where a consistent genotype/phenotype correlation exists. Investigators have found that the vast majority of cases with large *NF1* deletions encompassing all or most of the gene (often detectable by FISH analysis using intragenic cosmids and YAC's) have a distinctive and severe phenotype. The clinical picture is characterized by early onset of neurofibromas, facial anomalies, and learning disability or mental retardation. One explanation for this severe clinical course is that contiguous genes may be altered by the deletions, thereby adding to the number of different tissues affected. Alternatively, lack of a partially functional truncated gene product may predispose to more severe disease.

Exploring the hypothesis that other secondary genes are involved in the phenotypic expression of *NF1* may not be straightforward and may require the study of a large number of affected individuals. Genetic analysis of sibling-pairs with NF1 is one possible approach that may be used. Sibling-pair analysis has been employed in a limited number of diseases, including insulin dependent diabetes mellitus, multiple sclerosis, and psychiatric illnessess. This method of genetic analysis is discussed in detail in Chapter 7.

In contrast to NF1, there appears to be a much stronger correlation between the type of mutation in the NF2 gene and clinical outcome. Numerous investigators have noted that the severity of NF2 disease is generally quite consistent within families. Patients with very severe disease, often displaying a number of tumours associated with a high degree of morbidity and mortality, are more likely to be from kindreds where all or most of the cases developed severe disease. In some families this consistency of clinical severity is striking. Conversely, some kindreds may develop milder disease. Recently, we described an extremely mild NF2 family with 10 known mutation carriers (Ruttledge et al., 1996). Of these individuals five were asymptomatic at 29–74 years of age (mean = 55.2 years), while the other five carriers developed only vestibular schwannomas at ages between 22 and 54 years (mean = 38 years). This consistently mild clinical picture is almost certainly attributed to the type of mutation in the NF2 gene. This alteration is not predicted to result in the premature truncation of SCH, in contrast to the majority of mutations thus far identified in NF2 patients. It results in the duplication of a single leucine residue at codon 49 in SCH (exon 3). Presumably, this 'modest' structural modification does not completely inactivate SCH and residual protein activity is retained. This may account for the small number of tumours developing in these 10 mutation carriers even at a relatively late age. The absence of meningiomas and ependymomas in this kindred (despite CT and/or MRI examination in nearly every mutation carrier) may be a reflection of their slow growth rate. An alternative hypothesis is that in order for meningioma and ependymoma tumours to develop, another part of SCH needs to be disrupted. Two other families that we have studied, one with a missense mutation in exon 11 and the other with a splice-site mutation affecting exon 15 (families 256 and 779 in Ruttledge et al., 1996), support this latter possibility as none of the nine mutation carriers has developed meningiomas.

Another potential phenotype/genotype correlation has been identified in two NF2 families with large (> 500 kb) germline deletions encompassing the NF2 gene (Sanson et al., 1993; Watson et al., 1993). These germline deletions also inactivate a number of other known genes, including the NEFH gene, a recently cloned member of the β-adaptin gene family and the pK1.3 gene (Xie et al., 1993; Peyrard et al., 1994), and presumably several uncharacterized genes. Both of these families exhibit mild NF2 (Bourn et al., 1994a) with relatively late onset of disease, predominantly bilateral vestibular schwannomas and few if any meningiomas or other tumours. We propose that this mild NF2 phenotype is not only attributable to the inactivation of the NF2 gene, but also the deletion of one copy of other genes flanking the NF2 gene. In most NF2 individuals, an inactivating germline mutation exists within the NF2 gene and is unmasked by somatic loss of the remaining wild-type gene, often by total or partial chromosome loss, and tumour formation is initiated. Thus, loss of heterozygosity for chromosome 22 markers (LOH 22) is found in a large proportion of tumours from NF2 patients (Seizinger et al., 1987b; Wolff et al., 1992). In contrast, in the two families described above the first germline mutation is a large deletion encompassing the NF2 gene and several other genes. Presumably, inactivation of the remaining NF2 gene by LOH 22 cannot occur because one or more of the flanking deleted genes must be present in at least one copy for the cell to survive. This forces the 'second hit' of the NF2 gene to be a point mutation or small deletion which does not affect the surrounding genes. This occurs less frequently than LOH 22, and as a result the few tumours which form do so at a later age. Thus, we would expect to find inactivating mutations within the NF2 gene in tumours from these families. Furthermore, we would not expect to find LOH 22 for markers located proximal or distal to the constitutionally deleted region in these families. Confirmation of this explanation for the mild phenotype observed will require examination of tumour DNA from these and other families displaying large chromosome 22 deletions, in addition to extensive functional studies of the other genes affected by these deletions.

Alternative forms of neurofibromatosis

In addition to NF1 and NF2, a number of variant forms of neurofibromatosis have been suggested (Riccardi and Eichner, 1986; Riccardi 1992). These variants include mixed NF (NF3), segmental NF (NF5) and multiple *café au lait* macules in the absence of other NF features (NF6). Several independent groups have also described individuals that develop numerous Schwann cell tumours (but not bilateral vestibular schwannomas) in the absence of any other features of NF1 and NF2 (Shishiba et al., 1984; Daras et al., 1993; Honda et al., 1995; MacCollin et al., 1996). This condition has been alternatively named neurilemmomatosis or schwannomatosis, the latter term being most appropriate. In some cases the schwannomas are restricted to a particular limb or region of the body. This may be explained by a mutation in the NF2 gene in only a subset of cells, a situation referred to as 'segmental' disease (NF5) or somatic mosaicism. In other individuals, however, there is a more widespread distribution of tumours with the spinal nerve roots, cranial nerves and variuous peripheral nerves being affected. These latter cases are less likely to be somatic mosaics for mutations in the NF2 gene. It may be that bilateral vestibular schwannomas and other features of NF2 (such as meningiomas and ependymomas) have not yet developed in these individuals. Alternatively, this group of patients may represent a distinct syndrome where the NF2 gene is not involved. Interestingly, the vast majority of schwannomatosis patients have no family history of peripheral or CNS tumours; this is in contrast to NF2 where approximately half of all cases have an affected parent. Careful screening of the NF2 gene for mutations in constitutional DNA from these patients will determine whether schwannomatosis is part of NF2 or whether it represents a distinct genetic disease. Preliminary results suggest that some patients may harbour germline mutations in the NF2 gene (Honda et al., 1995).

274   M. Ruttledge and Guy Rouleau

Future management of neurofibromatosis patients

The neurofibromatoses are a complicated group of diseases displaying a wide range of clinical features. Management of these conditions therefore requires the cooperation of several different specialties, preferably located within one institution. The establishment of clinics specifically designed to evaluate and counsel neurofibromatosis patients should therefore be a priority of any modern health care system. Such clinics can benefit immensely from ongoing research into the genetic basis of these syndromes. It is now possible to perform predictive testing (based on genetic linkage analysis or direct mutation detection) for at-risk individuals in the vast majority of neurofibromatosis families, where at least two other affected members are available. Furthermore, in some kindreds (predominantly NF2) the severity of disease can be predicted from the type of mutation present in the predisposing gene. These advances do provide some benefits for counselling families with neurofibromatosis, but there is still a long way to go before we fully understand these complex syndromes and are equipped to provide a treatment.

Conclusion

NF1 is one of the commonest genetic conditions that features central and peripheral nervous system tumours. The gene for NF1 is exceptionally large and this has hindered both mutation analysis and functional studies. The neurofibromatosis type 2 gene (*NF2*) is considerably smaller and more headway has been made in genotype–phenotype analysis with *NF2* – missense mutations may be associated with a milder phenotype. Some alternate forms of NF1 and NF2 may be due to mosaicism. As yet, the identification of these genes has not resulted in large benefits for those at risk or already affected.

References

Barker, D., Wright, E., Nguyen, K. et al., 1987. Gene for von Recklinghausen neurofibromatosis is in the pericentromeric region of chromosome 17. *Science* **236**: 1100–2.

Bianchi. A.B., Hara, T., Ramesh, V. et al., 1994. Mutations in transcript isoforms of the neurofibromatosis 2 gene in multiple human tumour types. *Nature Genetics* **6**: 185–92.

Bourn, D., Carter, S.A., Evans, D.G.R., Goodship, J., Coakham, H. and Strachan, T. 1994a. A mutation in the neurofibromatosis type 2 tumor-suppressor gene, giving rise to widely different clinical phenotypes in two unrelated individuals. *American Journal of Human Genetics* **55**: 69–73.

Bourn, D., Carter, S.A., Mason, S., Evans, D.G.R. and Strachan, T. 1994b. Germline mutations in the neurofibromatosis type 2 tumor suppressor gene. *Human Molecular Genetics* **3**: 813–16.

Buchberg, A., Cleveland, L.S., Jenkins, N.A. and Copeland, N.G. 1990. Sequence homology shared by neurofibromatosis type-1 gene and IRA-1 and IRA-2 negative regulators of the RAS cyclic AMP pathway. *Nature* **347**: 291–4.

Carey, J.C., Laub, J.M. and Hall, B.D. 1979. Penetrance and variability of neurofibromatosis: a genetic study of 60 families. *Birth Defects* **15**: 271–81.

Cawthon, R., Weiss, R., Xu, G. et al., 1990a. A major segment of the neurofibromatosis type 1 gene: cDNA sequence, genomic structure and point mutations. *Cell* **62**: 193–201.

Cawthon, R., O'Connell, P., Buchberg, A.M. et al., 1990b. Identification and characterization of transcripts from the neurofibromatosis type 1 region: the sequence and genomic structre of EVI2 and mapping of other transcripts. *Genomics* **7**: 555–65.

Cawthon, R.M., Andersen, L.B., Buchberg, A.M. et al., 1991. cDNA sequence and genomic structure of EVI2B, a gene lying within an intron of the neurofibromatosis type 1 gene. *Genomics* **9**: 446–60.

Crowe, F.W., Schull, W.J. and Neel, J.V. 1956. *A Clinical, Pathological and Genetic Study of Multiple Neurofibromatosis*. Springfield: Charles C. Thomas.

Daras, M., Koppel, B., Heise, C., Mazzeo, M., Poon, T. and Duffy, K. 1993. Multiple spinal intradural schwannomas in the absence of von Recklinghausen's disease. *Spine* **18**: 2556–9.

Easton, D.F., Ponder, M.A., Huson, S.M. and Ponder, B.A.J. 1993. An analysis of variation in expression of NF1: evidence for modifying genes. *American Journal of Human Genetics* **53**: 305–13.

Eldridge, R. 1981. Central neurofibromatosis with bilateral acoustic neuroma. *Advances in Neurology* **29**: 57–65.

Eldridge, R., Parry, D.M. and Kaiser-Kupfer, M.I. 1991. Neurofibromatosis 2: clinical heterogeneity and natural history in 39 individuals in 9 families and 16 sporadic cases. *American Journal of Human Genetics* **49**: 32.

Evans, D.G.R., Birch, J.M. and Orton, C.I. 1991. Brain tumours and the occurrence of severe invasive basal cell carcinoma in first degree relatives with Gorlin syndrome. *British Journal of Neurosurgery* **5**: 643–6.

Evans, D.G.R., Huson, S.M., Donnai, D. et al., 1992a. A genetic study of type 2 neurofibromatosis in the United Kingdom. II. Guidelines for genetic counselling. *Journal of Medical Genetics* **29**: 847–52.

Evans, D.G.R., Huson, S.M., Donnai, D. et al., 1992b. A genetic study of type 2 neurofibromatosis in the United Kingdom. I. Prevalence, mutation rate, fitness and confirmation of maternal transmission effect on severity. *Journal of Medical Genetics* **29**: 841–6.

Friedman, H.S., Horowitz, M. and Oakes, W.J. 1991. Solid tumours in children. *Pediatrics Clinical North America* **38**: 381–91.

Gorlin, R.J. and Goltz, R.W. 1960. Multiple naevoid basal cell epithelioma, jaw cysts and bifid ribs; a syndrome. *New England Journal of Medicine* **262**: 908–12.

Honda, M., Arai, E., Sawada, S., Ohta, A. and Niimura, M. 1995. Neurofibromatosis 2 and neurilemmomatosis gene are identical. *Journal of Investigative Dermatology* **104**: 74–7.

Huson, S.M., Harper, P.S. and Compston, D.A.S. 1988. Von Recklinghausen neurofibromatosis: a clinical and population study in South East Wales. *Brain* **111**: 1355–81.

Huson, S.M., Clark, D., Compston, D.A.S. and Harper, P.S. 1989. A genetic study of von Recklinghausen neurofibromatosis in South East Wales. I: prevalence, fitness, mutation rate and effect of parental transmission on severity. *Journal of Medical Genetics* **26**: 704–11.

Irving, R.M., Moffat, D.A., Hardy, D.G., Barton, D.E., Xuereb, J.H. and Maher, E.R. 1994. Somatic NF2 gene mutations in familial and non-familial vestibular schwannoma. *Human Molecular Genetics* **3**: 347–50.

Jacoby, L.B., MacCollin, M., Louis, D.N. et al., 1994. Exon scanning for mutation of the NF2 gene in schwannomas. *Human Molecular Genetics* **3**: 413–19.

Kaiser-Kupfer, M.I., Friedlin, V., Datiles, M.B. et al., 1989. The association of posterior capsular lens opacities with bilateral acoustic neuromas in patients with neurofibromatosis type 2. *Archives of Ophthalmology* **107**: 541–4.

Kanter, W.R., Eldrige, R., Fabricant, R., Allen, J.C. and Koerber, T. 1980. Central neurofibromatosis with bilateral acoustic neuroma: genetic, clinical and biochemical distinctions from peripheral neurofibromatosis. *Neurology* **30**: 851–9.

Kepes, J.J. 1982. In *Meningiomas. Biology, Pathology, Differential Diagnosis*. New York: Masson.

Lekanne Deprez, R.H., Bianchi, A.B., Groen, N,A. et al., 1994. Frequent NF2 gene transcript mutations in sporadic meningiomas and vestibular schwannomas. *American Journal of Human Genetics* **54**: 1022–9.

Li, F.P. and Fraumeni, J.F. 1969. Soft tissue sarcomas, breast cancer, and other neoplasms. A familial syndrome? *Annals of Internal Medicine* **71**: 747–52.

Li, F.P. and Fraumeni, J.F. 1982. Prospective study of a family cancer syndrome. *Journal of the American Medical Association* **247**: 2692–4.

Li, F.P. Fraumeni, J.F. and Mulvihill, J.J. 1988. A cancer family syndrome in twenty-four kindreds. *Cancer Research* **48**: 5358–62.

MacCollin, M., Mohney, T., Trofatter, J., Wertelecki, W., Ramesh, V. and Gusella, J. 1993. DNA diagnosis of neurofibromatosis 2. *Journal of the American Medical Association* **270**: 2316–20.

MacCollin, M., Ramesh, V., Jacoby, L.B. et al., 1994. Mutational analysis of patients with neurofibromatosis 2. *American Journal of Human Genetics* **55**: 314–20.

MacCollin, M., Woodfin, W., Kronn, D. and Short, M.P. 1997. Schwannomatosis: a clinical and pathological study. *Neurology* **46**: 1072–9

Martuza, R.L. and Eldridge, R. 1988. Neurofibromatosis 2 (bilateral acoustic neurofibromatosis). *New England Journal of Medicine* **318**: 684–8.

McDowell, J.R. 1990. Familial meningioma. *Neurology* **40**: 312–14.

Memon, M.Y. 1980. Multiple and familial meningiomas without evidence of neurofibromatosis. *Neurosurgery* **7**(3): 262–4.

Merel, P, Hoang-Xuan, K., Sanson, M. et al. 1995. Screening for germ-line mutations in the NF2 gene. *Genes, Chromosomes and Cancer* **12**: 117–27.

Narod, S.A., Parry, D.M., Parboosingh, J. et al., 1992. Neurofibromatosis type 2 appears to be a genetically homogeneous disease. *American Journal of Human Genetics* **51**: 486–96.

O'Connell, P., Viskochil, D. and Buchberg, A.M. 1990. The human homolog of murine *Evi-2* lies between two von Recklinghausen neurofibromatosis translocations. *Genomics* **7**: 547–54.

Pastores, G.M., Michels, V.V. and Jack, C.R. 1991. Early childhood diagnosis of acoustic neuromas in presymptomatic individuals at risk for neurofibromatosis 2. *American Journal of Medical Genetics* **41**: 325–9.

Pearson-Webb, M.A., Kaiser-Kupfer, M.I. and Eldridge, R. 1986. Eye findings in bilateral acoustic (central) neurofibromatosis: association with presenile lens opacities and cataracts but absence of Lisch nodules. *New England Journal of Medicine* **315**: 1553-4.

Peyrard, M., Fransson, I., Xie, Y.G. et al., 1994. Characterization of a new member of the human beta-adaptin gene family from chromosome 22q12, a candidate meningioma gene. *Human Molecular Genetics* **3**(8): 1393-9.

Pulst, S.-M., Rouleau, G.A., Marineau, C., Fain, P. and Sieb, J.P. 1993. Familial meningioma is not allelic to neurofibromatosis 2. *Neurology* **43**: 2096-8.

Riccardi, V.M., Kleiner, B. and Lubs, M.I. 1979. Neurofibromatosis: variable expression is not intrinsic to the mutant gene. *Birth Defects* **15**: 283-9.

Riccardi, V.M. 1981. von Recklinghausen neurofibromatosis. *New England Journal of Medicine* **305**: 1617-27.

Riccardi, V. M. and Eichner, J.E. (Eds). 1986. *Neurofibromatosis: Phenotype, Natural History and Pathogenesis*. Baltimore: Johns Hopkins University Press.

Riccardi, V.M. and Lewis, R.A. 1988. Penetrance of von Recklinghausen neurofibromatosis; a distinction between predecessors and descendants. *American Journal of Human Genetics* **42**: 284-9.

Riccardi, V.M. (Ed.). 1992. *Neurofibromatosis: Phenotype, Natural History and Pathogenesis*. 2nd edn. Baltimore: Johns Hopkins University Press.

Robbins, S.L., Angell, M. and Kumar, V. (Eds). 1981. *Basic pathology*, 3rd edn. Philadelphia: Saunders.

Rouleau, G.A., Wertelecki, W., Haines, J.L. et al., 1987. Genetic linkage of bilateral acoustic neurofibromatosis to a DNA marker on chromosome 22. *Nature* **329**: 246-8.

Rouleau, G.A., Seizinger, B.R., Wertelecki, W., Haines, J.L., Superneau, D.W., Martuza, R.L. and Gusella, J.F. 1990. Flanking markers bracket the neurofibromatosis type 2 (NF2) gene on chromosome 22. *American Journal of Human Genetics* **46**: 323-8.

Rouleau, G.A., Merel, P., Lutchman, M. et al., 1993. Alteration in a new gene encoding a putative membrane-organizing protein causes neurofibromatosis type 2. *Nature* **363**: 515-21.

Russell, D.S. and Rubinstein, L.J. 1989. Tumours of the cranial, spinal and peripheral nerve sheaths. *Pathology of Tumours of the Nervous System*, 5th edn. Baltimore: Williams and Wilkins.

Ruttledge, M.H., Narod, S.A., Dumanski, J.P. et al., 1993. Pre-symptomatic diagnosis for neurofibromatosis 2 with chromosome 22 markers. *Neurology* **43**: 1753-60.

Ruttledge, M.H., Sarrazin. J., Rangaratnam, S. et al., 1994. Evidence for the complete inactivation of the NF2 gene in the majority of sporadic meningiomas. *Nature Genetics* **6**: 180-4.

Ruttledge, M.H., Andermann, A., Phelan, C.P. et al., 1996. Type of mutation in the neurofibromatosis type 2 (NF2) gene frequently determines severity of disease. *American Journal of Human Genetics* **59**: 331-42.

Sainz. J., Figueroa, C., Baser, M.E. and Pulst, S.-M. 1993. Mutations in the neurofibromatosis 2 gene in 31 vestibular schwannomas. *American Journal of Human Genetics* **53S**: 354.

Sanson, M., Marineau, C., Desmaze, C. et al., 1993. Germline deletion in a neurofibromatosis type 2 kindred inactivates the NF2 gene and a candidate meningioma locus. *Human Molecular Genetics* **2**(8): 1215-20.

278   *M. Ruttledge and Guy Rouleau*

Seizinger, B.R., Rouleau, G., Ozelius, L.J. et al., 1987a. Common pathogenic mechanism for three tumor types in bilateral acoustic neurofibromatosis. *Science* **236**: 317–19.
Seizinger, B.R., Rouleau, G.A., Ozelius, L.J. et al., 1987b. Genetic linkage of von Recklinghausen neurofibromatosis to the nerve growth factor receptor gene. *Cell* **49**: 589–94.
Sergeyev, A.S. 1975. On the mutation rate of neurofibromatosis. *Human Genetics* **28**: 129–38.
Shishiba, T., Niimura, M., Ohtsuka, F. and Tsura, N. 1984. Multiple cutaneous neurilemmomas as a skin manifestation of neurilemmomatosis. *Journal of the American Acadamy of Dermatology* **10**: 744–54.
Silverberg, E. and Lubera, J 1986. Cancer Statistics. *Ca–A Cancer Journal for Clinicians* **39**: 9.
Takeshima, H., Izawa, I., Lee, P.S.Y., Saldar, N., Levin, V.A. and Saya Hideyuki 1995. Detection of cellular proteins that interact with the NF2 tumor suppressor gene product. *Oncogene* **9**: 2135–44.
Trofatter, J.A., MacCollin, M.M., Rutter, J.L. et al., 1993. A novel moesin-, ezrin-, radixin-like gene is a candidate for the neurofibromatosis 2 tumor suppressor. *Cell* **72**: 791–800.
Twist, E.C., Ruttledge, M.H., Rousseau, M. et al., 1994. The neurofibromatosis type 2 gene is inactivated in schwannomas. *Human Molecular Genetics* **3**: 147–51.
Viskochil, D., Buchberg, A.M., Xu, G. et al., 1990. Deletions and a translocation interrupt a cloned gene at the neurofibromatosis type 1 locus. *Cell* **62**: 187–92.
Viskochil, D., Cawthon, R. and O'Connell, P. 1991. The oligodendrocyte myelin glycoprotein is embedded within the neurofibromatosis type 1 gene. *Molecular and Cellular Biology* **11**: 906–12.
Wallace, M.R., Marchuck, D.A., Anderson, L.B. et al., 1990. Type 1 neurofibromatosis gene: identification of a large transcript disrupted in three NF1 patients. *Science* **249**: 181–6.
Watson, C.J., Gaunt, J., Evans, G., Patel, K., Harris, R. and Strachan, T. 1993. A disease-associated germline deletion maps the type 2 neurofibromatosis (NF2) gene between the Ewing sarcoma region and the leukaemia inhibitory factor locus. *Human Molecular Genetics* **2**(6): 701–4.
Wellenreuther. R., Kraus, J.A., Lenartz, D. et al., 1995. Analysis of the neurofibromatosis 2 gene reveals molecular variants of meningiom. *American Journal of Pathology* **146**(4): 827–32.
Wolff, R.K., Frazer, K.A., Jackler, R.K., Lanser, M.J., Pitts, L.H. and Cox, D.R. 1992. Analysis of chromosome 22 deletions in neurofibromatosis type 2 related tumours. *American Journal of Human Genetics* **51**: 478–85.
Xie, Y.-G., Han, F.-Y., Peyrard, M. et al., 1993. Cloning of a novel, anonymous gene from a megabase-range YAC and cosmid contig in the neurofibromatosis type 2/meningioma region on human chromosome 22q12. *Human Molecular Genetics* **2**: 1361–8.
Xu, G., O'Connell, P., Viskochil, D., Cawthon, R.M. et al., 1990. The neurofibromatosis type 1 gene encodes a protein related to GAP. *Cell* **62**: 599–608.
Zulch, K.J. 1986. Tumors of nerve sheath cells. In *Brain Tumors; Their Biology and Pathology*. 3rd edn., ed. K.J Zulch. New York, Springer.

14

Malignant melanoma

NICHOLAS HAYWARD

Summary

This chapter considers cutaneous malignant melanoma from a molecular perspective, leading from the first results indicating linkage of a melanoma-prone phenotype to a locus on chromosome 1p. The subsequent linkage to chromosome 9p and the cloning of the *CDKN2A* gene (also known as *p16*) that followed is described in detail. Mutations in *CDKN2A* were found in some families with many cases of malignant melanoma. The effect of germline mutations on the function of the gene product and phenotype, and factors that could influence this, are considered. The spectrum of tumours to which such mutations predispose extends beyong melanoma, and evidence for this is discussed. The gene product appears to be a tumour suppressor, but in sporadic melanoma may act in tumour progression rather than initiation. The absence of *CDKN2A* mutations in some 9p-linked famjlies is intriguing – other candidate genes on this and other chromosomes are discussed.

Introduction

The first realization that melanoma may have a familial component came from a report by Norris (1820) who described development of the neoplasm in a father and son. More than a century passed before others reported the familial occurrence of melanoma (Cawley, 1952; Smith, 1966; Anderson et al., 1967; Andrews, 1968). Subsequent estimates of the proportion of melanomas that have a familial basis range from 8% to 12% (Greene and Fraumeni, 1979). Anderson and colleagues (Anderson et al., 1967; Anderson, 1971) noted that cases of familial melanoma generally had an earlier age of onset and were more likely to have multiple primary tumours than sporadically occurring cases. Anderson also concluded that familial melanoma was most likely transmitted in an autosomal dominant manner, although polygenic inheritance could not be ruled out. Further support for polygenic rather than mendelian inheritance came from studies by Wallace et al. (1973) and Duggleby et al. (1981). However, in 1983, Greene and coworkers (Greene et al., 1983) indicated that autosomal dominant inheritance, with incomplete penetrance, was the most likely mode of transmission from segregation analysis of a sample of 14 melanoma kindreds. In this study nonsignificant evidence for a melanoma predisposition gene linked to the rhesus blood group locus on the short arm of chromosome 1 (1p) was put forward. Six years later the same group (from the National Cancer Institute – NCI – in the US) reported statistically significant (logarithm of odds ratio – LOD – score of greater than 3) evidence for a locus (*MLM1*) on 1p, which was postulated to confer susceptibility to both familial melanoma (FM) and the dysplastic nevus syndrome (DNS) (Bale et al. 1989). There was considerable controversy over the validity of this finding based on the combined phenotype since there was no significant evidence for linkage if only those individuals with melanoma were considered affected (Goldstein et al., 1992). Furthermore, when dysplastic nevi (DN) were included in the disease phenotype of the original 14 families studied by Greene et al. (1983) (from which five of the six families reported in the study of Bale et al., 1989, were a subset), the segregation data were not consistent with a mendelian pattern of inheritance since the occurrence of nevi appeared to be too high and consequently the 'affected' phenotype over-segregated. Melanoma families from the Netherlands (Gruis et al., 1990), North America (Cannon-Albright et al. 1990) and Australia (Kefford et al., 1991; Nancarrow et al., 1992a) were typed for markers on 1p, but none of these cohorts provided confirmatory evidence for an FM susceptibility locus in this chromosomal region.

In an effort to search further for the location of an FM predisposition gene two groups attempted genome-wide linkage scans but neither provided statistical evidence to indicate the chromosomal position of a melanoma locus (Nancarrow et al., 1992b; Gruis et al., 1993). However, in the study of six Australian melanoma families (Nancarrow et al., 1992b) 13 different chromosomal regions (including 3p, 4q, 5q, 6p, 9p, 10q, 12q, 14q, 18q, and 21q) gave LOD scores of between 1 and 2.3 in individual families, providing very weak evidence of possible linkage of a melanoma gene to one or more of these loci.

The first real clues to the whereabouts of a major melanoma susceptibility gene came from molecular cytogenetic findings. Melanoma cell lines were found to have frequent heterozygous and homozygous deletions of the chromosome 9p21-p22 region (Fountain et al., 1992). In addition, Petty et al. (1993) identified a patient with eight primary melanomas and multiple atypical moles, who harbors an unbalanced germline 5p/9p translocation and consequently was shown to be hemizygous for several 9p21-p22 markers. Together, these data suggested that a melanoma gene mapped to 9p, near the interferon (*IFN*) gene cluster, and that the product of this gene normally functioned as a tumour suppressor.

Linkage to markers from 9p13-p22 in 11 melanoma families from Utah and Texas, USA, was subsequently reported (Cannon-Albright et al. 1992). The most likely position of the gene (*MLM2*) was determined to be between the markers *IFNA* and D9S126 by multipoint linkage analysis. This locus was confirmed in Australian (Nancarrow et al., 1993), Dutch (Gruis et al., 1993) and British families (MacGeoch et al., 1994). The NCI cohort of families has also been analysed with markers on 9p and there is strong evidence that some of them are linked to *MLM2* (Goldstein et al., 1994), however, there is also significant evidence for genetic heterogeneity with a number of families continuing to show linkage to *MLM1* (Goldstein et al., 1993).

Identification of a tumour suppressor gene on 9p

A combination of tumour deletion studies (Weaver-Feldhaus et al., 1994) and recombination mapping in melanoma families (Cannon-Albright et al., 1994a) was used to delimit further the location of the *MLM2* gene. Positional cloning of a candidate tumour suppressor gene from 9p21-p22, in the region centromeric of the *IFNA* gene cluster, was accomplished simultaneously by two groups (Kamb et al 1994a; Nobori et al., 1994). The gene thus isolated was found to be identical to a previously characterized cell cycle regulatory gene encoding the cyclin-dependent kinase (CDK)-inhibitor, p16 (Serrano et al., 1993). This gene has been variably called *INK4*, *INK4A*, *CDK4I*, and *MTS1*, but has been assigned the designation *CDKN2A* (for *c*yclin-*d*ependent *k*inase *i*nhibitor *2A*) by the Human Genome Organization nomenclature committee.

Initially, the *CDKN2A* gene was found to be homozygously deleted in a total of 161 (48%) out of 336 cell lines derived from various tumour types (Kamb et al., 1994a; Nobori et al., 1994), however, the frequency of deletion or intragenic mutation in uncultured tumour specimens was found subsequently to be considerably lower (Cairns et al., 1994; Spruck et al., 1994; reviewed in Elledge and Harper, 1994; Grana and Reddy, 1995; Sherr and Roberts, 1995), suggesting that many changes are induced (or selected for) by in vitro culturing. More recently, mutations have been found in vivo in a high proportion of a limited range of cancer subtypes, namely, pancreatic (Caldas et al., 1994), oesophageal (Mori et al., 1994; Zhou et al., 1994; Igaki et al., 1995) and non-small cell lung carcinomas (Hayashi et al., 1994; Okamoto et al., 1995; Washimi et al., 1995). In addition, homozygous deletions have also been reported at high frequency in bladder cancers (Cairns et al., 1995) and gliomas in vivo (Giani and Finocchiaro, 1994; Schmidt et al., 1994). These data clearly highlight the role this gene has as a universal suppressor of carcinogenesis (see Foulkes et al., 1997; Pollock et al., 1996 for databases of *CDKN2A* mutations in a wide variety of tumours and tumour cell lines, compiled from a comprehensive review of the literature). Moreover, melanoma cell lines (Kamb et al., 1994a; Ohta et al., 1994; Liu et al., 1995; Pollock et al., 1995; Flores et al., 1996; Pollock et al., 1996) and some fresh melanomas (Gruis et al., 1995c; Flores et al., 1996) show a high proportion of deletions or interstitial mutations of *CDKN2A*, indicating the central importance of *CDKN2A* in the development of this particular cancer. The majority of the nucleotide substitutions of *CDKN2A* seen in melanoma-derived DNA samples (Kamb et al., 1994a; Ohta et al., 1994; Gruis et al., 1995c; Liu et al., 1995; Pollock et al., 1995; Flores et al., 1996; Pollock et al., 1996) are C→T transitions or tandem base changes (predominantly CC→TT), which are highly characteristic of UV-induced mutagenesis (Brash et al., 1991 and references therein) and are thus likely to have occurred relatively early in the development of these tumours, prior to metastasis, and are also unlikely to have resulted during in vitro culturing. However, in a study of p16^{CDKN2A} expression in a series of 103 melanocytic lesions, the loss of this protein was clearly correlated with the invasive stage of tumour progression (Reed et al., 1995). p16^{CDKN2A} was detected in all melanomas in situ and the majority of primary invasive melanomas, whereas the protein was undetectable in 44% of metastatic lesions. This finding suggests that loss of p16^{CDKN2A} expression is not necessary for tumour initiation, but rather, is involved in progression to invasiveness and metastatic ability. Additional evidence for a role of p16^{CDKN2A} late in the development of some melanomas comes from the finding in a study of six autologous melanoma cell lines derived from separate metastases from the one individual, that only one of the cell lines carried a mutation of *CDKN2A* (Glendening et al., 1995). Fountain and colleagues have proposed a model for melanoma development based on haploinsufficiency for p16^{CDKN2A} in which loss or mutational inactivation of the first copy of *CDKN2A* is an initiating event, while loss/inactivation of the second copy either occurs late (e.g. during metastasis) or is unnecessary (Flores et al., 1996).

Whilst the body of data summarized above provides strong support for the notion that the *CDKN2A* gene is involved in melanoma tumourigenesis, proof of its role in melanoma predisposition required the identification of germline mutations in affected members of FM kindreds.

Identification of *CDKN2A* as the *MLM2* melanoma susceptibility locus

Nobori et al., (1994), sequenced the *CDKN2A* gene from a lymphoblastoid cell line derived from a patient with FM and DNS, and found that in one allele it had a nonsense mutation at amino acid position arginine-58. This individual was later identified as being a member of one of the NCI cohort of families (Hussussian et al., 1994) and provided the first evidence that the *CDKN2A* gene was indeed involved in predisposition to melanoma. Subsequently a diverse range of germline mutations was found in melanoma families from the US (Hussussian et al., 1994; Kamb et al., 1994b; Ohta et al., 1994; Goldstein et al., 1995; Whelan et al., 1995; Fitzgerald et al., 1996; Yarbrough et al., 1996), The Netherlands (Gruis et al., 1995a), Canada (Liu, L. et al., 1995; Sun et al., 1996), Australia (Walker et al., 1995a; Holland et al., 1995; G. Walker, 1996, pers. comm.), Sweden (Borg et al., 1996; Hansson et al., 1996), Italy (Ciotti et al., 1996) and the UK (N. Spurr, 1996, pers. comm.) (Table 14.1). A number of naturally occurring polymorphisms of this gene have also been identified, some of which result in amino acid substitution (reviewed in Pollock et al., 1996).

In the NCI cohort 9 out of 18 families were found to have mutations (Table 14.2). The alterations in this cohort comprised four missense mutations, one nonsense mutation and a presumed aberration of splicing (Table 14.1). All but one of the families with mutations have a conditional probability of greater than 0.7 of being linked to 9p (Hussussian et al., 1994). No mutations were found in the three families that have conditional probabilities of < 0.05 for linkage to the *IFNA* locus on 9p, two of which show linkage to 1p (Goldstein et al., 1993; Hussussian et al., 1994). From the Utah cohort, two out of eight families were found to have mutations and all but one showed 9p linkage by haplotype analysis

Table 14.1. CDKN2A *mutations in melanoma families*

Reference	Population	Base position[a]	Exon	Base change	Coding change[b]
Nobori et al. (1994); Hussussian et al. (1994)	USA	172	2	C→T	R58STOP
Hussussian et al. (1994)	USA	212	2	A→G	N71S[c]
Hussussian et al. (1994)	USA	260	2	G→C	R87P[d]
Hussussian et al. (1994)	USA	301[e]	2	G→T	G101W[d]
Hussussian et al. (1994)	USA	377[f]	2	T→A	V126D[d]
Hussussian et al. (1994)	USA	457+1[g]		G→T	splice
Kamb et al. (1994b)	USA	301	2	G→T	G101W[d]
Kamb et al. (1994b)	USA	377	2	T→A	V126D[d]
Goldstein et al. (1995)	USA	-h			no expression
Goldstein et al (1995)	USA	-16-8	1	24bp insertion	8 αα duplication
Ohta et al. (1994)	USA	240-253	2	14bp deletion	frameshift
Whelan et al. (1995)	USA	301	2	G→T	G101W[d]
FitzGerald et al. (1996)	USA	240-253[f]	2	14bp deletion	frameshift
FitzGerald et al. (1996)	USA	166-223	2	58bp deletion	frameshift
FitzGerald et al. (1996)	USA	44	1	G→A	W15STOP
FitzGerald et al. (1996)	USA	159	2	G→C	M53I[i]
Yarbrough et al. (1996)	USA	286-297	2	12 bp deletion	delete αα96-99
Walker et al. (1995a)	Australia	-16-8[f]	1	24bp insertion	8 αα duplication
Walker et al. (1995a)	Australia	46	1	1bp deletion	frameshift
Walker et al. (1995a)	Australia	95	1	T→C	L32P
Walker et al. (1995a)	Australia	104	1	G→C	G35A
Walker et al. (1995a)	Australia	149	1	A→G	Q50R[i]
Walker et al. (1995a)	Australia	159[e]	2	G→C	M53I[i]
Walker et al. (1995b)	Australia	322	2	G→A	D108N[j]
Holland et al. (1995)	Australia	71	1	G→C	R24P[i]
Gruis et al. (1995a)	Netherlands	225-243	2	19bp deletion	frameshift
Ciotti et al. (1996)	Italy	301	2	G→T	G101W[d]
Borg et al. (1996)	Sweden	337-3391	2	3bp insertion	insert R113
Hansson et al. (1996)	Sweden	337-339[l]	2	3bp insertion	insert R113
Hansson et al. (1996)	Sweden	143	1	C→T	P48L
Liu, L. et al. (1995)	Canada	310-315	2	6bp deletion	deletion L104/ D105[d]

Table 14.1. (*cont.*)

Reference	Population	Base position[a]	Exon	Base change	Coding change[b]
Sun et al. (1996)	Canada	159	2	G→C	M53I[i]
Spurr[k]	UK	-16-8	1	24 bp insertion	8 αα duplication

Note:

[a] Numbering begins with the A of the initiation codon.
[b] Aminoacids are numbered according to Okamoto et al. (1994).
[c] Mutant protein tested and found to be functionally normal, thus subsequently considered a neutral polymorphism (Ranade et al., 1995)
[d] Mutant protein tested and found to be functionally impaired.
[e] Found in three apparently unrelated kindreds from the same cohort.
[f] Found in two apparently unrelated families from the same cohort.
[g] Occurred at the first nucleotide of intron 2.
[h] Unspecified change that resulted in lack of expression from one allele.
[i] Not an ankyrin repeat consensus amino acid (Serrano et al., 1993).
[j] Possibly an acceptable amino acid substitution within an ankyrin repeat consensus (Serrano et al., 1993).
[k] Personal communication.
[l] The kindreds reported in Borg et al., 1996 and Hansson et al., 1996 are likely to share a common founder. It should be noted that the authors specified different positions for the inserted amino acid but this fact simply reflects whether they considered that the duplicated codon was placed before or after the original arginine codon. The numbering in Table 14.1 above is consistent with the latter since this is where the mutant sequence first deviates from wild type.

(Kamb et al., 1994b). The two mutations (G101W, V127D: numbering according to Okamoto et al. 1994) seen in these families were also observed in the NCI set of families (Hussussian et al., 1994). The relationship, if any, between the families in these two cohorts is unknown, thus the possibility of some common founders cannot be ruled out. This scenario seems particularly attractive for the G101W mutation, and may also suggest an Italian origin, since 7 out of 14 melanoma kindreds from a small geographic region of Italy were found to carry this alteration (Ciotti et al., 1996).

Several other germline mutations have been described in families from the US (Table 14.1). Yarbrough et al. (1996) reported a family with a deletion of amino acids 96–99, and Ohta et al., (1994) reported a family with a 14 bp deletion in exon 2, which results in a frameshift mutation leading to premature truncation of the protein. Interestingly, in a differ-

Table 14.2. *Proportion of families in different cohorts showing evidence of a 9p-linked melanoma gene*

Reference[a]	Population[b]	Number of families	Number 9p-linked	Number with CDKN2A mutation
Hussussian et al. (1994); Goldstein et al. (1995)	USA	19[c]	14	11[d]
Kamb et al. (1994b)	USA	8[e]	7	2
Walker et al. (1995a)	Australia	18	11[f]	7
Holland et al. (1995)	Australia	17	8	1
Gruis et al. (1995b,c)	Netherlands	3[g]	1[h]	1
MacGeoch et al. (1994)	UK	6	3[h]	1[i]

Note:
[a] Only the first author and year are given.
[b] Only those cohorts in which comprehensive 9p linkage, haplotype, and mutation analysis have been carried out on more than a single family are included.
[c] Two of these families were found subsequently to carry *CDK4* mutations (Zuo et al., 1996).
[d] Includes the N71S variant.
[e] The Dutch melanoma kindreds reported in Gruis et al., 1995b,c have not been included in this statistic.
[f] Includes those families which did not have a 9p marker haplotype that segregated but did have a *CDKN2A* mutation.
[g] Several kindreds were reported to share the same haplotype and *CDKN2A* mutation, indicating a common founder, thus have been considered here as different branches of the one large family.
[h] In one additional family 9p-linkage status could not be established.
[i] N. Spurr personal communication.

ent North American cohort two other independent melanoma cases with a reported family history of the disease were also found to have the same mutation (FitzGerald et al., 1996). Once again the possibility of common founders needs to be considered. In the latter study three other germline *CDKN2A* mutations were reported. These comprised a frameshift mutation caused by a 58 bp deletion in exon 2, a nonsense mutation at codon 15, and a missense mutation resulting in substitution of isoleucine for methionine at codon 53.

In a follow-up study of NCI families, Goldstein et al. (1995) reported two additional mutations. One was in a previously unreported family and comprised a 24 bp duplication in exon 1 that leads to an iteration of the first eight amino acids of p16^{CDKN2A}. The other mutation occurred in one

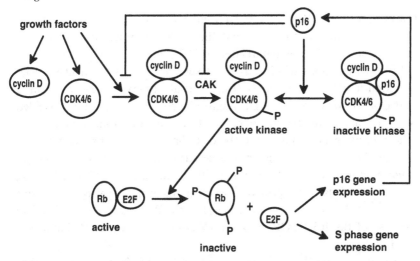

Figure 14.2. Role of CDK4 and p16^{CDKN2A} in regulation of progression through G1 phase of the cell cycle. Growth factor stimulation of cells results in increased levels of D-type cyclins and promotes assembly of CDK4 (or CDK6) and cyclin D complexes. An active kinase complex is then created through phosphorylation of CDK4/6 by a CDK-activating kinase (CAK). Active CDK4/6 phosphorylates the retinoblastoma (Rb) protein causing it to release bound transcription factors of the E2F family, which then activate transcription of a variety of genes required for S phase of the cell cycle. E2F also increases expression of the *CDKN2A* gene and the p16^{CDKN2A} protein then negatively regulates the action of the CDK4/6 kinase by (i) competing with cyclin D in binding to CDK4/6, (ii) inhibiting the phosphorylation of CDK4/6-cyclin D complexes by CAK, and (iii) inhibiting active CDK4/6-cyclin D complexes by binding to them and forming inactive ternary complexes.

Yang et al., (1995) to possess only 2% of the ability compared to wild-type p16^{CDKN2A} of inhibiting CDK4 from phosphorylating the retino-blastoma protein. However, Koh et al., (1995) did not replicate this finding, although they did show that this mutant protein failed to induce a G1 arrest when microinjected into mouse NIH3T3 cells. Subsequently, Parry and Peters (1996) showed that this variant was a temperature-sensitive mutant of p16, as was the V126D > variant.

The 24 bp in-frame duplication found in several melanoma kindreds to date (Goldstein et al., 1995; Walker et al., 1995a; N. Spurr, 1996, pers. comm.; G.Walker, 1996, pers. comm.) would lead to a duplication of the first eight amino acids of p16. Surprisingly, this difference does not appear to abolish the ability of the variant to bind to CDK4 or CDK6

(Parry and Peters, 1996). These data indicate that either this variant is a rare benign polymorphism or that the protein is functionally compromised in some subtle way unrelated to CDK binding.

In-frame deletions within *CDKN2A* such as the L104 and D105 deletion seen in a Canadian family (Liu, L. et al., 1995) and the four amino acid deletion observed in a US family (Yarbrough et al., 1996) yielded proteins that were unable to bind CDK4. In addition, a number of other germline mutations of *CDKN2A* that cause premature termination of the protein through nonsense substitutions (Hussussian et al., 1994; Nobori et al., 1994) or frameshifts (Ohta et al., 1994; Gruis et al., 1995a) would also be expected to yield significantly impaired or inactive p16^{CDKN2A}. Indeed, this has been confirmed (Parry and Peters, 1996) in the case of the R58STOP mutation (Hussussian et al., 1994; Nobori et al., 1994).

Moreover, several tumour-specific mutations (Koh et al., 1995; Lukas et al., 1995; Ranade et al., 1995; Yang et al., 1995; Parry and Peters, 1996) of *CDKN2A* have been shown to be functionally impaired, whereas the common germline polymorphisms (Koh et al., 1995; Ranade et al., 1995), and surprisingly some other tumour-specific changes (Koh et al., 1995; Yang et al., 1995; Parry and Peters, 1996), have little or no effect on p16^{CDKN2A} function. This finding should be treated with a degree of caution since it is possible that in vitro assays, in which the amounts of expressed proteins are usually far in excess of physiological levels, may not always reflect subtle differences in protein function that could be elucidated through more sensitive in vivo assay systems.

The finding that some mutations apparently did not result in functionally deficient p16^{CDKN2A} may be due in part to the relative positions of the substituted amino acids within the protein. p16^{CDKN2A} is comprised of four tandemly repeat ankyrin-like motifs and roughly about half of the amino acids in each repeat conform to the ankyrin consensus (Serrano et al., 1993). Mutations at one of the consensus residues invariably lead to aberrant p16^{CDKN2A}, however, mutations that occur at other positions e.g. G98S (Parry and Peters, 1996), A100P (Koh et al., 1995; Parry and Peters, 1996) or E120K (Yang et al., 1995) are often indistinguishable from wild type protein. In this regard it is noteworthy that all but three (R24P, Q50R, M53I) of the germline missense mutations found in melanoma families occur at ankyrin consensus residues (Table 14.1). Functional assays have not yet been carried out on these three mutations to determine whether they do in fact produce a protein with abrogated function.

Effect of *CDKN2A* mutations on phenotype

Development of melanoma

Naturally occurring human homozygous CDKN2A *knockouts*

An extremely valuable finding regarding the role of p16^{CDKN2A} in the development of melanoma is the identification of two individuals within one of the melanoma kindreds from The Netherlands that possess germline mutations of both copies of *CDKN2A* (Gruis et al., 1995b). Surprisingly, one of these homozygous 'knockouts' did not develop melanoma prior to her death at the age of 54 from an adenocarcinoma of uncharacterized origin. This individual did have 'three very mildly atypical nevi' which may have been the only phenotypic features bearing any relationship to the biological consequences of her lacking p16^{CDKN2A} (Gruis et al., 1995b). Although it could be argued that since *CDKN2A* is a tumour suppressor gene for a variety of cancer types (reviewed in Pollock et al., 1996), the adenocarcinoma in this person may well have developed through lack of functional p16^{CDKN2A}. In contrast, the second individual identified as carrying deletions within both alleles of *CDKN2A* had developed a large number of atypical moles by 11 years of age and also developed an invasive cutaneous melanoma and a melanoma in situ at the age of 15 (Gruis et al., 1995b). The first of these two cases indicates that simply lacking functional p16^{CDKN2A} is not sufficient for melanoma to develop. This situation has parallels with another tumour suppressor gene, *TP53*, which is responsible for the Li–Fraumeni cancer predisposition syndrome in humans (Malkin et al., 1990). Mice that are nullizygous for *TP53* do not usually develop tumours in utero, but they almost invariably develop some form of cancer during their lifespan (Donehower et al., 1992). These data tend to imply a certain degree of redundancy in the mechanisms that control normal cellular proliferation and tumourigenesis. The situation with regard to *CDKN2A* is complicated even further by the recent finding that mice homozygously deleted for this gene do not develop melanoma (Serrano et al., 1996). However, these *CDKN2A* null animals often spontaneously develop other tumours at a relatively young age and are highly sensitive to treatment with various carcinogens. The tumour spectrum in these mice is predominated by sarcomas and lymphomas.

Penetrance within families with CDKN2A *mutations*

It is pertinent to compare the penetrances for the development of melanoma in identified *CDKN2A* mutation carriers in different cohorts of families. In the NCI set of pedigrees, 33 (69%) out of 48 mutation carriers had developed melanoma (Hussussian et al., 1994), in the two Utah families (Kamb et al., 1994b), the value was 16 (73%) out of 22 and in the Australian cohort (Walker et al., 1995a) it was 47 (78%) out of 60. These values are remarkably similar even though the samples originate from diverse geographical regions. Furthermore, they imply that the life-time penetrance in *CDKN2A* mutation carriers could conceivably be as high as 90–100%. However, where penetrances have been reported for individual families with defined mutations they are generally lower e.g. 25% (1 out of 4: Whelan et al., 1995), 39% (9 out of 23: Holland et al., 1995), 50% (5 out of 10: Borg et al., 1996) or 60% (3 out of 5: Liu, L. et al., 1995) of carriers and obligate carriers had developed melanoma at the time of sampling.

Interaction of CDKN2A *mutations with other genetic and environmental factors*

In three Utah–Texas families analyzed by Cannon-Albright et al. (1994b), mutation carriers with melanoma generally had lighter skin and had more cumulative sunlight exposure than carriers who had not developed melanoma, suggesting that development of melanoma in these families depended on other genetic (genes controlling pigmentation) and environmental (sunlight) factors. Additional evidence for a role of UV radiation in modulating the phenotypic penetrance of *CDKN2A* mutations has been reported by Battistutta et al. (1994) in which 151 putative mutation carriers from 18 melanoma families were analysed according to year of birth cohort. The cumulative incidence of melanoma was found to be 21-fold higher among those born after 1959 than those born before 1900 and the expected age of onset was 24 years earlier (21 versus 45 years) in the more recent cohort. These findings support the hypothesis that the phenotypic penetrance of *CDKN2A* mutations is increasing possibly as a result of increased sun exposure to carriers due to lifestyle changes. In presumptive mutation carriers born after 1959 more than half have already developed melanoma, consistent with the high penetrances observed in families with identified mutations (Hussussian et al., 1994; Kamb et al., 1994b; Liu, Q. et al., 1995; Walker et al., 1995a).

Development of dysplastic nevi

Since the linkage study of Bale et al., (1989) there has been considerable speculation that the melanoma predisposition genes are also likely to be responsible for predisposition to atypical/dysplastic nevi. However, analysis of phenotype in known carriers of *CDKN2A* mutations does not readily support the notion that the genes controlling melanoma and dysplastic nevi are necessarily the same. In the nine NCI pedigrees with *CDKN2A* mutations only 10 out of 33 individuals with dysplastic nevi (but not melanoma) carried mutations (Hussussian et al., 1994). Similar findings were seen in the kindreds from The Netherlands in which 5 out of 37 melanoma cases did not have the mutant haplotype, i.e. were sporadic cases, yet all possessed multiple atypical moles (Gruis et al., 1995a). Both studies imply the existence of additional genes for predisposition to and/or development of atypical/dysplastic nevi. However, this should not be interpreted to mean that the *CDKN2A* gene has no role to play in nevus development. When more quantitative measures of nevi are considered, such as an individual's total nevus number (TNN) or total nevus density (TND), correlations with mutation carrier status are apparent (Cannon-Albright et al., 1994b). For instance, when 124 presumed mutation carriers (by haplotype analysis) from three 9p-linked Utah–Texas families were analysed, carriers were found to have higher TNN and TND than non-carriers, although it should be stressed that melanoma risk did not increase proportionately relative to either of these variables (Cannon-Albright et al., 1994b).

Development of other cancers in CDKN2A *mutation carriers*

Considering the involvement of the *CDKN2A* gene in the development of a wide variety of tumours (reviewed in Foulkes et al., 1997; Pollock et al., 1996), it is tempting to speculate that the incidence of a number of different neoplasms will be higher in *CDKN2A* mutation carriers. Whilst presentation of such data has been sparse to date, it is interesting to note that several *CDKN2A* mutation carriers have developed second cancers other than melanoma. In particular, several cases of pancreatic cancer have been observed (Goldstein et al., 1995; Gruis et al., 1995a; Whelan et al., 1995; Ciotti et al., 1996; Hayward et al., unpub. obs.). This finding is intriguing in light of the high frequency of mutations and deletions of *CDKN2A* that have been found in sporadically occurring pancreatic carcinomas (Caldas et al., 1994). Other tumours observed in *CDKN2A* mutation carriers include an adenocarcinoma of unspecified type (Gruis et al., 1995a), a smoking-related laryngeal carcinoma (Liu, L. et al., 1995), an early onset breast carcinoma and a prostate carcinoma (Kamb et al., 1994b), cancers of the cervix and breast, as well as a non-Hodgkin's lymphoma (Borg et al., 1996), and carcinomas of the colon, breast, and mouth (Sun et al., 1996). Moreover, several second tumours including bowel cancer, multiple myeloma, squamous cell carcinoma of the mandible, squamous cell carcinoma of the vocal chord, and two cases of lung cancer, have also occurred in known *CDKN2A* mutation carriers in Australian melanoma families (Hayward et al., unpub. obs.). A member of a North American family with a defined mutation was noted to have developed a squamous cell carcinoma of the tongue (Whelan et al., 1995) and members of another US family with a *CDKN2A* mutation have been reported to have non-small cell lung cancers as well as head and neck carcinomas (Yarbrough et al., 1996). These data, taken together, suggest that individuals who inherit mutant *CDKN2A* alleles are not only predisposed to develop melanoma but are also at increased risk of developing pancreatic cancer or squamous cell carcinoma of the head and neck. It is noteworthy that these cancer types do not appear to be over-represented in mice that are nullizygous for *CDKN2A* (Serrano et al., 1996).

Another intriguing finding is that in some families from The Netherlands (Lynch et al., 1981) and Australia (Hayward et al., unpub. obs.) cases of ocular melanoma have been found, thus suggesting that mutations within *CDKN2A* may lead to the development of both cutaneous and ocular forms of this neoplasm. However, molecular analysis of a limited number of sporadically occurring uveal melanomas has so far failed to identify any somatic mutations or deletions of this gene (Ohta et al., 1994).

9-linked melanoma families without *CDKN2A* mutations

There is now considerable evidence to indicate that the *CDKN2A* gene is the *MLM2* locus on 9p. What is intriguing however, is that mutations have only been identified in about half of the families that show linkage to 9p (Hussussian et al., 1994; Kamb et al., 1994b; Gruis et al., 1995a; Walker et al., 1995a) (Table 14.2). This would suggest that mutations in the remaining families must occur outside the coding region of the gene, or that another gene lying in close proximity to *CDKN2A* is responsible for susceptibility in some families. A strong candidate for the latter is the *CDKN2B* gene, encoding p15, another CDK-inhibitor that is highly homologous to p16^{CDKN2A}. These two proteins share a region of 81 amino acids with 97% identity (Hannon and Beach, 1994). The *CDKN2B* gene is located within 20 kb of *CDKN2A* (Stone et al.,

1995a) and is comprised of only two exons, which correspond to exons 1(α) and 2 of the *CDKN2A* gene (Kamb et al., 1994a). So far no germline mutations within *CDKN2B* have been found in melanoma families (Stone et al., 1995a; G. Walker, 1996, pers. comm.).

When initially characterised the *CDKN2A* gene was thought to be comprised of only three exons (Serrano et al., 1993), however, recent studies have discovered the existence of an alternately spliced form of the gene that includes a novel exon at its proximal end, termed exon 1β (Mao et al., 1995; Stone et al., 1995b). Exon 1β is alternatively spliced on to exons 2 and 3 and creates a translation product with an open reading frame that is out of frame with respect to p16. There is evidence that the alternative protein is translated in vivo in mice (but not as yet in humans) and that when ectopically expressed in murine cells in vitro it is capable of inducing cell cycle arrest (Quelle et al., 1995). Sequence analysis of exon 1β in several 9p-linked melanoma kindreds (Stone et al., 1995b; G. Walker pers. comm.) and various tumour samples (Mao et al., 1995; Stone et al., 1995b) has not revealed any mutations. Its significance to the development or progression of melanoma at this stage is thus enigmatic.

An alternative mechanism for inactivation of *CDKN2A* is through transcriptional repression by methylation of critical cytosine residues in the 5' CpG island of the gene (Merlo et al., 1995). Somatic changes in the methylation status of *CDKN2A* have been been reported in a diverse range of cancer cell lines and primary tumours (Gonzalez-Zulueta et al., 1995; Herman et al., 1995; Merlo et al., 1995; Otterson et al., 1995) and reactivation of *CDKN2A* expression could be achieved by treatment of the cell lines with the demethlyating agent 5-aza 2'-deoxycytidine (Merlo et al., 1995; Otterson et al., 1995). Potentially, germline mutations which affect the methylation pattern of the *CDKN2A* gene, and hence eliminate expression from one allele, could be responsible for melanoma predisposition in some 9p-linked families which do not carry mutations within the protein coding region of the gene. Indeed one family has already been described which lacks expression of *CDKN2A* from one allele, however, the mechanism responsible for this defect has not yet been characterized (Goldstein et al., 1995).

Germline mutations of the *CDK4* gene

Whilst *CDKN2A* is likely to account for the majority of FM cases (Table 14.2), one other gene *CDK4*, which encodes cyclin-dependent kinase 4, has recently been shown to be involved in predisposition to

melanoma (Zuo et al., 1996). A cohort of 11 melanoma families from
North America and 22 families from Australia were screened for germline mutations within each of the coding exons of the *CDK4* gene. The
same mutation, which results in substitution of an arginine residue for a
cysteine residue at amino acid position 24, was observed in two apparently unrelated families from North America (Zuo et al., 1996). The
mutant allele segregated in all 11 melanoma patients and 2 out of 22
unaffected individuals within these two pedigrees. In all, 11 out of 14
carriers and obligate carriers of the mutation had developed melanoma,
giving a penetrance value of 79% at the time of sampling. This value is
very similar to the values observed for mutations within *CDKN2A*
(Hussussian et al., 1994; Kamb et al., 1994b; Liu, Q. et al., 1995;
Walker et al., 1995a). Of note is the fact that whilst the two families
with a germline *CDK4* mutation appeared strongly linked to chromosome 1p by linkage analysis (Goldstein et al., 1993; Hussussian et al.,
1994), the *CDK4* gene has been mapped to chromosome band 12p13
(Demetrick et al, 1994). It is therefore looking increasingly unlikely that
a melanoma predisposition gene actually exists on the short arm of
chromosome 1. However, it is still too early to rule out the possibility
that a gene on 1p may be involved in development of nevi/dysplastic
nevi, since the original linkage data indicated that this locus segregated
better with nevi than with melanoma (Bale et al., 1989; Goldstein et al.,
1992).

Interestingly, the R24C change in *CDK4* had been found previously to
occur as a somatic mutation in 2 out of 29 melanomas tested (Wolfel et
al., 1995). In one of the two patients whose melanoma developed this
mutation, the R24C variant of *CDK4* was found to be a tumour-specific
antigen recognized by HLA-A2.1-restricted autologous T lymphocytes.
Binding of mutant CDK4 to either $p16^{CDKN2A}$ or $p15^{CDKN2B}$ was dramatically impaired, indicating that the arginine-24 residue may be
directly involved in the binding of CDK4 to these proteins. The CDK4
mutation had no effect on the binding of $p21^{CDKN1A}$ or $p27^{CDKN1B}$, nor
did it alter the catalytic activity in the presence of cyclin D1 (Wolfel et al.,
1995). Thus, melanomas may have arisen in these cases with the R24C
mutation as a result of cellular CDK4 kinase activity being less sensitive
to inhibition/regulation by $p16^{CDKN2A}$ (and/or $p15^{CDKN2B}$). Hence, in
contrast to mutations within *CDKN2A*, mutations within *CDK4* are
likely to result in the kinase acting as a dominant oncogenic protein.

Other candidate melanoma genes

A number of other genes involved in regulation of the cell cycle, particularly those involved in progression through G1 phase, are attractive candidates for additional melanoma predisposition genes. A brief synopsis and what is currently known about some of these genes in relation to development of melanoma or other cancers is given below.

CDK6

The *CDK6* gene is localized to chromosome band 7q21 (Demetrick et al., 1994), a region that commonly shows rearrangement in melanoma cell lines and fresh tumours (reviewed in Walker et al., 1995b). Given these data and the finding that some melanoma families have germline mutations within the *CDK4* gene, a functional homolog of *CDK6*, it would appear that the *CDK6* gene is a very good candidate for a melanoma predisposition gene.

CDKN2C

The gene (*CDKN2C*) encoding the CDK-inhibitor, p18 (reviewed in Elledge and Harper, 1994; Grana and Reddy, 1995; Sherr and Roberts, 1995), was found to map to 1p32, near the putative *MLM1* locus (Guan et al., 1994). However, its location appears to be centromeric of the region of strongest linkage in the NCI families.

CDKN2D

The *CDKN2D* gene, codes for the CDK-inhibitor, p19 (Okuda et al., 1995), which shares approximately 44% amino acid homology with p16^{CDKN2A}. *CDKN2D* maps to chromosome band 19p13, a region that has been found to be involved in chromosome translocations in some melanomas (Parmiter et al., 1986). Recent analysis of the *CDKN2D* gene in acute lymphoblastic leukaemia showed that it was not rearranged nor deleted in 41 cases (Okuda et al., 1995).

CDKN1A

The *CDKN1A* gene, encoding p21, another CDK-inhibitor (reviewed in Elledge and Harper, 1994; Grana and Reddy, 1995; Sherr and Roberts, 1995), intriguingly maps to 6p21.2 (El-Deiry et al., 1993), a region that has indicated a weak suggestion of linkage in some melanoma families (Walker et al., 1994 and references therein). However, mutation analysis of this gene in a limited number of kindreds did not detect any germline alterations and mutations in melanoma cell lines were rare, occurring only in lines with a 'mutator' phenotype (Vidal et al., 1995).

CDKN1B

The gene (*CDKN1B*) for the CDK-inhibitor, p27 (reviewed in Elledge and Harper, 1994; Grana and Reddy, 1995; Sherr and Roberts, 1995), maps to 12p12-p13.1 (Ponce-Casteneda et al., 1995), a chromosomal region not frequently altered in melanomas. Somatic mutations of this gene were not found upon analysis of 147 primary solid tumours of various types (Ponce-Casteneda et al., 1995).

CDKN1C

Another member of the p21/p27 family is p57, the gene for which is located on chromosome 11p15.5, close to the Beckwith–Wiedemann cancer predisposition locus (Matsuoka et al., 1995). The mouse homolog of *CDKN1C* is known to be genomically imprinted, with the paternally derived allele being transcriptionally repressed by methylation (Hatada and Mukai, 1995). Interestingly, development of certain human cancers appears to proceed through relaxation of the imprinted signal on other genes from this chromosomal region (Ogawa et al., 1993; Rainer et al., 1993).

Conclusions

Over the last few years there have been considerable advances in our understanding of the molecular genetic basis of melanoma. The most significant findings have clearly been the identification in some melanoma families of germline mutations within either the *CDKN2A* or *CDK4* genes. However, in the majority of melanoma families analyzed so far, mutations have not been identified within these genes. Thus the search for additional susceptibility genes is continuing, with the major focus on analysis of genes involved in cell cycle regulation such as those encoding the CDKs or CDK-inhibitors listed above. In addition, it seems likely that further detailed analysis of chromosomal regions showing frequent karyotypic abnormalities (reviewed in Fountain et al., 1990; Walker et al., 1995b), or those regions showing a high rate of loss of somatic heterozygosity (Healey et al., 1995; Walker et al., 1995b) in melanoma-derived specimens, are likely to yield the location of other melanoma susceptibility loci and even point to possible candidate predisposition genes.

In those families with defined mutations of *CDKN2A* or *CDK4*, correlates can now be sought between genotype and phenotype. Specifically, it will be of great interest to see whether mutations of these genes have any effect on the development of nevi and whether mutations predispose individuals to cancers other than melanoma.

Acknowledgements

The author is supported by a Research Fellowship from the National Health and Medical Research Council of Australia and is grateful to Pamela Pollock for critical reading of this article and helpful discussions. Work carried out in the author's laboratory was funded by the NH&MRC and the Queensland Cancer Fund.

References

Anderson, D.E. 1971. Clinical characteristics of the genetic variety of cutaneous malignant melanoma in man. *Cancer* **28**: 721–5.

Anderson, D.E., Smith, J.L. Jr. and McBride, C.M. 1967. Hereditary aspects of malignant melanoma. *Journal of the American Medical Association* **200**: 741–6.

Andrews, J.C. 1968. Malignant melanoma in siblings. *Archives of Dermatology* **98**: 282–3.

Bale, S., Dracopoli, N., Tucker, M. et al. 1989. Mapping the gene for hereditary cutaneous melanoma-dysplastic naevus to chromosome 1p. *New England Journal of Medicine* **320**: 1367–72.

Battistutta, D., Palmer, J.M., Walters, M.K., Walker, G.J., Nancarrow, D.J., and Hayward, N.K. 1994. Incidence of familial melanoma and MLM2 gene. *Lancet* **344**: 1607–8.

Borg, A., Johansson, U., Johansson, O. et al. 1996. Novel germline *p16* mutation in familial malignant melanoma in Southern Sweden. *Cancer Research* **56**: 2497–500.

Brash, D.E., Rudolph, J.A., Simon, J.A. et al. 1991. A role for sunlight in skin cancer: UV-induced p53 mutations in squamous cell carcinoma. *Proceedings of the National Academy of Sciences, USA* **88**: 10124–8.

Cairns, P., Mao, L., Merlo, A. et al. 1994. Rates of p16 (MTS1) mutations in primary tumours with 9p loss. *Science* **265**: 415–6.

Cairns, P., Polascik, T.J., Eby, Y. et al. 1995. Frequency of homozygous deletion at *p16/CDKN2* in primary tumours. *Nature Genetics* **11**: 210–12.

Caldas, C., Hahn, S.A., da Costa, L.T. et al. 1994. Frequent somatic mutations
and homozygous deletions of the p16 (MTS1) gene in pancreatic
adenocarcinoma. *Nature Genetics* **8**: 27–32.

Cannon-Albright, L., Goldgar, D.E., Meyer, L.J. et al. 1992. Assignment of a
locus for familial melanoma, MLM, to chromosome 9p13-p22. *Science* **258**:
1148–52.

Cannon-Albright, L.A., Goldgar, D.E., Neuhausen, S. et al. 1994a. Localisation
of the 9p melanoma susceptiblity locus (MLM) to a 2-cM region between
D9S736 and D9S171. *Genomics* **23**: 265–8.

Cannon-Albright, L., Goldgar, D., Wright, E. et al. 1990. Evidence against the
reported linkage of cutaneous melanoma-dysplastic nevus syndrome locus to
chromosome 1p36. *American Journal of Human Genetics* **46**: 912–18.

Cannon-Albright, L.A., Meyer, L., Goldgar, D.E. et al. 1994b. Penetrance and
expressivity of the chromosome 9p melanoma susceptibility locus (MLM).
Cancer Research **54**: 6041–4.

Cawley, E.P. 1952. Genetic aspects of malignant melanoma. *Archives of
Dermatology and Syphilis* **65**: 440–50.

Ciotti, P., Strigini, P. and Bianchi-Scarra, G. 1996. Familial melanoma and
pancreatic cancer. *New England Journal of Medicine* **334**: 469–70.

Demetrick, D.J., Zhang, H., and Beach, D.H. 1994. Chromosomal mapping of
human CDK2, CDK4 and CDK6 cell cycle kinase genes. *Cytogenetics and
Cell Genetics* **66**: 72–4.

Donehower, L.A., Harvey, M., Slagle, B.L., McArthur, M.J., Montgomery, C.A.
Jr, Butel, J.S. and Bradley, A. 1992. Mice deficient for p53 are
developmentally normal but susceptible to spontaneous tumours. *Nature*
356: 215–21.

Duggleby, W.F., Stoll, H., Priore, R.L., Greenwald, P., and Graham, S. 1981. A
genetic analysis of melanoma – polygenic inheritance as a threshold trait.
American Journal of Epidemiology **114**: 63–72.

El-Deiry, W.S., Tokino, T., Velculescu, V.E. et al. 1993. WAF1, a potential
mediator of p53 tumour suppression. *Cell* **75**: 817–25.

Elledge, S. and Harper, J.W. 1994. Cdk inhibitors: on the threshold of
checkpoints and development. *Current Opinions in Cell Biology* **6**: 847–52.

FitzGerald, M.G., Harkin, D.P., Silva-Arrieta, S., et al. 1996. Prevalence of germline mutations in p16, p19ARF, and CDK4 in familial melanoma: analysis of
a clinic-based population. *Proceedings of the National Academy of Sciences,
USA* **93**: 8541–5.

Flores, J.F.,Walker, G.J., Glendening, J.M. et al. 1996. Loss of the p16INK4a
and p15INK4B genes, as well as neighboring 9p21 markers, in sporadic
melanoma. *Cancer Research* **56**: 5023–32.

Foulkes, W.D., Flanders, T.Y., Pollock, P.M. and Hayward, N.K. 1997.
CDKN2A and cancer. *Molecular Medicine* **3**: 5–20.

Fountain, J.W., Bale, S.J., Housman, D.E. and Dracopoli, N.C. 1990. Genetics of
melanoma. In *Cancer Surveys: Advances and Prospects in Clinical,
Epidemiological and Laboratory Oncology*, ed. L.M. Franks, pp. 645–71.
London: Oxford University Press.

Fountain, J.W., Karayiorgou, M., Ernstoff, M.S. et al. 1992. Homozygous
deletions within human chromosome band 9p21 in melanoma. *Proceedings
of the National Academy of Sciences, USA* **89**: 10557–61.

Giani, C. and Finocchiaro, G. 1994. Mutation rate of the CDKN2 gene in
malignant gliomas. *Cancer Research* **54**: 6338–9.

Glendening, J.M., Flores, J.F., Walker, G.J., Stone, S., Albino, A.P. and Fountain, J.W. 1995. Homozygous loss of the $p15^{INK4B}$ gene (and not the $p16^{INK4A}$ gene) during tumour development in a sporadic melanoma patient. *Cancer Research* **55**: 5531–5.

Goldstein, A.M., Bale, S.J. and Tucker, M.A. 1992. Linkage analysis of melanoma alone and chromosome 1p markers PND, D1S47, and LMYC. *Cytogenetics and Cell Genetics* **59**: 203–5.

Goldstein, A., Dracopoli, N., Ho, E. et al. 1993. Further evidence for a locus for cutaneous malignant melanoma-dysplastic naevus (CMM/DN) on chromosome 1p, and evidence for genetic heterogeneity. *American Journal of Human Genetics* **52**: 537–50.

Goldstein, A., Dracopoli, N., Engelstein, M., Fraser, M., Clark, W.H. Jr. and Tucker, M. 1994. Linkage of cutaneous malignant melanoma/dysplastic nevi to chromosome 9p, and evidence for genetic heterogeneity. *American Journal of Human Genetics* **54**: 489–96.

Goldstein, A., Fraser, M., Struewing, J.P. et al. 1995. Increased risk of pancreatic cancer in melanoma-prone kindreds with $p16^{INK4}$ mutations. *New England Journal of Medicine* **333**: 970–4.

Gonzalez-Zulueta, M., Bender, C.M., Yang, A.S., Nguyen, T., Beart, R.W., Van Tornout, J.M. and Jones, P.A. 1995. Methylation of the 5' CpG island of the $p16/CDKN2$ tumour suppressor gene in normal and transformed human tissues correlates with gene silencing. *Cancer Research* **55**: 4531–5.

Grana, X., and Reddy, E.P. 1995. Cell cycle control in mammalian cells: role of cyclins, cyclin dependent kinases (CDKs), growth suppressor genes and cyclin-dependent kinase inhibitors (CKIs). *Oncogene* **11**: 211–19.

Greene, M.H. and Fraumeni, J.F. Jr. 1979. The hereditary variant of malignant melanoma. In *Human Malignant Melanoma*, ed. W.H. Clark Jr, L.I. Golman and M.J. Mastrangelo, pp. 139–66. New York: Grune Stratton.

Greene, M.H., Goldin, L.R., Clark, W.H. et al. 1983. Familial cutaneous melanoma: autosomal dominant trait possibly linked to the Rh locus. *Proceedings of the National Academy of Sciences, USA* **80**: 6071–5.

Gruis, N., Bergman, W. and Frants, R. 1990. Locus for susceptibility to melanoma on chromosome 1p. *New England Journal of Medicine* **322**: 853–4.

Gruis, N., Sandkuijl, L., Weber, J., Van der Zee, A., Borgstein, A-M., Bergman, W. and Frants, R. 1993. Linkage analysis in Dutch familial atypical mole-melanoma (FAMMM) syndrome families. Effect of naevus count. *Melanoma Research* **3**: 271–7.

Gruis, N.A., Sandkuijl, L.A., van der Velden, P.A., Bergman, W. and Frants, R.R. 1995b. CDKN2 explains part of the clinical phenotype in Dutch familial atypical multiple-mole melanoma (FAMMM) syndrome families. *Melanoma Research* **5**: 169–77.

Gruis, N.A., van der Velden, P.A., Sandkuijl, L.A. et al. 1995c. Homozygotes for CDKN2 (p16) germline mutation in Dutch familial melanoma kindreds. *Nature Genetics* **10**: 351–3.

Gruis, N.A., Weaver-Feldhaus, J.M., Liu, Q. et al. 1995a. Genetic evidence in melanoma and bladder cancers that p16 and p53 function in separate pathways of tumour suppression. *American Journal of Pathology* **146**: 1199–206.

Guan, K-L., Jenkins, C.W., Li, Y. et al. 1994. Growth suppression by p18, a p16INK4/MTS1- and p14INK4B/MTS2-related CDK6 inhibitor, correlates with wild-type pRb function. *Genes and Development* **8**: 2939–52.

Hannon, G.J. and Beach, D. 1994. p15INK4B is a potential effector of TGFβ-induced cell cycle arrest. *Nature* **371**: 257–61.

Hansson, J., Platz, A., Linder, S. et al. 1996. Germline *p16* mutations are rare in Swedish melanoma families. *Proceedings of the American Association of Cancer Research* **37**: 186, Abstract No. 1270.

Hatada, I. and Mukai, T. 1995. Genomic imprinting of p57^KIP2, a cyclin-dependent kinase inhibitor, in mouse. *Nature Genetics* **11**: 204–6.

Hayashi, N., Sugimoto, Y., Tsuchiya, E., Ogawa, M. and Nakamura, Y. 1994. Somatic mutations of the MTS (multiple tumour suppressor) 1/CDK4I (cyclin dependent kinase-4 inhibitor) gene in human primary non-small cell lung carcinomas. *Biochemical and Biophysics Research Communcations* **202**: 1426–30.

Hayward, N. 1996. The current situation with regard to human melanoma and genetic inferences. *Current Opinions in Oncology* **8**: 136–42.

Healey, E., Rehman, I., Angus, B. and Rees, J.L. 1995. Loss of heterozygosity in sporadic primary cutaneous melanoma. *Genes, Chromosomes and Cancer* **12**: 152–6.

Herman, J.G., Merlo, A., Mao, L. et al. 1995. Inactivation of the *CDKN2/p16/MTS1* gene is frequently associated with aberrant DNA methylation in all common human cancers. *Cancer Research* **55**: 4525–30.

Holland, E.A., Beaton, S.C., Becker, T.M. et al. 1995. Analysis of the p16 gene, CDKN2, in 17 Australian melanoma kindreds. *Oncogene* **11**: 2289–94.

Hussussian, C.J., Struewing, J.P., Goldstein, A.M. et al. 1994. Germline p16 mutations in familial melanoma. *Nature Genetics* **8**: 15–21.

Igaki, H., Sasaki, H., Tachimori, Y. et al. 1995. Mutation frequency of the p16/CDKN2A gene in primary cancer in the upper digestive tract. *Cancer Research* **55**: 3421–3.

Kamb, A., Gruis, N.A., Weaver-Feldhaus, J. et al. 1994a. A cell cycle regulator potentially involved in genesis of many tumour types. *Science* **264**: 436–40.

Kamb, A., Shattuck-Eidens, D., Eeles, R. et al. 1994b. Analysis of the p16 gene (CDKN2A) as a candidate for the chromosome 9p melanoma susceptibility locus. *Nature Genetics* **8**: 22–6.

Kefford, R., Salmon, J., Shaw, H., Donald, J. and McCarthy, W. 1991. Hereditary melanoma in Australia: variable association with dysplastic naevi and absence of genetic linkage to chromosome 1p. *Cancer Genetics and Cytogenetics* **51**: 45–55.

Koh, J., Enders, G.H., Dynlacht, B.D. and Harlow, E. 1995. Tumour-derived p16 alleles encoding proteins defective in cell-cycle inhibition. *Nature* **375**: 506–10.

Liu, L., Lassam, N.J., Slingerland, J.M., Bailey, D., Cole, D., Jenkins, R., and Hogg, D. 1995. Germline p16INK4A mutation and protein dysfunction in a family with inherited melanoma. *Oncogene* **11**: 405–12.

Liu, Q., Neuhausen, S., McClure, M. et al., 1995. CDKN2A (MTS1) tumour suppressor gene mutations in human tumour cell lines. *Oncogene* **10**: 1061–7.

Lukas, J., Parry, D., Aagaard, L. et al. 1995. Retinoblastoma-protein-dependent cell-cycle inhibition by the tumour suppressor p16. *Nature* **375**: 503–6.

Lynch, H.T., Fusaro, R.M., Pester, J. et al. 1981. Tumour spectrum in the FAMMM syndrome. *British Journal of Cancer* **44**: 553–60.

MacGeoch, C., Newton Bishop, J.A., Bataille, V. et al. 1994. Genetic heterogeneity in familial malignant melanoma. *Human Molecular Genetics* **3**: 2195–200.

Malkin, D., Li, F.P., Strong, L.C. et al. 1990. Germline p53 mutations in a familial syndrome of breast cancer, sarcomas, and other neoplasms. *Science* **250**: 1233–8.

Mao, L., Merlo, A., Bedi, G., Shapiro, G.I., Edwards, C.D., Rollins, B.J., and Sidransky, D. 1995. A novel p16INK4A transcript. *Cancer Research* **55**: 2995–7.

Matsuoka, S., Edwards, M.C., Bai, C. et al. 1995. p57^{KIP2}, a structurally distinct member of the p21^{CIP1} Cdk inhibitor family, is a candidate tumour suppressor gene. *Genes and Development* **9**: 650–62.

Merlo, A., Herman, J.G., Mao, L et al. 1995. 5'CpG island methylation is associated with transcriptional silencing of the tumour suppressor *p16/CDKN2/MTS1* in human cancers. *Nature Medicine* **1**: 686–92.

Mori, T., Miura, K., Nishihira, T., Mori, S. and Nakamura, Y. 1994. Frequent somatic mutation of the MTS1/CDK4I (multiple tumour suppressor/cyclin-dependent kinase 4 inhibitor) gene in esophageal squamous cell carcinomas. *Cancer Research* **54**: 3396–7.

Nancarrow, D.J., Palmer, J.M., Walters, M.K. et al. 1992a. Exclusion of the familial melanoma locus (MLM) from the PND/D1S47 regions of chromosome arm 1p in 7 Australian families. *Genomics* **12**: 18–25.

Nancarrow, D., Mann, G., Holland, E. et al. 1993. Confirmation of chromosome 9p linkage to melanoma. *American Journal of Human Genetics* **53**: 936–42.

Nancarrow, D.J., Walker, G.J., Weber, J.L., Walters, M., Palmer, J. and Hayward, N. 1992b. Linkage mapping of melanoma (MLM) using 172 microsatellite markers. *Genomics* **14**: 939–47.

Nobori, T., Miura, K., Wu, D.J., Louis, A., Takabayashi, K., and Carson, D.A. 1994. Deletions of the cyclin-dependent kinase-4 inhibitor gene in multiple human cancers. *Nature* **368**: 753–6.

Norris, W. 1820. A case of fungoid disease. *Edinburgh Medical and Surgical Journal* **16**: 562–5.

Ogawa, O., Eccles, M.R., Szeto, J. et al. 1993. Relaxation of insulin-like growth factor II gene imprinting implicated in Wilms' tumour. *Nature* **362**: 749–51.

Ohta, M., Nagai, H., Shimizu, M. et al. 1994. Rarity of somatic and germline mutations of the cyclin-dependent kinase 4 inhibitor gene, CDK4I, in melanoma. *Cancer Research* **54**: 5269–72.

Okamoto, A., Demetrick, D.J., Spillare, E.A. et al. 1994. Mutations and altered expression of p16INK4 in human cancer. *Proceedings of the National Academy of Sciences, USA* **91**: 11045–9.

Okamoto, A., Hussain, S.P., Hagiwara, K. et al. 1995. Mutations in the p16INK4/MTS1/CDKN2A, p15INK4B/ MTS2, and p18 genes in primary and metastatic lung cancer. *Cancer Research* **55**: 1448–51.

Okuda, T., Hirai, H., Valentine, V. et al. 1995. Molecular cloning, expression pattern, and chromosomal localization of human CDKN2D/*INK4d*, an inhibitor of cyclin D-dependent kinases. *Genomics* **29**: 623–30.

Otterson, G.A., Khleif, S.N., Chen, W., Coxon, A.B. and Kaye, F.J. 1995. *CDKN2* gene silencing in lung cancer by DNA hypermethylation and kinetics of p16^{INK4} protein induction by 5-aza 2'deoxycytidine. *Oncogene* **11**: 1211–16.

Parmiter, A.H., Balaban, G., Herlyn, M., Clark, W.H. Jr. and Nowell, P.C. 1986. A t(1;19) chromosome translocation in three cases of human malignant melanoma. *Cancer Research* **46**: 1526–9.

Parry, D. and Peters, G. 1996. Temperature-sensitive mutants of p16^{CDKN2} associated with familial melanoma. *Molecular and Cellular Biology* **16**: 3844–52.

Petty, E.M., Gibson, L.H., Fountain, J.W., Bolognia, J.L., Yang-Feng, T.L., Housman, D.E. and Bale, A.E. 1993. Molecular definition of a chromosome 9p21 germ-line deletion in a woman with multiple melanomas and a plexiform neurofibroma; implications for 9p tumour-suppressor gene(s). *American Journal of Human Genetics* **53**: 96–104.

Pollock, P., Pearson, J. and Hayward, N.K. 1996. Compilation of somatic mutations of the CDKN2 gene in human cancers: non-random distribution of base substitutions. *Genes, Chromosomes and Cancer* **15**: 77–88.

Pollock, P.M., Yu, F., Qiu, L., Parsons, P.G. and Hayward, N.K. 1995. Evidence for UV induction of CDKN2A mutations in melanoma cell lines. *Oncogene* **11**: 663–8.

Ponce-Casteneda, M.V., Lee, M-H., Latres, E. et al. 1995. p27Kip1: Chromosomal mapping to 12p12-12p13.1 and absence of mutations in human tumours. *Cancer Research* **55**: 1211–14.

Quelle, D.E., Zindy, F., Ashmun, R.A. and Sherr, C.J. 1995. Alternative reading frames of the *INK4a* tumour suppressor gene encode two unrelated proteins capable of inducing cell cycle arrest. *Cell* **83**: 993–1000.

Rainier, S., Johnson, L.A., Dobry, C.J., Ping, A.J., Grundy, P.E. and Feinberg, A.P. 1993. Relaxation of imprinted genes in human cancer. *Nature* **362**: 747–9.

Ranade, K., Hussussian, C.J., Sikorski, R.S. et al. 1995. Mutations associated with familial melanoma impair p16INK4 function. *Nature Genetics* **10**: 114–16.

Reed, J.A., Loganzo, F. Jr., Shea, C.R. et al. 1995. Loss of expression of the *p16/* cyclin-dependent kinase inhibitor 2 tumour suppressor gene in melanocytic lesions correlates with invasive stage of tumour progression. *Cancer Research* **55**: 2713–18.

Reymond, A. and Brent, R. 1995. p16 proteins from melanoma-prone families are deficient in binding to Cdk4. *Oncogene* **11**: 1173–8.

Schmidt, E.E., Ichimura, K., Reifenberger, G. and Collins, V.P. 1994. CDKN2 (p16/MTS1) gene deletion or CDK4 amplification occurs in the majority of glioblastomas. *Cancer Research* **54**: 6321–4.

Serrano, M., Hannon, G.J. and Beach, D. 1993. A new regulatory motif in cell-cycle control causing specific inhibition of cyclin D/CDK4. *Nature* **366**: 704–7.

Serrano, M., Lee, H-W., Chin, L., Cordon-Carlo, C., Beach, D. and DePinho, A. 1996. Role of the *INK4a* locus in tumour suppression and cell mortality. *Cell* **85**: 27–37.

Sherr, C. and Roberts, J.M. 1995. Inhibitors of mammalian G1 cyclin-dependent kinases. *Genes and Development* **9**: 1149–63.

Spruck, C.H. III, Gonzalez-Zulueta, M., Shibata, A. et al. 1994. p16 gene in uncultured tumours. *Nature* **370**: 183–4.

Smith, F.E. 1966. Familial melanoma. *Archives of Internal Medicine* **117**: 820–3.

Stone, S., Dayananth, P., Jiang, P., Weaver-Feldhaus, J.M., Tavtigian, S.V., Cannon-Albright, L. and Kamb, A. 1995a. Genomic structure, expression and mutational analysis of the P15 (MTS2) gene. *Oncogene* **11**: 987–91.

Stone, S., Jiang, P., Dayananth, P. et al. 1995b. Complex structure and regulation of the p16 (MTS1) locus. *Cancer Research* **55**: 2988–94.

Sun, S., Narod, S.A. and Foulkes, W.D. 1996. A p16 mutation in a family with multiple cancers. *European Journal of Human Genetics* **4**(Suppl. 1): 13.

Vidal, M.J., Loganzo, F., de Oliveira, A.R., Hayward, N.K. and Albino, A.P. 1995. Mutations and defective expression of the WAF1 p21 tumour-suppressor gene in malignant melanomas. *Melanoma Research* **5**: 243–50.

Walker, G.J., Nancarrow, D.J., Walters, M.K., Palmer, J.M., Weber, J. and Hayward, N.K. 1994. Linkage analysis in familial melanoma kindreds to markers on chromosome 6p. *International Journal of Cancer* **59**: 771–5.

Walker, G.J., Hussussian, C.J., Flores, J.F. et al. 1995a. Mutations of the CDKN2/p16INK4 gene in Australian melanoma kindreds. *Human Molecular Genetics* **4**: 1845–52.

Walker, G.J., Palmer, J.M., Walters, M.K. and Hayward, N.K. 1995b. A genetic model of melanoma tumorigenesis based on allelic losses. *Genes, Chromosomes and Cancer* **12**: 134–41.

Wallace, D.C., Beardmore, G.L. and Exton, L.A. 1973. Familial malignant melanoma. *Annals of Surgery* **177**: 15–20.

Washimi, O., Nagatake, M., Osada, H. et al. 1995. In vivo occurrence of p16 (MTS1) and p15 (MTS2) alterations preferentially in non-small cell lung cancers. *Cancer Research* **55**: 514–17.

Weaver-Feldhaus, J.M., Gruis, N.A., Neuhausen, S. et al. 1994. Localization of a putative tumour suppressor gene by using homozygous deletions in melanomas. *Proceedings of the National Academy of Sciences, USA* **91**: 7563–7.

Whelan, A.J., Bartsch, D. and Goodfellow, P.J. 1995. A familial syndrome of pancreatic cancer and melanoma with a mutation in the *CDKN2* tumour-suppressor gene. *New England Journal of Medicine* **333**: 975–7.

Wolfel, T., Hauer, M., Schneider, J. et al. 1995. A p16INK4a-insensitive CDK4 mutant targeted by cytolytic T lymphocytes in a human melanoma. *Science* **269**: 1281–4.

Yang, R., Gombart, A.F., Serrano, M. and Koeffler, H.R. 1995. Mutational effects on the p16INK4a tumour suppressor protein. *Cancer Research* **55**: 2503–6.

Yarbrough, W.G., Aprelikova, O., Pei, H., Olshan, A.F. and Liu, E.T. 1996. Familial tumour syndrome associated with a germline non-functional p16[INK4a] allele. *Journal of the National Cancer Institute* **88**: 1489–91.

Zhou, X., Tarmin, L., Yin, J. et al. 1994. The MTS1 gene is frequently mutated in primary human esophageal tumours. *Oncogene* **9**: 3737–41.

Zuo, L., Weger, J., Yang, Q. et al. 1996. Germline mutations in the p16[INK4a] binding domain of CDK4 in familial melanoma. *Nature Genetics* **12**: 97–9.

15

Non-melanoma skin cancer

DAVID GOUDIE

Summary

This chapter discusses hereditary aspects of non-melanoma skin cancers, which at least numerically, form an important group of tumours. Although familial conditions only account for a small proportion of non-melanoma skin cancers, genetic defects involved in the pathogenesis of both familial and sporadic tumours have been identified and characterized through investigations of affected families. There are many familial genodermatoses associated with non-melanoma skin cancer. Some of these conditions, in which the primary genetic defect has been characterized or the disease gene located, are described in more detail. The role of these genes in the genesis of common sporadic skin tumours is also discussed.

Introduction

Non-melanoma skin cancers are among the most frequent malignancies in humans (Miller, 1991a,b; Kwa et al., 1992). The most common malignant lesions are basal cell and squamous cell carcinomas. The morphology and clinical behaviour of these tumours differ despite their common origin in the epidermis. In basal cell carcinomas, the malignant cells are similar in appearance to cells in the normal basal cell layer of the skin. Although these ulcerating lesions are locally invasive and may be very destructive, metastasis is very rare. Squamous cell carcinomas echo the appearances of the upper layers of the epidermis but in a disordered and invasive fashion. They can metastasize but metastases are infrequent and tend to occur late. There are many other cutaneous tumours with patterns of differentiation similar to the various skin appendages such as

306

eccrine (sweat producing) glands, apocrine (scent producing) glands and hair follicles. Not only can differences in the propensity of skin tumours to invade locally or to metastasize be observed but in situ lesions (such as actinic keratoses, Miller, 1991b) and some invasive lesions (Marks et al., 1988) can regress spontaneously. The elucidation of the molecular pathology of the various forms of non-melanoma skin cancer should provide important clues to the understanding of mechanisms controlling cellular proliferation and differentiation.

There is considerable genetic variability in susceptibility to development of skin tumours. Susceptibility may be affected by normal variation in skin pigmentation and by diseases associated with alterations in the normal resistance of the skin to the carcinogenic effects of sunlight and other environmental mutagens. Skin tumours are more common in conditions such as albinism where production of melanin is impaired. They are also more common in the porphyrias (Ferguson-Smith, 1934) where deposition of sensitizing agents in the skin promotes sunlight induced DNA damage. Defects in the ability of cells to repair or replicate past damaged DNA such as occurs in xeroderma pigmentosum greatly increase susceptibility to skin cancer. It has also been suggested that variants of polymorphic enzyme systems involved in the metabolism of carcinogens may contribute to susceptibility to non-melanoma skin cancer (Kappas et al., 1995). Squamous cell carcinoma may arise in scars or as a consequence of chronic ulceration. Skin tumours may therefore complicate genetic disorders like epidermolysis bullosa. Skin neoplasia may also occur in individuals with abnormal susceptibility to cutaneous viral infections (Heagerty et al., 1994) or be associated with immunological impairment (Jablonska et al., 1979). Germline defects in genes regulating growth and differentiation of cutaneous keratinocytes may also result in the development of skin tumours.

Skin pigmentation

Although non-melanoma skin cancer can be associated with exposure to a variety of carcinogens such as cigarette smoke, soot, arsenic, tar, and machine oil (Mukhtar and Bickers, 1993; Glover et al., 1994) the most ubiquitous carcinogenic agent associated with skin neoplasia is ultraviolet (UV) radiation. Both squamous and basal cell carcinomas are closely associated with chronic exposure to sunlight. Sporadic skin tumours commonly arise in the elderly on sun exposed areas and are particularly common in fair skinned individuals who tan poorly (Aubry and

MacGibbon, 1985). The incidence of both melanoma and non-melanoma skin cancer is highest in areas like Australia where fair-skinned people are exposed to intense sunlight. Excessive exposure in childhood is associated with the highest risks although tumours do not usually develop until middle or old age (Marks et al., 1990; Kricker et al., 1991).

Melanin pigmentation protects the skin from the damaging effects of UV radiation. Single gene defects resulting in impaired melanin synthesis such as those associated with the various forms of oculocutaneous albinism (King et al., 1995) may therefore predispose to actinic skin damage, squamous cell carcinoma, and basal cell carcinoma.

Hair and skin colour are thought to be polygenic traits (King et al., 1995). Recently relatively common variants of the melanocyte stimulating hormone receptor gene (*MC1R*) have been identified which have an important effect on skin pigmentation and hair colour (Valverde et al., 1995). Black eumelanin is photoprotective while red phaeomelanin may contribute to UV-induced skin damage because of its ability to generate free radicals in response to UV radiation (Ranadive et al., 1986). Individuals with red hair and fair skin have a predominance of phaeomelanin in hair and skin and/or a reduced ability to produce eumelanin and therefore are at increased risk when exposed to UV radiation (Aubry and MacGibbon, 1985). The relative proportions of phaeomelanin and eumelanin in mammals are regulated in part by melanocyte stimulating hormone (Burchill et al., 1993; Hunt et al., 1995). Mutations in *MC1R* have been found in a high proportion of individuals with red hair who tan poorly and less frequently in individuals with brown or black hair (Valverde et al., 1995). The mouse homologue of *MC1R* is the extension (e) locus. Alleles at this locus resulting in yellow mice (with predominant production of phaeomelanin) are recessive (Robbins et al., 1993).The pattern of inheritance of red hair and fair skin in humans remains unclear. Many red-haired/ fair-skinned individuals are apparent heterozygotes for variant *MC1R* alleles. A minority carry two variant alleles. Family studies correlating skin colour with segregation of *MCIR* variants have not yet been reported.

DNA repair defects and non-melanoma skin cancer

The various types of xeroderma pigmentosum and related conditions associated with autosomal recessive defects in DNA repair pathways are described in the Chapter 18. The great increase in the frequency of skin cancers including melanoma, actinic keratoses, basal cell carcinoma, squamous cell carcinoma, and keratoacanthoma in patients with xeroderma pigmentosum demonstrates the key role of nucleotide excision repair in preventing skin tumours resulting from DNA damage induced by sunlight and other mutagens.

Defects in the mismatch repair pathway implicated in the pathogenesis of colon cancer and other internal neoplasms may be associated with some non-melanoma skin tumours. Muir–Torre syndrome is a rare autosomal dominant disorder in which internal maligancies including colon, stomach, oesophageal, breast, ovarian, bladder, and laryngeal cancer are associated with skin neoplasia. In women, endometrial tissue is a primary site of carcinoma. The skin lesions include sebaceous hyperplasia, sebaceous adenoma, sebaceous carcinoma, and keratoacanthoma (a spontaneously resolving tumour with similar morphology to squamous cell carcinoma of the skin) (Schwartz and Torre, 1995). Not all affected individuals develop skin tumours (Hall et al., 1994). True sebaceous tumours are relatively rare. Their frequent association with other maligancies suggests that a significant proportion of patients with true sebaceous skin tumours have Muir–Torre syndrome (Finan and Connolly, 1984). Patients with sebaceous adenomas or carcinomas and their families may therefore benefit from screening for other neoplasms such as colon cancer which is the most common associated malignancy. The overlap between Muir–Torre syndrome and what was originally referred to as Lynch II cancer family syndrome (Lynch et al., 1985) suggested that this disorder might be attributable to defects in DNA mismatch repair. This possibility is supported by genetic linkage between cancer susceptibility in families with Muir–Torre syndrome and the *MSH2* gene on chromosome 2 (Hall et al., 1994) and by identification of mutations in this gene in several affected families (Kruse et al., 1996; Liu et al., 1994; Kolodner et al., 1994). This and other genes implicated in hereditary non-polyposis colorectal cancer (HNPCC) code for components of the DNA mismatch repair pathway and is implicated in the pathogenesis of HNPCC (Fishel et al., 1994), discussed in chapters 9 and 18. Simple sequence repeat instability, a characteristic feature of DNA mismatch repair defects, has been reported in Muir–Torre associated skin tumours (Honchel et al., 1994; Kruse et al., 1996). Interestingly, this simple sequence repeat instability has also been found in some sporadic squamous cell carcinomas of the skin suggesting defective mismatch repair (Zaphiropoulos et al., 1994) although this phenomenon was not described in another study of simple sequence repeat polymorphisms in cutaneous squamous cell carcinoma (Quinn et al., 1994).

The nevoid basal cell carcinoma syndrome (Gorlin syndrome)

The nevoid basal cell carcinoma syndrome (NBCCS) is an autosomal dominant disorder characterized by the development of multiple basal cell carcinomas, jaw cysts (odontogenic keratocysts), skeletal abnormalities, and intracranial calcification (Gorlin, 1987). The condition was first reported as early as 1894 (White, 1894; Jarisch, 1894) but was not clearly delineated until 1960 (Gorlin and Goltz, 1960). A minimum estimate of its prevalence is about 1 per 56,000 (Evans et al., 1993). One in 200 patients with one or more basal cell carcinomas has the syndrome, but the proportion is much higher in younger patients (Springate, 1986).

At around puberty, affected individuals develop cutaneous tumours. By 20 years of age over 95% have some tumours (Evans et al., 1993). Severely affected individuals may have many hundreds. Most of these tumours do not change in size and usually only a few grow and become locally invasive (Farndon et al., 1992). The invasive lesions have the same morphology and behaviour as ordinary sporadic basal cell carcinomas but may occur on both non-exposed as well as sun-exposed skin. Tumours are most common on the face, neck, and upper trunk. Basal cell carcinomas are infrequent before puberty but tumours have been reported in young children (Gilhuus-Moe et al., 1968). The frequency of basal cell carcinomas in affected individuals increases in their third and forth decades. By 40 years of age 90% of patients will have had at least one basal cell carcinoma (Gorlin, 1987; Evans et al., 1993). Tumours may occur earlier and are more frequent and aggressive in patients who have had radiotherapy. Small pathognomonic dyskeratotic pits (1–2 mm in diameter) are present on the palms and soles in about 70% of affected individuals (Evans et al., 1993).

Odontogenic keratocysts may first develop in the first decade of life but appear most frequently in the second or third decades (Evans et al., 1993). They may arise in both jaws but are more frequent in the mandible. They may occasionally cause pathological fractures. Jaw malignancy is rare in NBCCS.

Progressive intracranial calcification most frequently involving the falx cerebri is common (occurring in at least 85%) usually becoming evident during the second decade. The calcification is typically lamellar in pattern. Macrocephaly with frontal bossing is also characteristic. Cleft palate occurs in about 5% of patients (Evans et al., 1993). Up to a quarter of affected individuals have been found to have eye problems

(Evans et al., 1993) including strabismus, nystagmus, iris coloboma, and cataracts.

Skeletal defects including rib, vertebral and shoulder abnormalities, and pectus excavatum, are frequent (Gorlin, 1987). Polydactyly of the hands or feet occurs occasionally. Pseudolytic hamartomatous bone lesions composed of fibrous tissue are seen particularly in the hands and feet (Dunnick, 1978) but may occur at other sites.

Medulloblastoma may affect up to 5% of children with NBCCS. This tumour tends to develop unusually early in affected children with a mean age of onset of two years (Evans et al., 1991). Patients with the condition are also at increased risk from cardiac fibromas (which may develop in childhood), ovarian fibromas and calcification, meningiomas fibrosarcomas, rhabdomyosarcomas, and ovarian desmoids (Gorlin, 1995). The condition may also be associated with lymphomesenteric cysts.

Management of families with NBCCS may be facilitated by regular screening of affected and 'at risk' individuals. Echocardiography in early infancy may detect cardiac fibromas which have been reported in up to 3% of patients. Regular neurological examination of children below seven years of age who are at risk has been recommended, to facilitate early diagnosis of medulloblastoma. Dental examinations starting at around eight years have also been recommended, as jaw cysts may arise in the first decade of life. Jaw cysts are rarely symptomatic but may result in loss of teeth if not detected early. Dermatological assessments from puberty may be beneficial (Evans et al., 1993). Radiotherapy should be avoided if possible because increased numbers of basal cell carcinomas occur in areas of skin exposed to irradiation.

The condition is virtually fully penetrant (Farndon et al., 1992), but there is considerable variation in severity both within and between families. It is thought to arise as a consequence of a new mutation in between a third and a half of affected individuals (Gorlin, 1995).

The disease locus (NBCCS) was mapped to 9q22.3 in family studies (Farndon et al., 1992; Gailani et al., 1992; Reis et al., 1992; Goldstein et al., 1994; Wicking et al., 1994). There was no evidence of locus heterogeneity. Mutations in the human homologue of the Drosophila *patched* gene, which lies in this chromosomal region, have been found in affected patients (Johnson et al., 1996; Echelard et al., 1993). The *patched* gene codes for a transmembrane glycoprotein protein which, in *Drosophila*, antagonizes the induction of several genes by the hedgehog protein that are involved in intercellular signalling. This signalling system was originally identified in *Drosophila* through its role in determining segment patterning during development (Nakano et al., 1989; Hooper and Scott, 1989). The patterns of expression of *hedgehog* and *patched* in vertebrates indicate that they are likely to be involved in organizing many tissues including the neural tube, skeleton, limbs craniofacial structures, and skin (Echelard et al., 1993; Riddle et al., 1993; Goodrich et al., 1996; Iseki et al., 1996). These findings are consistent with the developmental anomalies associated with *patched* mutations in patients with nevoid basal cell carcinoma syndrome.

Patched functions as a tumour suppressor gene in humans. Of the eight mutations described in patients with NBCCS seven truncate the open reading frame and would therefore be inactivating. In patients with the condition, the normal NBCCS/*patched* allele inherited from their unaffected parent is lost in basal cell carcinomas (Bonifas et al., 1994; Gailani et al., 1992). The tumours therefore have no functional copy of the gene. Loss of the normal copy of the gene has also been observed in the epithelial lining of jaw cysts demonstrating that they are of clonal origin and develop as a consequence of loss of the tumour suppressor function (Levanat et al., 1996). Mutations involving the gene are also found in a high proportion of sporadic basal cell carcinomas (Gailani et al., 1996a).

Bazex–Dupré–Christol syndrome

This is another rare familial disorder associated with the development of multiple basal cell carcinomas in which the primary genetic defect has been localized. In Bazex syndrome basal cell carcinomas, which typically occur on the face from the second decade, are associated with follicular atrophoderma and impaired sweating and hair growth (Bazex et al., 1966). Follicular atrophoderma appears as funnel-shaped follicular depressions on the face, dorsa of the hands, extensor surfaces and back which are said to resemble multiple ice pick marks. These lesions, which are characterized by follicular dilatation and plugging associated with malformed and poorly developed follicular structures, do not occur in NBCCS while palmar and plantar pits do not occur in Bazex syndrome. Facial hyperpigmentation and milia also occur in affected individuals. The condition is not associated with skeletal or other developmental anomalies seen in the NBCCS. It is inherited as an X-linked dominant trait with both males and females being affected. Linkage studies in three affected families indicate that the disease gene lies on the long arm of the X-chromosome (Xq14-q27) adjacent to the polymorphic marker locus DXS1192 (Vabres et al., 1995).

Multiple self-healing squamous epithelioma (Ferguson-Smith disease)

Multiple self-healing squamous epithelioma is a rare autosomal dominant trait (Ferguson-Smith et al., 1971; Marks et al., 1988). Mapping of
the disease gene (*ESS1*) to chromosome 9q22 indicated that the disorder
could be related to NBCCS. The condition is characterized by the development of multiple skin tumours which are morphologically indistinguishable from sporadic well differentiated squamous carcinomas.
Despite invading deep into the dermis and along local lymphatics the
lesions regress spontaneously leaving deep pitted scars. Over 80 cases
have been reported. The majority of affected families that have been
described are of Scottish origin and most are descended from a common
ancestor (Goudie et al., 1993; Ferguson-Smith et al., 1971). (See Figures
15.1 and 15.2.)

Lesions start as small red macules or papules. Initially they may be
more easily felt than seen and have been described as being 'small hard
and millet-seed-like' (Wright et al., 1988). The lesions enlarge, ulcerate,
and heal leaving pitted scars with irregular, overhanging crenellated bor-
ders (particularly when they occur on the face). Lesions on the limbs tend
to be larger but heal with flatter, less punched out, scars. The lesions grow
rapidly for a period of weeks and may persist for months or occasionally
for years. As the lesions develop a central plug of keratin often forms in
their centre. This keratin plug is extruded as the lesion resolves. The

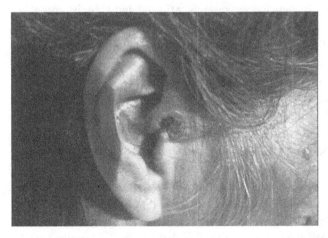

Figure 15.1. A typical ulcerated self-healing squamous epithelioma affecting the
external ear.

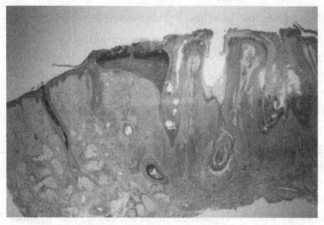

Fgure 15.2. H&E section of a self-healing epithelioma with tumour keratinocytes invading deep into the dermis.

lesions may become inflamed and infected. They can be itchy and occasionally painful. Metastasis is very rare. Lesions arising in areas previously exposed to radiotherapy may be more numerous, persistent and aggressive (Ferguson-Smith et al., 1971). One such lesion metastasized to a local lymph gland.

The age of onset of a first tumour is variable ranging from 8–62 years of age (Goudie et al., 1993). Mean age of onset is about 26 years (Ferguson-Smith et al., 1971). Tumour numbers are variable. The condition can be very disfiguring in severely affected individuals, some of whom have had over 100 tumours. Lesions occur predominantly on the exposed skin of the head and neck, implicating sunlight in their aetiology. They are less frequent on the limbs and rarely occur on the trunk. It has been suggested that tumours may arise within pilosebaceous follicles (Currie and Ferguson-Smith, 1952; Wright et al., 1988). In familial cases of Scottish ancestry, only one tumour has been reported to arise on palmar or plantar surfaces where pilosebaceous follicles do not occur (Sommerville and Milne, 1950). Some patients reported to have multiple epitheliomas of the 'Ferguson-Smith type' have had lesions with an atypical anatomical distribution (large numbers of lesions on the trunk and limbs or multiple plantar lesions; Tarnowski, 1966; Ereaux et al., 1955; Haydey et al., 1981; Hilker and Winterscheidt, 1987). It is unlikely that these patients have the same condition as that originally described by J. Ferguson-Smith although the conditions may be related.

No consistent dysmorphic features or developmental anomalies have been reported in patients with this condition. It does not appear to be associated with a significant increase in the incidence of other forms of neoplasia.

Although most lesions will resolve spontaneously, the residual scars can be disfiguring. Good cosmetic results can be achieved if lesions are treated with cryotherapy in their earliest stages (Wright et al., 1988). Larger lesions may require surgical excision. Oral etretinate (a retinoic acid derivative) has been found to reduce tumour numbers in some severely affected individuals (Wright et al., 1988). Radiotherapy should be avoided.

The primary genetic defect associated with multiple self-healing squamous epithelioma (*ESS1*) has been mapped to 9q22.3 using polymorphic markers in linkage studies within affected families and by comparing disease associated haplotypes between affected families of Scottish ancestry (Goudie et al., 1993). The *ESS1* gene is flanked by the marker loci D9S180 and D9S197 (Goudie et al., 1994) and therefore lies in the same 4 cM interval on the long arm of chromosome 9 as the *patched* gene (Hahn et al., 1996). There is no increase in the frequency of basal cell carcinomas in patients with multiple self-healing squamous epithelioma and they do not have other cutaneous or skeletal stigmata of the NBCCS. If mutations in *patched* cause self-healing epitheliomas, these mutations must result in a subtle alteration in the pattern of expression of the gene or production of an abnormal protein since inactivating mutations are associated with NBCCS. It remains to be determined whether the multiple self-healing squamous epithelioma syndrome is attributable a mutation affecting the function of the *patched* gene or if the condition is caused by mutations in another gene adjacent to *patched*. No mutations have been identified within the *patched* gene in affected individuals. Somatic allele losses for marker loci in 9q22.3 have not been found in self-healing epitheliomas but it has been difficult to obtain adequate quantities of pure tumour material for analysis. Nucleated tumour cells tend to lie adjacent to the tumour margins and to be closely associated with inflammatory cells infiltrating the underlying dermis.

Other conditions associated with a predisposition to non-melanoma skin cancer

Genes associated with two other familial conditions in which squamous cell carcinomas of the skin occur have been mapped.

Huriez syndrome

There is inconclusive evidence that the genetic defect associated with sclerotylosis (Huriez syndrome) lies on the long arm of chromosome 4 (Delaporte et al., 1995). This autosomal dominant condition is characterized by scleroatrophic lesions predominantly of the hands, hypoplastic nail changes, and palmoplantar keratodermia. Squamous cell carcinomas often arise in scleroatrophic areas and bowel cancer may occur in affected individuals.

Dyskeratosis congenita

The gene for this X-linked recessive condition has been mapped to Xq28 in the region of D9S52 (Arngrimsson et al., 1993). This condition is characterized by reticulate skin hyperpigmentation, mucosal leukoplakia, and nail dystrophy. Pancytopaenia predisposes affected individuals to opportunistic infections. Squamous cell carcinomas usually arise in the leukoplakia on mucous membranes but may occur in the skin (Davidson and Connor, 1988).

Genes associated with familial skin appendage tumours

Cylindromas are cutaneous tumours which originate in skin appendages (van Balkom and Hennekam, 1994). In familial cylindromatosis, which is inherited as an autosomal dominant trait, tumours arise predominantly in hairy areas of the body, with approximately 90% on the head and neck (Crain and Helwig, 1961). In severely affected individuals tumours on the scalp may become confluent leading to the designation 'turban tumours syndrome'. The scalp tumours are hairless, firm and nodular. The tumours have morphological features reminiscent of both sweat and apocrine glands (Hashimoto and Lever, 1969; Cotton and Braye, 1984). Occasionally other skin appendage tumours, such as trichoepitheliomas (which show hair follicle differentiation) and eccrine spiradenomas (arising from the secretory coils of the sweat gland), are observed in affected families. The condition is not associated with basal or squamous cell carcinomas. Tumours first appear in adolescence and gradually increase in size and number thereafter. Expression of the condition is variable with some obligate carriers having few or no signs of the disorder. The tumours very rarely become malignant or metastasize. The condition can be very disfiguring in severely affected individuals. Lesions involving the external ear may cause deafness.

The genetic defect associated with the condition in two families with common ancestry has been found to lie on the long arm of chromosome 16 (16q12-q13) in linkage studies (Biggs et al., 1995). The disease gene is most likely to lie in a 6 cM interval between the polymorphic marker loci D16S411 and D16S416. Tumours from affected individuals have consistently lost heterozygosity for polymorphic markers from this chromosomal region with the allele inherited from their affected parent being retained. It is therefore likely that familial cylindromatosis is due to a defect in a tumour suppressor gene with specificity for keratinocytes derived from skin appendages.

Trichoepithelioma is a benign skin tumour originating in hair follicles. A gene associated with this condition has been mapped to 9p21, a chromosomal region involved in the pathogenesis of sporadic skin tumours (Quinn et al., 1994) and other forms of neoplasia (Kamb et al., 1994). The majority of these tumours are solitary and occur sporadically, but a predisposition to the development of multiple trichoepitheliomas can be inherited as a dominant trait (van Balkom and Hennekam, 1994). Affected individuals develop multiple small flesh coloured, translucent, cutaneous tumours, which may first appear in childhood. The majority of lesions occur on the face. These tumours may sometimes degenerate into basal cell carcinomas.

In view of the occurrence of trichoepitheliomas in familial cylindromatosis it has been suggested that these conditions might be associated with different mutations at the same locus (Gerretsen et al., 1995). However, in three affected families multiple familial trichoepithelioma was found to segregate with polymorphic markers for the short arm of chromosome 9 (9q21) suggesting that a second gene involved in the pathogenesis of skin appendage tumours may lie in this region (Harada et al., 1996). The disease gene is most likely to be located between IFNA and the marker locus D9S126. Typing of these families for 16q markers was not reported.

Genetic alterations in common sporadic non-melanoma skin cancers

The development of non-melanoma skin cancer is a multistep process. Several genes and chromosome regions implicated in the pathogenesis of common basal and squamous cell carcinomas have been identified.

Ha-*ras* (*RASH*) gene activation is an early event in the development of mouse skin tumours induced by exposure to chemical carcinogens (Balmain et al., 1984; Brown et al., 1990). Mutations in members of the *RAS* oncogene family (Harvey *RAS* and Kirsten *RAS*) have been found in both basal and squamous cell carcinomas but estimates of the frequency of these mutations are variable and they have been infrequent in some studies (van der Schroeff et al., 1990; Pierceall et al., 1991; Campbell et al., 1993a).

Mutations in the *TP53* gene on chromosome 17p are common in both basal and squamous cell carcinomas (Brash et al., 1991; Rady et al., 1992; Ziegler et al., 1993). The *TP53* mutations occur early in tumour development being found frequently in pre-invasive lesions (actinic keratoses and Bowen disease; Campbell et al., 1993b; Ziegler et al., 1994). Most mutations occur at adjacent pyrimidines and are C → T substitutions or CC → TT double base changes, implicating sunlight in their pathogenesis. Ultraviolet radiation characteristically damages DNA by inducing formation of covalent bonds between adjacent pyrimidines on the same DNA strand.

TP53 has a key role in the removal of potentially neoplastic cells that have sustained genetic damage. High levels of *TP53* protein are induced in normal skin by exposure to the genotoxic effects of ultraviolet light (Hall et al., 1993). In mice that are unable to produce *TP53* the programmed cell death that normally occurs in skin keratinocytes that have been damaged by ultraviolet-irradiation is suppressed (Ziegler et al., 1994). A skin keratinocyte that has previously sustained genetic damage resulting in loss of the normal *TP53* response to ultraviolet-induced injury will therefore be more likely to survive the effects of sunburn than its neighbours resulting in selective growth of potentially neoplastic cells (Ziegler et al., 1994).

The most frequent genetic abnormality observed in basal cell carcinomas is loss of heterozygosity for polymorphic marker loci for the region of chromosome 9 (9q22) which contains the *patched* gene (Gailani et al., 1992, 1996b; Quinn et al., 1994; Stanley et al., 1995). Inactivating mutations have been found within remaining copy of the *patched* gene in several sporadic basal cell carcinomas which have lost heterozygosity for 9q22, confirming that inactivation of this tumour suppressor gene is a principal cause of both sporadic and familial tumours. Paradoxically, levels of patched mRNA have been found to be elevated in some basal cell carcinomas with mutations within the *patched* gene (Gailani et al., 1996b). In Drosophila, *patched* interacts with the *hedgehog* signalling pathway repressing the expression of various genes which are expressed in response to exposure of cells to hedgehog protein including *wingless*, *decapentaplegic*, and *patched* itself (Ingham and Hidalgo, 1993; Chen and Struhl, 1996). Failure of this negative feedback loop may result in production of large amounts of mutant patched mRNA which cannot be translated into functional protein (Gailani et al., 1996b).

Loss of genetic material from other chromosomal regions is relatively infrequent in basal cell carcinomas (Quinn et al., 1994). Despite the involvement of *TP53* mutations in the development of basal cell carcinoma loss of heterozygosity for 17p is rare.

In contrast, widespread allelic losses are common in squamous cell carcinomas of the skin. Losses of heterozygosity have been most frequent from 9p, 13q, 17p, 17q and 3p (Quinn et al., 1994). Loss of 9q is not particularly common.

Surprisingly widespread allelic loss is also common in actinic keratoses. Actinic keratoses are premalignant lesions associated with sun exposure. Only a small proportion of these lesions develop into invasive squamous carcinomas and many resolve spontaneously (Miller, 1991a). In one report over half of actinic keratoses examined were found to show loss of heterozygosity at four or more loci (Rehman et al., 1996). Losses were most frequent from 17p,17q,13q, 9p, 9q. Genetic instability appears to be an early feature of the genesis of some skin tumours. It is of note that *TP53* mutations are also common in these lesions.

The allelic losses for 9p markers in squamous cell carcinomas and their precursors indicates a possible relationship between the pathogenesis of these tumours and familial trichoepitheliomas. This chromosomal region, containing the *CDKN2A* (*p16*) tumour suppressor gene and its homologue *CDKN2B* (*p15*), is implicated in the pathogenesis of many types of cancer (see also Chapter 14). Whether or not non-melanoma skin tumours are associated with defects in either of these genes is not firmly established.

Some of the genetic factors determining predisposition to non-melanoma skin cancer and the molecular pathology associated with different patterns of tumour differentiation are beginning to emerge. Although the role of the genes associated with many of the familial skin and skin appendage tumours in sporadic skin cancer is as yet unknown, it is likely that an understanding of the genetic pathology of these diverse lesions will provide new insights into the pathways involved in the development of common skin cancers and other forms of neoplasia.

Conclusions

Although the skin is often exposed to carcinogens such as sunlight, cigarette smoke and machine oil, in most instances cancer does not develop. In

certain individuals, non-melanomatous skin cancer occurs at a young age
and at numerous sites. Pedigree studies have shown that in many cases,
these persons belong to families with defined genetic disorders such as
Gorlin syndrome or xeroderma pigmentosum. Many of the genes responsible for these conditions have now been isolated. Alterations in the
human homologue of *patched*, mutated in Gorlin syndrome, are also
found in sporadic basal cell carcinomas. Mutations in *TP53* and *RAS*
are seen in both basal and squamous cell carcinomas. Skin carcinogenesis
is in many ways a useful model system for studying the steps leading from
normal epithelium to frank malignancy.

References

Arngrimsson, R., Dokal, I., Luzzatto, L. and Connor, J.M. 1993. Dyskeratosis
    congenita: three additional families show linkage to a locus in Xq28. *Journal
    of Medical Genetics* **30**: 618–19.
Aubry, F. and MacGibbon, B. 1985. Risk factors for squamous carcinoma of the
    skin, a case control study in the Montreal region. *Cancer* **55**: 907–11.
Balmain, A., Ramsden, M., Bowden, G.T. and Smith, J. 1984. Activation of the
    mouse cellular Harvey-ras gene in chemically induced benign skin
    papillomas. *Nature* **307**: 658–60.
Bazex, A., Dupre, A. and Christol, B. 1966. Atrophodermie folliculaire,
    proliferations basocellulaires et hypotrichose. *Archives of Dermatology and
    Syphilis* **93**: 241–54.
Biggs, P.J., Wooster, R., Ford, D. et al. 1995. Familial cylindromatosis (turban
    tumour syndrome) gene localised to chromosome 16q12-q13: evidence for its
    role as a tumour suppressor gene. *Nature Genetics* **11**: 441–3.
Bonifas, J.M., Bare, J.W., Kerschmann, R.L., Master, S.P. and Epstein, E.H., Jr.
    1994. Parental origin of chromosome 9q22.3-q31 lost in basal cell carcinomas
    from basal cell nevus syndrome patients. *Human Molecular Genetics* **3**: 447–
    8.
Brash, D.E., Rudolph, J.A., Simon, J.A., Lin, A. et al. 1991. A role for sunlight in
    skin cancer: UV-induced p53 mutations in squamous cell carcinoma.
    Proceedings of the National Academy of Sciences, USA **88**: 10124–8.
Brown, K., Buchmann, A. and Balmain, A. 1990. Carcinogen-induced mutations
    in the mouse c-Ha-ras gene provide evidence of multiple pathways for tumor
    progression. *Proceedings of the National Academy of Sciences, USA* **87**: 538–
    42.
Burchill, S.A., Ito, S. and Thody, A.J. 1993. Effects of melanocyte-stimulating
    hormone on tyrosinase expression and melanin synthesis in hair follicular
    melanocytes of the mouse. *Journal of Endocrinology* **137**: 189–95.
Campbell, C., Quinn, A.G. and Rees, J.L. 1993a. Codon 12 Harvey-ras mutations
    are rare events in non-melanoma human skin cancer. *British Journal of
    Dermatology* **128**: 111–14.
Campbell, C., Quinn, A.G., Ro, Y.S., Angus, B. and Rees, J.L. 1993b. p53
    mutations are common and early events that precede tumor invasion in
    squamous cell neoplasia of the skin. *Journal of Investigative Dermatology*
    100: 746–8.

Chen, Y. and Struhl, G. 1996. Dual roles for patched in sequestering and transducing hedgehog. *Cell* **87**: 553–63.

Cotton, D.W.K. and Braye, S.G. 1984. Dermal cylindromas originate from the eccrine sweat gland. *British Journal of Dermatology* **111**: 53–61.

Crain, R.C. and Helwig, E.B. 1961. Dermal cylindroma (dermal eccrine cylindroma). *American Journal of Clinical Pathology* **6**: 504–15.

Currie, A. and Ferguson-Smith, J. 1952. Multiple primary spontaneous-healing squamous cell carcinomata of the skin. *Journal of Pathology and Bacteriology* **64**: 827–39.

Davidson, H.R. and Connor, J.M. 1988. Dyskeratosis congenita. *Journal of Medical Genetics* **25**: 843–6.

Delaporte, E., N'guyen-Mailfer, C., Janin, A. et al. 1995. Keratoderma with scleroatrophy of the extremities or sclerotylosis (Huriez syndrome): a reappraisal. *British Journal of Dermatology* **133**: 409–16.

Dunnick, N.R. 1978. Nevoid basal cell carcinoma syndrome. *Radiology* **127**: 331–4.

Echelard, Y., Epstein, D.J., St-Jacques, B., Shen, L., Mohler, J., McMahon, J.A. and McMahon, A.P. 1993. Sonic hedgehog, a member of a family of putative signaling molecules, is implicated in the regulation of CNS polarity. *Cell* **75**: 1417–30.

Ereaux, L.P., Schopflocher, P. and Fournier, C.J. 1955. Keratoacanthomata. *Archives of Dermatology* **71**: 73–9.

Evans, D.G., Farndon, P.A., Burnell, L.D., Gattamaneni, H.R. and Birch, J.M. 1991. The incidence of Gorlin syndrome in 173 consecutive cases of medulloblastoma. *British Journal of Cancer* **64**: 959–61.

Evans, D.R.G., Ladusans, E.J., Rimmer, S., Burnell, L.D., Thakker, N. and Farndon, P.A. 1993. Complications of the nevoid basal cell carcinoma syndrome: results of a population based study. *Journal of Medical Genetics* **30**: 460–4.

Farndon, P.A., Mastro, R.G.D., Evans, D.R.G. and Kilpatrick, M.W. 1992. Location of the gene for Gorlin syndrome. *Lancet* **339**: 581–2.

Ferguson-Smith, J. 1934. A case of multiple primary squamous-celled carcinomata in a young man, with spontaneous healing. *British Journal of Dermatology* **46**: 267.

Ferguson-Smith, M.A., Wallace, D.C., James, Z.H. and Renwick, J.H. 1971. Multiple self-healing squamous epithelioma. *Birth Defects Original Articles Series* **VII**: 157–63.

Finan, M.C. and Connolly, S.M. 1984. Sebaceous gland tumors and systemic disease: a clinicopathologic analysis. *Medicine* **63**: 232–42.

Fishel, R., Lescoe, M.K., Rao, M.R. et al. 1994. The human mutator gene homolog MSH2 and its association with hereditary nonpolyposis colon cancer. *Cell* **77**: 167.

Gailani, M.R., Bale, S.J., Leffell, D.J. et al. 1992. Developmental defects in Gorlin syndrome related to a putative tumor suppressor gene on chromosome 9. *Cell* **69**: 111–17.

Gailani, M.R., Leffell, D.J., Ziegler, A., Gross, E.G., Brash, D.E. and Bale, A.E. 1996a. Relationship between sunlight exposure and a key genetic alteration in basal cell carcinoma. *Journal of the National Cancer Institute* **88**: 349–54.

Gailani, M.R., Stahle-Backdahl, M., Leffell, D.J. et al. 1996b. The role of the human homologue of Drosophila patched in sporadic basal cell carcinomas *Nature Genetics* **14**: 78–81.

Gerretsen, A.L., Beemer, F.A., Deenstra, W., Hennekam, F.A. and van Vloten, W.A. 1995. Familial cutaneous cylindromas: investigations in five generations of a family. *Journal of the American Academy of Dermatology* **33**: 199–206.

Gilhuus-Moe, O., Haugen, L.K. and Dee, P.M. 1968. The syndrome of multiple cysts of the jaws, basal cell carcinomata and skeletal anomalies. *British Journal of Oral Surgery* **5**: 211–22.

Glover, M.T., Niranjan, N., Kwan, J.T. and Leigh, I.M. 1994. Non-melanoma skin cancer in renal transplant recipients: the extent of the problem and a strategy for management. *British Journal of Plastic Surgery* **47**: 86–9.

Goldstein, A.M., Stewart, C., Bale, A.E., Bale, S.J. and Dean, M. 1994. Localization of the gene for the nevoid basal cell carcinoma syndrome. *American Journal of Human Genetics* **54**: 765–73.

Goodrich, L.V., Johnson, R.L., Milenkovic, L., McMahon, J.A. and Scott, M.P. 1996. Conservation of the hedgehog/patched signaling pathway from flies to mice: induction of a mouse patched gene by Hedgehog. *Genes and Development* **10**: 301–12.

Gorlin, R.J. 1987. Nevoid basal cell carcinoma syndrome. *Medicine* **66**: 99–109.

Gorlin, R.J. 1995. Nevoid basal cell carcinoma syndrome. *Dermatologic Clinics* **13**: 113–25.

Gorlin, R.J. and Goltz, R.W. 1960. Multiple nevoid basal cell epithelioma, jaw cysts and bifid rib syndrome. *New England Journal of Medicine* **262**: 908–12.

Goudie, D.R., Yuille, M.A., Leversha, M.A., Furlong, R.A., Carter, N.P., Lush, M.J., Affara, N.A. and Ferguson-Smith, M.A. 1993. Multiple self-healing squamous epitheliomata (ESS1) mapped to chromosome 9q22-q31 in families with common ancestry. *Nature Genetics* **3**: 165–9.

Goudie, D.R., Yuille, M.A.R., Barroso, I. and Ferguson-Smith, M.A. 1994. Mapping of the gene for multiple self-healing squamous epithelioma in families with common ancestry. *Annals of Human Genetics* **58**: 213.

Hahn, H., Wicking, C., Zaphiropoulous, P.G. et al. 1996. Mutations of the human homolog of Drosophila patched in the nevoid basal cell carcinoma syndrome. *Cell* **85**: 841–51.

Hall, N.R., Williams, M.A., Murday, V.A., Newton, J.A. and Bishop, D.T. 1994. Muir–Torre syndrome: a variant of the cancer family syndrome. *Journal of Medical Genetics* **31**: 627–31.

Hall, P.A., McKee, P.H., Menage, H.D., Dover, R. and Lane, D.P. 1993. High levels of p53 protein in UV-irradiated normal human skin. *Oncogene* **8**: 203–7.

Harada, H., Hashimoto, K. and Ko, M.S. 1996. The gene for multiple familial trichoepithelioma maps to chromosome 9p21. *Journal of Investigative Dermatology* **107**: 41–3.

Hashimoto, K. and Lever, W.L. 1969. Histiogenesis of skin appendage tumors. *Archives of Dermatology* **100**: 356–69.

Haydey, R.P., Reed, M.L., Dzubow, L.M. and Schupack, J.L. 1981. Treatment of keratoacanthomas with oral 13-cis-retinoic acid. *New England Journal of Medicine* **303**: 560–2.

Heagerty, A.H., Fitzgerald, D., Smith, A., Bowers, B., Jones, P., Fryer, A.A., Zhao, L., Alldersea, J. and Strange, R.C. 1994. Glutathione S-transferase GSTM1 phenotypes and protection against cutaneous tumours. *Lancet* **343**: 266–8.

Hilker, O. and Winterscheidt, M. 1987. Familial multiple keratoacanthomas. *Zeitschrift fur Hautkrankheiten* **62**: 280–9.

Honchel, R., Halling, K.C., Schaid, D.J., Pittelkow, M. and Thibodeau, S.N. 1994. Microsatellite instability in Muir-Torre syndrome. *Cancer Research* **54**: 1159–63.

Hooper, J.E. and Scott, M.P. 1989. The Drosophila patched gene encodes a putative membrane protein required for segmental patterning. *Cell* **59**: 751–65.

Hunt, G., Kyne, S., Wakamatsu, K., Ito, S. and Thody, A.J. 1995. Nle4DPhe7 alpha-melanocyte-stimulating hormone increases the eumelanin:phaeomelanin ratio in cultured human melanocytes. *Journal of Investigative Dermatology* **104**: 83–5.

Ingham, P.W. and Hidalgo, A. 1993. Regulation of wingless transcription in the Drosophila embryo. *Development* **117**: 283–91.

Iseki, S., Araga, A., Ohuchi, H., Nohno, T., Yoshioka, H., Hayashi, F. and Noji, S. 1996. Sonic hedgehog is expressed in epithelial cells during development of whisker, hair, and tooth. *Biochemical and Biophysical Research Communications* **218**: 688–93.

Jablonska, S., Orth, G., Jarzabek-Chorzelska, M. et al. 1979. Twenty-one years of follow-up studies of familial epidermodysplasia verruciformis. *Dermatologica* **158**: 309–27.

Jarisch, W. 1894. Zur Lehre von den Hautgeschwulsten. *Archives of Dermatology and Syphilis* **28**: 162–222.

Johnson, R.L., Rothman, A.L., Xie, J. et al. 1996. Human homolog of patched, a candidate gene for the basal cell nevus syndrome. *Science* **272**: 1668–71.

Kamb, A., Gruis, N.A., Weaver-Feldhaus, J. et al. 1994. A cell cycle regulator potentially involved in genesis of many tumor types. *Science* **264**: 436–40.

Kappas, A., Sassa, S., Galbraith, R.A. and Normand, Y. 1995. The porphyrias. In *The Metabolic and Molecular Bases of Inherited Disease*, ed. C.R. Scriver, A.L. Beaudet, W.S. Sly and D. Valle, 7th edn., pp. 2103–60. New York: McGraw-Hill Inc.

King, R.A., Hearing, V.J., Creel, D.J. and Oetting, W.S. 1995. Albinism. In *The Molecular and Molecular Bases of Inherited Disease*, ed. C.R. Scriver, A.L. Beaudet, W.S. Sly and D. Valle, 7th edn., pp. 4353–92. New York: McGraw-Hill Inc.

Kolodner, R.D., Hall, N.R., Lipford, J. et al. 1994. Structure of the human MSH2 locus and analysis of two Muir-Torre kindreds for msh2 mutations. *Genomics* **24**: 516–26.

Kricker, A., Armstrong, B.K., English, D.R. and Heenan, P.J. 1991. Pigmentary and cutaneous risk factors for non-melanocytic skin cancer – a case-control study. *International Journal of Cancer* **48**: 650–62.

Kruse, R., Lamberti, C., Wang, Y. et al. 1996. Is the mismatch repair deficient type of Muir–Torre syndrome confined to mutations in the hMSH2 gene? *Human Genetics* **98**: 747–50.

Kwa, R.E., Campana, K. and Moy, R.L. 1992. Biology of cutaneous squamous cell carcinoma. *Journal of the American Academy of Dermatology* **26**: 1–26.

Levanat, S., Gorlin, R.J., Fallet, S., Johnson, D.R., Fantasia, J.E. and Bale, A.E. 1996. A two-hit model for developmental defects in Gorlin syndrome. *Nature Genetics* **12**: 85–7.

Liu, B., Parsons, R.E., Hamilton, S.R. et al. 1994. hMSH2 mutations in hereditary nonpolyposis colorectal cancer kindreds. *Cancer Research* **54**: 4590–4.

324   D. Goudie

Lynch, H.T., Fusaro, R.M., Roberts, L., Voorhees, G.J. and Lynch, J.F. 1985.
    Muir–Torre syndrome in several members of a family with a variant of the
    Cancer Family Syndrome. *British Journal of Dermatology* **113**: 295–301.
Marks, R., Rennie, G. and Selwood, T.S. 1988. Malignant transformation of
    solar keratoses to squamous cell carcinoma. *Lancet* **1**: 795–7.
Marks, R., Jolley, D., Lectsas, S. and Foley, P. 1990. The role of childhood
    exposure to sunlight in the development of solar keratoses and non-
    melanocytic skin cancer. *Medical Journal of Australia* **152**: 62–6.
Miller, S.J. 1991a. Biology of basal cell carcinoma (Part I). *Journal of the
    American Academy of Dermatology* **24**: 1–13.
Miller, S.J. 1991b. Biology of basal cell carcinoma (Part II). *Journal of the
    American Academy of Dermatology* **24**: 161–75.
Mukhtar, H. and Bickers, D.R. 1993. Environmental skin cancer: mechanisms,
    models and human relevance. *Cancer Research* **53**: 3439–42.
Nakano, Y., Guerrero, I., Hidalgo, A., Taylor, A., Whittle, J.R. and Ingham,
    P.W. 1989. A protein with several possible membrane-spanning domains
    encoded by the Drosophila segment polarity gene patched. *Nature* **341**:
    508–13.
Pierceall, W.E., Goldberg, L.H., Tainsky, M.A., Mukhopadhyay, T. and
    Ananthaswamy, H.N. 1991. *Ras* gene mutation and amplification in human
    nonmelanoma skin cancers. *Molecular Carcinogenesis* **4**: 196–202.
Quinn, A.G., Sikkink, S. and Rees, J.L. 1994. Basal cell carcinomas and
    squamous cell carcinomas of human skin show distinct patterns of
    chromosome loss. *Cancer Research* **54**: 4756–9.
Rady, P., Scinicariello, F., Wagner, R.F., Jr. and Tyring, S.K. 1992. p53
    mutations in basal cell carcinomas. *Cancer Research* **52**: 3804–6.
Ranadive, N.S., Shirwadkar, S., Persad, S. and Menon, I.A. 1986. Effects of
    melanin induced free radicals on the isolated rat peritoneal mast cells.
    Journal of Investigative Dermatology **86**: 303–7.
Rehman, I., Takata, M., Wu, Y.Y. and Rees, J.L. 1996. Genetic change in actinic
    keratoses. *Oncogene* **12**: 2483–90.
Reis, A., Kuster, W., Linss, G., Gebel, E. et al. 1992. Localisation of gene for the
    naevoid basal-cell carcinoma syndrome. *Lancet* **339**: 617.
Riddle, R.D., Johnson, R.L., Laufer, E. and Tabin, C. 1993. Sonic hedgehog
    mediates the polarizing activity of the ZPA. *Cell* **75**: 1401–16.
Robbins, L.S., Nadeau, J.H., Johnson, K.R. et al. 1993. Pigmentation phenotypes
    of variant extension locus alleles result from point mutations that alter MSH
    receptor function. *Cell* **72**: 827–34.
Schwartz, R.A. and Torre, D.P. 1995. The Muir–Torre syndrome: a 25-year
    retrospect. *Journal of the American Academy of Dermatology* **33**: 90–104.
Shanley, S.M., Dawkins, H., Wainwright, B.J. et al. 1995. Fine deletion mapping
    on the long arm of chromosome 9 in sporadic and familial basal cell
    carcinomas. *Human Molecular Genetics* **4**: 129–33.
Sommerville, J. and Milne, J.A. 1950. Familial primary self-healing squamous
    epithelioma of the skin (Ferguson-Smith type). *British Journal of
    Dermatology and Syphilis* **62**: 485–90.
Springate, J.E. 1986. The nevoid basal cell carcinoma syndrome. *Journal of
    Pediatric Surgery* **21**: 908–10.
Tarnowski, W.M. 1966. Multiple keratoacanthomata. *Archives of Dermatology*
    94: 74–80.

Vabres, P., Lacombe, D., Rabinowitz, L.G. et al. 1995. The gene for Bazex–Dupre-Christol syndrome maps to chromosome Xq. *Journal of Investigative Dermatology* **105**: 87–91.

Valverde, P., Healy, E., Jackson, I., Rees, J.L. and Thody, A.J. 1995. Variants of the melanocyte stimulating hormone receptor gene are associated with red hair and fair skin in humans. *Nature Genetics* **11**: 328-30.

van Balkom, I.D. and Hennekam, R.C. 1994. Dermal eccrine cylindromatosis. *Journal of Medical Genetics* **31**: 321–4.

van der Schroeff, J.G., Evers, L.M., Boot, A.J. and Bos, J.L. 1990. Ras oncogene mutations in basal cell carcinomas and squamous cell carcinomas of human skin. *Journal of Investigative Dermatology* **94**: 423–5.

White, J.C. 1894. Multiple benign cystic epitheliomas. *Journal of Cutaneous and Genitourinary Diseases* **12**: 477–84.

Wicking, C., Berkman, J., Wainwright, B. and Chenevix-Trench, G. 1994. Fine genetic mapping of the gene for nevoid basal cell carcinoma syndrome. *Genomics* **22**: 505–11.

Wright, A.L., Gawkrodger, D.J., Branford, W.A., McLaren, K. and Hunter, J.A. 1988. Self-healing epitheliomata of Ferguson-Smith: cytogenetic and histological studies, and the therapeutic effect of etretinate. *Dermatologica* **176**: 22–8.

Zaphiropoulos, P.G., Soderkvist, P., Hedblad, M.A. and Toftgard, R. 1994. Genetic instability of microsatellite markers in region q22.3-q31 of chromosome 9 in skin squamous cell carcinomas. *Biochemical and Biophysical Research Communications* **201**: 1495–501.

Ziegler, A., Leffell, D.J., Kunala, S. et al. 1993. Mutation hotspots due to sunlight in the p53 gene of nonmelanoma skin cancers. *Proceedings of the National Academy of Sciences, USA* **90**: 4216–20.

Ziegler, A., Jonason, A.S., Leffell, D.J. et al. 1994. Sunburn and p53 in the onset of skin cancer. *Nature* **372**: 773–6.

16

Endocrine cancers

HARRIET FEILOTTER and LOIS MULLIGAN

Summary

This chapter introduces several examples of inherited predisposition to endocrine cancer. The focus is primarily on the multiple endocrine neoplasia syndromes which have been well investigated genetically and represent excellent models for genetic analyses in detection and management of hereditary endocrine cancer. First, multiple endocrine neoplasia type 1 (MEN 1), a rare, autosomal dominant disease is discussed, and then MEN 2 and its causative gene, *RET*, is considered in detail. Other rarer endocrine-related cancer syndromes such as hereditary paraganglionoma and Carney complex are introduced.

Introduction

Tumours of the endocrine system represent a dual health risk for the affected individual. These diseases span a broad range of lesions from benign adenoma or hyperplasia with little risk of invasion or metastases to highly aggressive, metastatic disease. In addition to the cancer itself, endocrine tumours have the accompanying risk of complications caused by endocrine expression which can lead to secondary tumours or other, non-neoplastic effects such as acromegaly and hypertensive crisis. Thus, detection and treatment are particularly important to management of the patient with endocrine cancer.

Hereditary endocrine tumours occur primarily in the context of multicancer syndromes. These may be principally associated with endocrine manifestations as seen in the multiple endocrine neoplasia syndromes, types 1 and 2 (MEN 1 and MEN 2). Alternatively, an endocrine component may represent an integral part of a cancer syndrome which affects multiple systems, such as von Hippel–Lindau disease, neurofibromatosis type 1, or familial adenomatous polyposis. The endocrine involvement in the latter syndromes will not be further discussed here.

Multiple endocrine neoplasia type 1

MEN 1 is an inherited disorder characterized by hyperplasia and/or benign or malignant tumours of the parathyroid glands, the endocrine pancreatic cells and the anterior pituitary gland. It is a rare disease with a predicted prevalence of 2–20 in 100,000 (Brandi et al., 1987) although no long-term population studies have yet confirmed this estimate. MEN 1 is transmitted as an autosomal dominant predisposition to neoplasms of the tissues mentioned above. Thus, offspring of affected individuals are at 50% risk of inheriting the familial mutation that leads to MEN 1. The penetrance of the disease phenotype is high, approaching 80% by the fifth decade (reviewed in Mallette, 1994). Typically, onset of clinically significant disease is in the fourth decade although, more recently, prospective screening of at-risk members of MEN 1 kindreds has lowered the age of detection to the second decade (Skogseid et al., 1991). Although MEN 1-like tumours also occur sporadically, these are usually isolated tumours that occur later in life than those associated with MEN 1.

Lesions associated with MEN 1

Tumours associated with MEN 1 are frequently bilateral or multifocal, and often functional, secreting one or more peptides that cause a variety of biochemical imbalances (Öberg *et al.*, 1982; Klöppel et al., 1986). In individuals with MEN 1, any combination of the target glands may be affected; however, the pattern of glands involved and the type of peptide secreted is often consistent within families. Three major types of lesions are associated with MEN 1, although several others occur less frequently.

Parathyroid lesions

Hyperparathyroidism is observed in 87–97% of MEN 1 patients and is often the first clinical manifestation of the disease (Benson et al., 1987; Skogseid et al., 1991). Parathyroid hyperplasia results in increased production of parathyroid hormone, leading to the primary presenting symptom of hypercalcaemia (reviewed in Mallette, 1994).

328 _H. Feilotter and L. Mulligan_

Endocrine pancreatic lesions

Adenomas or carcinomas of the endocrine pancreas are observed in 65–80% of MEN 1 patients (reviewed in Skogseid et al., 1994). These tumours may secrete gastrin, insulin, glucagon, vasoactive intestinal peptide, pancreatic polypeptide, somatostatin or neurotensin (Klöppel et al., 1986). Gastrin-secreting pancreatic tumours, seen in Zollinger–Ellison syndrome, and insulin-secreting tumours which lead to hypoglycaemia, are the most common. Approximately 50% of MEN 1 patients with pancreatic involvement display an aggressive, metastatic tumour phenotype (Donow et al., 1991), which constitutes a major cause of death among MEN 1 patients (Wilkinson et al., 1993).

Pituitary lesions

Lesions of the anterior pituitary gland are seen in 50–65% of MEN 1 patients (reviewed in McCutcheon, 1994; Skogseid et al., 1994). Approximately 40% of these are prolactin-secreting, while the rest may secrete growth hormone, corticotrophin, thyrotrophin, gonadotrophin or may be non-secretory (reviewed in McCutcheon, 1994).

Other lesions

Adrenocortical tumours are found in about one-third of MEN 1 patients (Skogseid et al., 1994). It is not clear whether these tumours are a result of the same genetic event which predisposes to the more typical MEN 1 neoplasms, or whether they are a consequence of the biochemical anomalies associated with the more common MEN 1 tumours (Beckers et al., 1992; Skogseid et al., 1992). Other lesions that are overrepresented in MEN 1 patients include bronchic, thymic or gastric carcinoids; carcinoid-like tumours of the duodenum; thyroid adenomas and carcinomas; colloid goiters; lipomas and pinealomas (Skogseid et al., 1994).

MEN 1-related syndromes

There are at least two syndromes with phenotypes that overlap that of classical MEN 1.

Familial isolated hyperparathyroidism (FIHP)

This is a rare autosomal, dominantly inherited syndrome characterized by hypercalcaemia, elevated levels of parathyroid hormone, and isolated parathyroid tumours (Goldsmith et al., 1976). In these families, there is no evidence for other endocrinopathies normally associated with MEN 1, although some families, initially diagnosed with FIHP, have later been shown to have classical MEN 1 symptoms (Larsson et al., 1995). About half of the FIHP families tested show linkage to the *MEN1* locus (Larsson et al., 1995), while the rest are unlinked (Wassif et al., 1993; Larsson et al., 1995). These results are consistent with either genetic heterogeneity of FIHP, or phenotypic overlap between two genetically distinct syndromes, FIHP and MEN 1.

Familial pituitary tumours (FPT)

These tumours generally lead to acromegaly (Yausa et al., 1990), represent another MEN 1-related syndrome. Linkage to the *MEN1* locus has been excluded in the small number of FPT families tested so far (Benlian et al., 1995; Larsson et al., 1995), suggesting that FPT may be genetically distinct from MEN 1.

Genetics of MEN 1

The *MEN1* gene has been mapped to the long arm of chromosome 11, at 11q13, using the complementary approaches of deletion mapping in MEN 1-associated tumours and linkage analysis in MEN 1 families. The combination of these approaches provides important information regarding not only the location but also the nature of the *MEN1* gene.

Investigation of the specific loss of alleles in tumours from MEN 1 patients provided the first clues to both the localization of the *MEN1* gene and the general mechanism by which it might give rise to cancer. The initial study of allele loss in insulinomas from two siblings in an MEN 1 family demonstrated that both tumours had lost one copy of chromosome 11, and that the deleted copy, in each case, was that inherited from the unaffected parent (Larsson et al., 1988). Thus, a germline defect in one allele would be present in all cells in an affected individual, and functional loss of the normal allele would be acquired as a somatic event, leading to tumour development. Subsequent linkage analysis in this family suggested that the *MEN1* gene mapped close to the muscle glycogen phosphorylase gene (*PYGM*) on 11q (Larsson et al., 1988). Together these data suggested that *MEN1* was a tumour suppressor gene on chromosome 11q.

Allele loss studies have shown that more than 50% of informative MEN 1 tumours tested have lost chromosomal material from 11q (Table 16.1a) (Friedman et al., 1989, 1992; Thakker et al., 1989, 1993a; Byström et al., 1990; Radford et al., 1990; Bale et al., 1991; Beckers et al., 1992, 1994; Morelli et al., 1995; Lubensky et al., 1996; Emmert-Buck et al., 1997; Heppner et al., 1997). The smallest common deleted region is telomeric of the *PYGM* locus and centormeric marker of D11S4936, which places the *MEN1* gene in chromosome band 11q13 (Figure 16.1). Studies of sporadic parathyroid tumours (Table 16.1b) (Friedman et al., 1989, 1992; Byström et al., 1990; Bale et al., 1991; Falchetti et al., 1993; Heppner et al., 1997), thyroid adenomas (Matsuo et al., 1991), pituitary lesions (Bale et al., 1991; Thakker et al., 1993a), and pancreatic tumours (Ding et al., 1992) have shown that loss of chromosome 11 material in the region of the *MEN1* locus occurs in a percentage of sporadic cases, but not in the majority of them. This suggests that while some sporadic tumours may involve the inactivation of the *MEN1* gene, a significant percentage may develop through different genetic routes.

The localization of the *MEN1* locus was further refined by linkage analyses in a large number of MEN 1 families. These studies placed the *MEN1* gene within the region between the microsatellite marker loci *D11S1883* and *D11S807* (Figure 16.1) (Fujimori et al., 1992; Larsson et al., 1992a,b; Thakker et al., 1993b; Debelenko et al., 1997; The European Consortium on MEN 1, 1997).

Finally, the *MEN1* gene was identified from amongst several candidates within a 300 Kilobase (kb) interval. *MEN1* spans 10 exons and encodes a 610 amino acid ubiquitously expressed protein, MENIN, with little homology to other known proteins (Chandrasekharappa et al., 1997). It has no identifiable motifs and lacks both signal peptide and nuclear localization signals. Hence, the function of MENIN remains to be determined. Mutations including missense and nonsense point mutations, deletions, frameshifts, and insertions have been reported (Agarwal et al., 1997; Chandrasekharappa et al., 1997; The European Consortium on MEN1, 1997) in the majority of MEN 1 families and in sporadic MEN1. Similar somatic mutations of MEN 1 have been detected in sporadic parathyroid tumours (Heppner et al., 1997).

Table 16.1a. *Allele loss at 11q13 in MEN 1-associated tumours*

Lesion	No. cases*	Allele loss** (%)	References
insulinoma	2	100	Larsson et al., 1988
parathyroid	16	63	Friedman et al., 1989
parathyroid	6	50	Thakker et al., 1989
parathyroid	11	82	Radford et al., 1990
parathyroid	5	90	Byström et al., 1990
pituitary	1	0	Byström et al., 1990
VIPoma	1	100	Bale et al., 1991
insulinoma	1	100	Bale et al., 1991
adrenal	1	100	Beckers et al., 1992
parathyroid	41	58	Friedman et al., 1992
pituitary	1	100	Thakker et al., 1993a
pituitary	1	100	Beckers et al., 1994
parathyroid	1	100	Beckers et al., 1994
lipoma	6	17	Morelli et al., 1995

Note:
* Number of informative cases.
** Percentage of informative cases that showed allele loss in the *MEN1* region.

Table 16.1b *Allele loss at 11q13 in sporadic endocrine tumours*

Lesion	No. cases *	Allele loss** (%)	References
parathyroid	34	21	Friedman et al., 1989
parathyroid	24	29	Byström et al., 1990
parathyroid	33	39	Heppner et al., 1997
pituitary	26	8	Byström et al., 1990
pancreas	8	0	Bale et al., 1991
pituitary	3	0	Bale et al., 1991
thyroid	27	15	Matsuo et al., 1991
parathyroid	61	26	Friedman et al., 1992
pancreas	1	100	Ding et al., 1992
pituitary	12	33	Thakker et al., 1993a
parathyroid	12	17	Falchetti et al., 1993

Note;
* Number of informative cases.
** Percentage of informative cases that showed allele loss in the *MEN1* region.

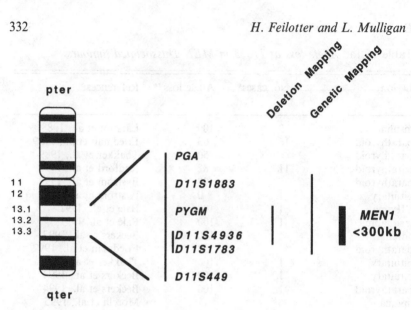

Figure 16.1. Schematic representation of human chromosome 11 showing a detail from band 11q13. Genes and polymorphic DNA markers from this interval are listed with genetic distances in centiMorgans (cM) between them indicated where known. The minimum regions containing the *MEN1* gene predicted from deletion mapping studies and from linkage studies are indicated. At right, the solid bar indicates the 900 kb region that contains the *MEN1* gene.

MEN 1: management and screening

Although not documented, it is likely that early detection of MEN 1-related lesions might lead to decreased morbidity. Biochemical screening to look for early signs of disease is carried out using radioimmunoassays for the products that are hypersecreted by the various tumour cells (parathyroid hormone, prolactin, insulin-like growth factor, insulin, proinsulin, glucagon, pancreatic peptide and gastrin) or consequences thereof (serum glucose and calcium) (reviewed in Skogseid et al., 1994; Skogseid and Öberg, 1995). In addition, meal stimulation tests are commonly used with high accuracy to identify pancreatic lesions (Skogseid et al., 1994). All of these tests are performed at intervals on unaffected individuals with a family history of the disease, and periodically on MEN 1 patients because of the probability that multiple tumours of various histologic types will develop over time.

Once a lesion has been identified, several courses of action can be taken, depending on the type and tumour stage. Hyperplastic lesions of the parathyroid generally require surgical intervention (Mallette, 1994; Thompson, 1995). With pancreatic lesions, resection and enucleation of accessible lesions in the pancreatic head is the treatment of choice (Thompson, 1995). Pituitary lesions may be treatable with drug therapy in some cases, but may require surgery in others (McCutcheon, 1994).

While the biochemical tests described can identify early lesions in MEN 1, they do not have the capacity to detect at-risk individuals prior to the development of any signs of the disease. Following the identification of numerous polymorphic markers that mapped close to the *MEN1* locus (Larsson *et al.*, 1992b, 1995; Kytölä et al., 1995), DNA-based presymptomatic testing was applied to MEN 1 with a high degree of confidence. However, this type of diagnostic testing requires the analysis of samples from multiple family members so that the segregation of the disease allele and several linked markers can be followed. The identification of the *MEN1* gene and of the disease related mutations now makes direct mutation detection and disease prediction possible with improved efficiency and accuracy. Identification of at-risk individuals is important so that biochemical testing protocols and schedules can be optimized to ensure the earliest possible detection, and therefore treatment, of MEN 1-associated lesions.

Multiple endocrine neoplasia type 2

MEN 2 comprises a triad of inherited cancer syndromes characterized by the presence of medullary thyroid carcinoma (MTC) or its presumed precursor lesion, C-cell hyperplasia (CCH) (Schimke, 1984). Clinically significant C-cell disease is detected in approximately 70% of cases (Easton et al., 1989). In addition, patients with MEN 2 subtype A (MEN 2A) may also have phaeochromocytoma (phaeo), a tumour of the adrenal chromaffin cells, in 40–50% of cases and/or parathyroid hyperplasia or adenoma (HPT) in 10–35% of cases (Schimke, 1984; Howe *et al.*, 1993). Patients with MEN 2B have a similar incidence of phaeo; however, parathyroid involvement is rare. MEN 2B is associated with other, more diffuse anomalies including Marfanoid habitus, buccal neuromas, diffuse intestinal ganglioneuromatosis and thickened corneal nerves (Schimke, 1984; Vasen et al., 1992). In the final MEN 2 subtype, familial MTC (FMTC), the presence of MTC is the only disease phenotype (Farndon et al., 1986).

Like MEN 1, MEN 2 is an autosomal, dominantly inherited cancer syndrome. The age of onset of disease signs in affected individuals is variable but occurs earlier than for similar sporadic tumours (Easton *et al.*, 1989). As with other inherited cancer syndromes, the disease frequently presents with multifocal or bilateral tumours (Schimke, 1984). In patients with MEN 2, penetrance is incomplete and more than 30% of gene carriers do not display clinically significant symptoms by age 70 (Gagel et al., 1982; Easton et al., 1989). However, biochemical manifestations of C-cell disease, detected as increased calcitonin release in response to stimulation, are detectable in more than 93% of cases by age 31 (Easton et al., 1989).

The RET proto-oncogene

The underlying cause of all three MEN 2 syndromes is mutation of the RET proto-oncogene. RET is a member of the transmembrane receptor tyrosine kinase family (Figure 16.2) (Takahashi et al., 1988; 1989). The gene encodes a large extracellular domain with cysteine rich dimerization and putative ligand-binding domains that contains a region with homology to the cadherin family of cell interaction molecules (Takahashi et al., 1988, 1989; Schneider, 1992). RET spans the cell surface membrane and, intercellularly, consists of a tyrosine kinase domain involved in transduction of signals initiated by ligand binding (Figure 16.2).

RET is expressed primarily in cells and lineages derived from the branchial arches, neural crest and ureteric bud. Expression is detected in the thyroid C-cells, adrenal chromaffin cells, parasympathetic and sympathetic ganglia, enteric ganglia, parathyroid and in tissues of the urogenital system (Tahira et al., 1988; Pachnis et al., 1993; Nakamura et al., 1994). In addition, RET is expressed at high levels in tumours arising from neural crest-derived precursors including MTC, phaeo and neuroblastoma (Ikeda et al., 1990; Santoro et al., 1990; Tahira et al., 1991; Nakamura et al., 1994). The spatial and temporal pattern of RET expression has suggested a role in neural crest cell migration and kidney induction (Pachnis et al., 1993; Schuchardt et al., 1994). This role is supported by the phenotype of RET null mice, which lack functional RET protein and have no enteric ganglia and dysgenic or agenic kidneys (Schuchardt et al., 1994).

The RET ligand has been identified as a multicomponent complex comprising both a soluble protein and a non-signalling, extracellular cell surface-bound molecule. The first identified soluble component, glial cell line-derived neurotrophic factor (GDNF), is distantly related to the transforming growth factor-β superfamily, although it shares less than 20% homology with other family members (Lin et al., 1993). A second, closely related member of the GDNF family, neurturin (NTN),

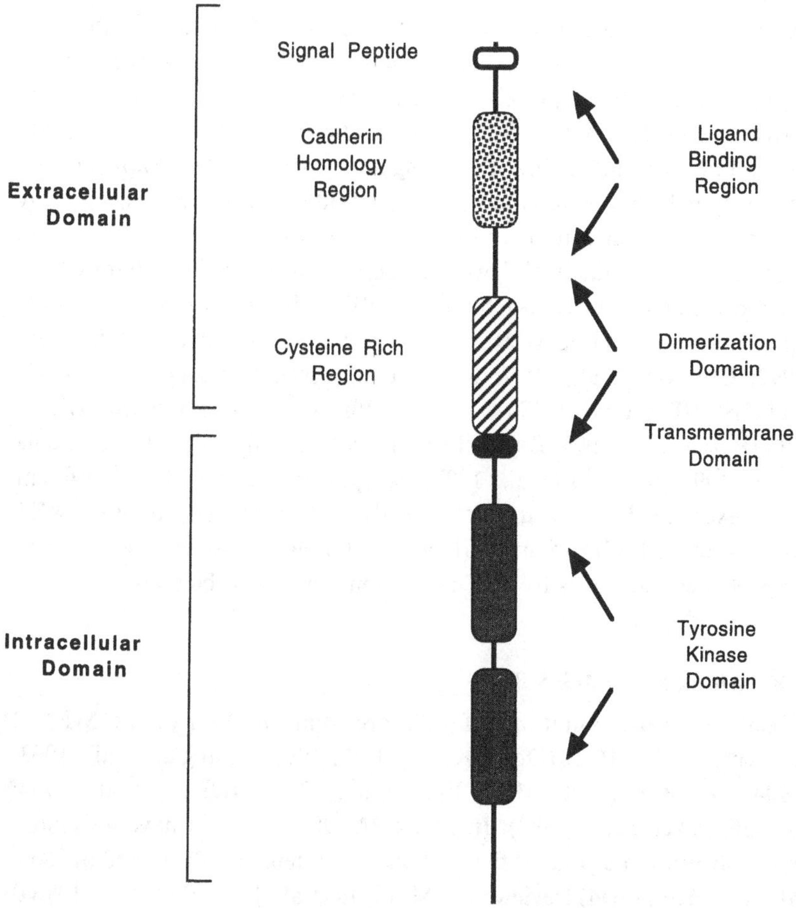

Figure 16.2. A schematic diagram of the RET tyrosine kinase cell surface receptor. The protein domains predicted from the DNA sequence are shown.

has recently been identified (Kotzbauer et al., 1996). GDNF and NTN exhibit selective neurotrophic properties and are strong promoters of neurite outgrowth and survival of peripheral neurons (Lin et al., 1993; Mount et al., 1995; Trupp et al., 1995; Kotzbauer et al., 1996; Buj-Bello et al., 1997). This role is consistent with the predicted function of the RET ligand which is required for neural crest cell migration, innervation of the hind gut, and survival or proliferation of the enteric neuroblasts (Schuchardt et al., 1994, 1995; Durbec et al., 1996a,b; Trupp et al., 1996).

Members of the GDNF family are required for RET activation but apparently are unable to bind to and activate RET alone. A second, extracellular cell surface-bound molecule is required to mediate this process. The GDNF receptor alpha (GDNFR-α) family comprises a novel group of extracellular proteins attached to the cell membrane by a gly-cosyl-phosphatidylinositol (GPI)-linkage (Jing et al., 1996; Treanor et al., 1996). Family members bear no strong homologies to other known receptors although they do contain a group of 30 cysteine residues, similarly spaced to those in cytokine receptors (Jing et al., 1996; Treanor et al., 1996; Sanicola et al., 1997) Two members of the GDNFR-α family have been described. GDNFR-α binds GDNF with high affinity and NTN with low affinity (Jing et al., 1996; Treanor et al., 1996; Baloh et al., 1997; Creedon et al., 1997; Klein et al., 1997; Sanicola et al., 1997) while NTNR-α binds NTN with high affinity and GDNF with low affinity (Baloh et al., 1997; Buj-Bello et al., 1997; Klein et al., 1997; Sanicola et al., 1997; Suvanto et al., 1997). It appears that all of the different complexes can bind to and activate RET. It is likely that other RET ligands, in both GDNF and GDNFR-α families, exist but the relationship of such molecules to RET activation remains to be seen.

RET *Mutations in MEN 2*

Specific missense mutations of *RET* are found in each of the MEN 2 subtypes (Table 16.2) (Donis-Keller et al., 1993; Mulligan et al., 1993; 1994b; Carlson et al., 1994; Eng et al., 1994; Hofstra et al., 1994; Schuffenecker et al., 1994). In MEN 2A, 98% of cases have an amino acid substitution at one of five codons for cysteine residues (codons 609, 611, 618, 620 or 634) (reviewed in Mulligan et al., 1995; Eng et al., 1996a) which lie within the cysteine-rich dimerization domain (Takahashi et al., 1988). In the majority (83%) of cases these mutations lie in codon 634, where all seven of the possible base changes, which would result in a novel amino acid, have been identified. The most frequent substitutions at codon 634 result in a cysteine→arginine (52%) or a cysteine→tyrosine (26%) change (Mulligan et al., 1995; Eng et al., 1996a).

MEN 2B is exclusively associated with an ATG→ACG mutation in codon 918, which results in a substitution of threonine for methionine (Carlson et al., 1994; Eng et al., 1994; Hofstra et al., 1994). This change has been detected in 95% of MEN 2B cases and, to date, no other *RET* mutations have been found associated with this phenotype (reviewed in Mulligan et al., 1995; Eng et al., 1996a).

In FMTC, *RET* mutations are more dispersed (Table 16.2). MEN 2A-like mutations, affecting the same five cysteine residues (609, 611, 618,

Table 16.2 **RET** *mutations detected in MEN 2**

	Mutations in *RET* codon (%)									
	609	611	618	620	634	768	804	918	None Detected
MEN 2A	<1	2	5	7	83	0	0	0	2
MEN 2B	0	0	0	0	0	0	0	95	5
FMTC	6	3	29	15	26	9	2.5 (2.5)**	0	12

Note;
* Data compiled from Bolino et al., 1995; Mulligan et al., 1995; Eng et al., 1996.
** Cases reported by Bolino *et al.* (1995). One of the reported families was small, with only two confirmed cases of MTC and thus the definition of FMTC rather than MEN 2A was tentative.
MEN: multiple endocrine neoplasia (type 1/type 2); FMTC: familial medullary thyroid carcinoma.

620, 634), are also found associated with this phenotype (Donis-Keller et al., 1993; Mulligan et al., 1994b; Schuffenecker et al., 1994). However, the distribution of these mutations is quite different with approximately equal representation of mutations at codons 618, 620 and 634 (Mulligan et al., 1994b, 1995; Eng et al., 1996a). In addition, mutations of two codons within the tyrosine kinase domain, codon 768 in exon 13 and codon 804 in exon 14, have been identified. In five families with FMTC, missense mutations of codon 768 (GAG→GAC or GAT), resulting in an aspartic acid for glutamic acid substitution, have been seen (Eng et al., 1995; Bolino et al., 1995; Boccia et al., 1997). Bolino *et al.* (1995) have also reported two families with a GTG→TTG mutation at codon 804 which would result in the substitution of a leucine for the normal valine at that position in RET.

The relationship of the MEN 2 disease phenotype and specific *RET* mutations indicates a strong genotype–phenotype association. Several large studies have shown that the presence of phaeo and HPT in MEN 2A families is correlated with mutation of codon 634 (Mulligan et al., 1994b; Schuffenecker et al., 1994; Eng et al., 1996a). In two studies the presence of the cysteine→arginine mutation at that codon was correlated with the presence of HPT (Mulligan et al., 1994b; Eng et al., 1996a), although this has not been confirmed by other groups (Schuffenecker et al., 1994; Frank-Raue et al., 1996).

Sporadic tumours

RET mutations have also been detected in a subset of presumed sporadic MEN 2-type tumours. In a subset of these cases, *RET* mutations have been found in both tumour and non-tumour tissue. This suggests that these represent de novo cases of MEN 2A rather than true sporadic tumours. In fact, it has been predicted that 5% of sporadic MTC may truly represent such de novo cases of MEN 2 (Cote et al., 1995). These cases have been excluded from the following discussion of sporadic disease. In the remainder of cases, representing true sporadic disease, *RET* mutations are present only in the tumour, not in other unaffected tissues.

In sporadic MTC the most frequently detected mutation is a methionine to threonine change at codon 918, identical to that seen in MEN 2B, which is found in approximately 43% of all sporadic MTC examined (Table 16.3) (reviewed in Eng and Mulligan, 1997). In addition, rare mutations including insertion/deletion mutations of codon 634, deletion of codon 630 and missense mutations of codons 768 and 883 have been

Table 16.3 RET *mutations in sporadic tumours**

				Mutations in RET codon					
	609	618	620	634	768	883	918	Other	
MTC	0/150	1**/150	0/150	4***/131	4/72	4/111	89/208	del codon 630	
Phaeo	1/129	0/129	2/129	1/129	0/55	0/55	6/129	codon 925	
								del AG exon 9	
								del 632-3	
HPT	0/73	0/73	0/73	0/73	0/34	ND	0/73		

Note:

* Table compiled using data from studies reviewed in Eng and Mulligan (1997).

** This case represents a germline mosaic for codon 618 mutation (Komminoth et al., 1994).

*** Includes three simple missense mutations (Romei et al., 1996) and one complex insertion/deletion change which also disrupts codon 634 (Marsh et al., 1997).

MTC: medullary-thyroid cancer; Phaeo: phaeochromocytoma; HPT: parathyroid hyperplasia/adenoma.

reported (Table 16.3) (Eng et al., 1994, 1995; Donis-Keller, 1995; Marsh et al., 1997). Somatically occuring MEN 2A-type mutations of codons 609, 611 and 620 occur infrequently, if at all, in sporadic MTC. Missense mutations of codon 634 have been confirmed only rarely in sporadic MTC (Romei et al., 1996).

Although *RET* mutations are much less frequent in sporadic phaeo than MTC, they occur at a broader range of codons (Table 16.3). Mutations are found in codons 918 (5%), and 620 (< 2%) and, as unique events, in codons 609, 634, 632-633 and 925 and at the 3' splice acceptor site of exon 9 (reviewed in Eng and Mulligan, 1997). Finally, several studies have been unable to identify *RET* mutations of exons 10, 11, 13, 14 or 16 (Figure 16.3) in sporadic parathyroid lesions including hyperplasia, adenoma and carcinoma (reviewed in Eng and Mulligan, 1997).

RET *mutations in Hirschsprung disease*

RET mutations are also found in approximately 50% of familial and 15–35% of sporadic cases of Hirschsprung disease (HSCR), a congenital abnormality resulting from absence of the enteric nerve plexes from all or part of the lower gut. Deletions of the entire *RET* coding sequence, missense and nonsense mutations, interstitial deletions and splice junction mutations have been reported (reviewed in Attié et al., 1995; Chakravarti, 1996; Eng and Mulligan, 1997). The nature of many of these mutations has suggested that, in the case of HSCR, *RET* mutations are inactivating and the disease phenotype arises from haploinsufficiency for RET. This is supported by the observation that introduction of *HSCR* mutations can abrogate the transforming ability of rearranged oncogenic *RET* constructs in vitro (Pasini et al., 1995) and that mutations of the *RET* extracellular domain result in reduced transport to the cell surface (Carlomagno et al., 1996; Iwashita et al., 1996).

A limited number of families in which both HSCR and either MEN 2A or FMTC co-segregate have been identified (Mulligan et al., 1994a; Borst et al., 1995; Landsvater et al., 1996). In each case, this phenotype is associated with a single missense mutation resulting in a cysteine→arginine substitution at codon 618 or 620 (Mulligan et al., 1994a; Landsvater et al., 1996), or a cysteine→serine change at codon 618 (Borst et al., 1995). Sequence analysis of the remaining *RET* coding sequence has detected no further mutations in at least three of these families (Mulligan et al., 1994a). Recent studies have shown that the mutant RET forms in these cases are not efficiently transported to the cell surface (Carlomagno et al.,

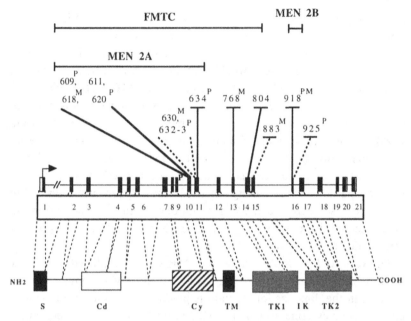

Figure 16.3. Location of *RET* mutations found in MEN 2 (multiple endocrine neoplasia type 2) and related sporadic tumours. A schematic diagram of the *RET* intro/exon structure is shown and the positions of known *RET* activating mutations in MEN 2 are indicated. The codon positions of somatic mutations unique to sporadic tumours are shown by dashed lines. The locations of mutations in sporadic phaeo (P) or MTC (M) are shown. The location of the deletion of a splice junction in a sporadic phaeo is similarly indicated (P). FMTC: familial-medullary thyroid carcinoma.

1997; Ito et al., 1997). These data suggest different sensitivity to RET in the neural crest precursors of the enteric ganglia and those of the thyroid C-cells or adrenal chromaffin cells. Several studies have detected rare mutations of the gene for the RET-ligand, *GDNF,* in HSCR patients (Angrist et al., 1996; Ivanchuk et al., 1996; Salomon et al., 1996). While such mutations may lead to HSCR by themselves (Ivanchuk et al., 1996) the majority occur in conjunction with other factors, such as *RET* mutations, which are implicated in the disease phenotype.

Functional significance of RET mutations

It is now generally accepted that *RET* mutations in MEN 2 are activating. This hypothesis is supported by three major types of evidence. First, only a single *RET* mutation is necessary for tumourigenesis in tumours from MEN 2 patients. The normal *RET* allele is almost always present and expressed in these tumours but does not suppress the disease phenotype as is the case described for MEN 1 above. Secondly, expression of *RET* constructs with MEN 2A (codon 634) or MEN 2B (codon 918) mutations in NIH 3T3 cells results in transformation which is not seen if normal *RET* constructs are used (Borrello et al., 1995; Santoro et al., 1995). Finally, transfection of similar mutant *RET* constructs can result in differentiation of the rat phaeo cell line PC12 (Borrello et al., 1995). The presence of normal *RET* constructs has no such effect. Thus MEN 2 represents a novel entity among inherited cancer syndromes described to date as it results from activating mutations of an oncogene where all other such syndromes arise through inactivation of a tumour suppresser gene as described above for MEN 1.

The various *RET* mutations seen in MEN 2 are predicted to activate RET by different mechanisms. In MEN 2A and FMTC, mutation of a cysteine in the dimerization domain is predicted to result in RET molecules where a cysteine, usually involved in intramolecular interactions, is unpaired and becomes available for intermolecular interaction (Santoro et al., 1995). As a consequence, RET molecules are predicted to dimerize in the absence of RET-ligand with resultant autophosphorylation and activation of the normal downstream signal transduction pathway (Santoro et al., 1995). This model is supported by in vitro studies which demonstrate dimerization and phosphorylation of MEN 2A-RET products in transfected cells where normal RET fails to dimerize or become phosphorylated (Asai et al., 1995; Borrello et al., 1995). The MEN 2B mutation appears to activate RET by a different mechanism. Unlike those seen in MEN 2A, MEN 2B-RET mutations do not lead to ligand-independent RET dimerization but appear to result in active monomers (Santoro et al., 1995), although in vitro studies suggest dimerization may increase their transforming potential (Borrello et al., 1995). Codon 918 encodes a portion of the substrate recognition pocket of the tyrosine kinase domain (Songyang et al., 1995). The amino acid substitution at this site alters the substrate selectivity of RET such that it recognizes substrates similar to those of cytoplasmic tyrosine kinases rather than its own normal substrates (Borrello et al., 1995; Santoro et al., 1995; Songyang et al., 1995). Thus the MEN 2B mutation alters the downstream signal transduction pathways of RET leading to transformation.

Codon 768 encodes a glutamic acid residue within an α helix with a stabilizing effect on residues involved in ATP binding (Eng et al., 1995).

The FMTC mutations of this codon are predicted to destabilize the region resulting in activation of the kinase. Codon 804 encodes a valine in the tyrosine kinase domain which is conserved among species. As yet, the functional significance of mutations at this codon has not been determined.

Although a single mutation of *RET* is sufficient to initiate tumourigenesis, two recent studies have demonstrated that additional *RET* mutations may occur in MEN 2-type tumours as progressional events (Eng et al., 1996b; Marsh et al., 1996). In sporadic and MEN 2-MTC and metastases the codon 918 mutation has been recognized in subpopulations of tumour cells. These events are apparently progressional and their significance in tumourigenesis is unclear.

MEN 2: diagnosis and management

The advent of genetic testing for *RET* mutations in MEN 2 has made early diagnosis and improved disease management possible. Previously, screening of individuals at risk for MEN 2 was performed biochemically by measurement of calcitonin release after pentagastrin stimulation. The presence of CCH or MTC results in increased levels of calcitonin release. As this method detects the early stage of C-cell disease, a negative result indicates only that there is currently no C-cell hyperplasia but makes no predictions as to future development of the MEN 2 phenotype. Thus, the test must be repeated at regular intervals. Interpretation of calcitonin tests has been complicated by the recent recognition that CCH occurs outside the context of MEN 2, affecting approximately 5% of individuals (Landsvater et al., 1993).

Direct mutation testing in MEN 2 has greatly improved diagnosis of the disease. In families with known *RET* mutations, at-risk individuals may now be genetically tested at a very early age. Those who have not inherited the characteristic *RET* mutation present in their family may then be excluded from further study. Individuals identified as carrying the MEN 2-RET mutations would undergo stringent biochemical monitoring and early surgical intervention, offered before overt signs of the disease were manifested. With this combination of genetic and biochemical screening, coupled with early surgery, it should be possible to reduce morbidity and mortality associated with MEN 2.

Mutation-based diagnosis of MEN 2 also impacts on recognition of truly sporadic MTC and phaeo. Several studies have suggested that a proportion of of sporadic MTCs represent de novo cases of MEN 2 (reviewed in Cote et al., 1995). *RET* mutations are found in germline DNA from these individuals and thus they remain at risk of other MEN 2 phenotypes (phaeo, HPT). As a corollary, individuals with sporadic MTC with no detectable germline *RET* mutations are at low risk of these MEN 2 phenotypes as are their family members. These individuals and their families could be exempted from further biochemical screening programmes although, as a caveat, low level germline mosaicism for *RET* mutations would not be excluded,[1] this confirming a theoretical risk for *RET* mutations in their offspring.

Other hereditary endocrine cancers

A number of rare hereditary endocrine cancers that are distinct from the multiple endocrine neoplasias have been reported. Because of the small numbers of families in which they have been found, these disorders are less well characterized than either MEN 1 or MEN 2. However, recent reports of linkage to specific chromsomal regions for three of these diseases suggest that identification of the underlying genes may soon be possible.

Hereditary paragangliomas

Hereditary paragangliomas, also known as chemodectomas or familial glomus tumours, are benign tumours of chemoreceptor structures derived from the neural crest. The most clinically significant tumours are of the carotid, vagal, and jugular bodies of the neck, inner ear, and skull respectively (reviewed in Brenton et al., 1995). The tumours are usually multifocal, and, like other inherited cancers, occur at an earlier age than their sporadic counterparts. The segregation of the tumours in families is consistant with an autosomal dominant mode of inheritance. Interestingly, expression of the disease is exclusively in individuals with the paternally

---

1 International *RET* Mutation Consortium. The International *RET* Mutation Consortium (IRMC) was convened in 1994 with the goal of investigating the relationship between *RET* mutation genotype and MEN 2 phenotype. The consortium currently includes more than 20 centres worldwide from which a pooled set of data from 477 MEN 2 families has recently been collected for these analyses. The consortium is currently soliciting information on *RET* mutations in sporadic tumours and welcomes the interest and participation of other investigators. Contact Lois M. Mulligan, PhD, Dept. of Paediatrics, Queens University, 20 Barrie Street, Kingston, ON K7L 3N6, Canada, Fax: +1 613 548 1348, E-mail: mulligaL@qucdn.queensu.ca or Charis Eng, Md, PhD, Dana-Farber Cancer Institute, D920C, 44 Binney Street, Boston, MA 02115-6084, USA, Fax: +1 617 632 4280, E-mail: chariseng@macmailgw.dfci.harvard.edu.

inherited disease, suggesting that an imprinted gene might be responsible for the syndrome (van der Mey et al., 1989). Two non-overlapping regions of chromosome 11, 11q22.2-q23.3 (Heutink et al., 1992, 1994; Baysal et al., 1997) and 11q13.1 (Mariman et al., 1993, 1995), show linkage to the disease phenotype in small numbers of families. This has raised the possibility that two different imprinted genes on the long arm of chromosome 11 are involved in the development of familial glomus tumours.

Hereditary hyperparathyroidism and jaw tumours (HPT-JT)

This syndrome is a rare autosomal dominant trait consisting of early onset recurring parathyroid adenomas, accompanied by fibro-osseous tumours of the mandible and/or maxilla (Jackson et al., 1990). The parathyroid adenomas may occur in the absence of the jaw tumours in some family members, although the jaw tumours are not seen alone (Szabó et al., 1995). Parathyroid carcinomas and Wilms' tumour may also be associated with this syndrome in some families (Kakinuma et al., 1994; Szabó et al., 1995). Linkage studies on five families have mapped the gene for the disorder, designated *HRPT2*, to chromosome 1q21-q31 (Szabó et al., 1995).

Carney complex

This rare autosomal dominant disorder comprises neoplasias of mesenchymal or neural crest derivatives. The complex manifests as myxomas of the heart, skin and breast, peripheral nerve tumours, spotty pigmentation, and adrenal, pituitary and testicular neoplasias and ductal adenomas of the breast (reviewed in Carney, 1995; Carney and Stratakis, 1996). Recently, the locus for Carney complex has been mapped to chromosome 2p16 (Stratakis et al., 1996). Involvement of the adjacent mismatch repair gene *hMSH2* has been excluded.

Conclusion

Hereditary endocrine cancers occur within the context of a diverse group of disorders. Although biochemical screening tests have greatly increased our ability to identify individuals at risk for some of these disorders, accurate and early diagnosis remains problematic because of the variety of presenting symptoms and the variability of the age of onset. It is clear that the identification of the genes underlying these disorders will lead to improved screening, diagnosis and treatment of affected individuals. This is already evident for MEN 2, where identification of RET mutations has been useful in the modification of screening programmes and treatment protocols. In addition to such immediate gains, characterization of the relevent genes and their products will increase our understanding of the molecular basis of hereditary endocrine cancers. In the long-term, a greater understanding of the genetic events underlying these diseases may lead to non-invasive treatments directed at the biochemical defect, and perhaps preventive therapies for at-risk individuals.

References

Agarwall, S.K., Kester, M.B., Debelenko, L.V. et al. 1997. Germline mutations of the *MEN1* gene in familial multiple endocrine neoplasia type 1 and related states. *Human Molecular Genetics* 6: 1169–75.

Angrist, M., Bolk, S., Halushka, M., Lapchak, P.A. and Chakravarti, A. 1996. Germline mutations in glial cell line-derived neurotrophic factor (*GDNF*) and *RET* in a Hirschsprung disease patient. *Nature Genetics* 14: 341–3.

Asai, N., Iwashita, T., Matsuyama, M. and Takahashi, M. 1995. Mechanism of activation of the *ret* proto-oncogene by multiple endocrine neoplasia 2A mutations. *Molecular Cell Biology* 15: 1613–19.

Attié, T., Pelet, A., Edery, P. et al. 1995. Diversity of *RET* proto-oncogene mutations in familial and sporadic Hirschsprung disease. *Human Molecular Genetics* 4: 1381–6.

Bale, A.E., Norton, J.A., Wong, E. L. et al. 1991. Allelic loss on chromosome 11 in hereditary and sporadic tumors related to familial multiple endocrine neoplasia type 1. *Cancer Research* 51: 1154–7.

Baloh, R.H., Tamsey, M.G., Golden, J.P. et al. 1997. TmR2, a novel receptor that mediates neurturin and GDNF signalling through Ret. *Neuron* 18: 793–802.

Baysal B.E., Farr, J.E., Rubinstein, W.S. et al. 1997. Fine mapping of an imprinted gene for familial nonchromaffin paragangliomas, on chromosome 11q23. *American Journal of Human Genetics* 60: 121–32.

Beckers, A., Abs, R., Reyniers, E. et al. 1994. Variable regions of chromosome 11 loss in different pathological tissues of a patient with the multiple endocrine neoplasia type 1 syndrome. *Journal of Clinical Endocrinology and Metabolism* 79: 1498–502.

Beckers, A., Abs, R., Willems, P.J., van der Auwera, B., Kovacs, K., Reznik, M. and Stevenaert, A. 1992. Aldosterone-secreting adrenal adenoma as part of multiple endocrine neoplasia type 1 (MEN 1): loss of heterozygosity for polymorphic chromosome 11 deoxyribonucleic acid markers, including the *MEN1* locus. *Journal of Clinical Endocrinology and Metabolism* 75: 564–70.

Benlian, P., Giraud, S., Lahlou, N. et al. 1995. Familial acromegaly: a specific clinical entity- further evidence from the genetic study of a three-generation family. *European Journal of Endocrinology* 133: 451–6.

Benson, L., Ljunghall, S., Åkerström, G. and Öberg, K. 1987. Hyperparathyroidism presenting as the first lesion in multiple endocrine neoplasia type 1. *American Journal of Medicine* 82: 731–7.

Boccia, L.M., Green, J.S., Joyce, C., Eng, C., Taylor, S.A.M. and Mulligan, L.M. 1997. Mutation of *RET* codon 768 is associated with the FMTC phenotype. *Clinical Genetics* **51**: 81–5.

Bolino, A., Shuffenecker, I., Luo, Y. et al. 1995. RET mutations in exons 13 and 14 of FMTC patients. *Oncogene* **10**: 2415–19.

Borrello, M.G., Smith, D.P., Pasini, B. et al. 1995. *RET* activation by germline *MEN2A* and *MEN2B* mutations. *Oncogene* **11**: 2419–27.

Borst, M.J., VanCamp, J.M., Peacock, M.L. and Decker, R.A. 1995. Mutational analysis of multiple endocrine neoplasia type 2A associated with Hirschsprung's disease. *Surgery* **117**: 386–91.

Brandi, M.L., Marx, S.J., Aurbach, G.D. and Fitzpatrick, L.A. 1987. Familial multiple endocrine neoplasia type 1: a new look at pathophysiology. *Endocrine Reviews* **8**: 391–405.

Brenton, J.D., Viville, S. and Surani, M.A. 1995. Genomic imprinting and cancer. *Cancer Survey* **25**: 161–71.

Buj-Bello, A., Adu, J., Piñón, L.G.P. et al. 1997. Neurturin responsiveness requires a GPI-linked receptor and the RET receptor tyrosine kinase. *Nature* **387**: 721–4.

Byström, C., Larsson, C., Blomberg, C. et al. 1990. Localization of the *MEN1* gene to a small region within chromosome 11q13 by deletion mapping in tumors. *Proceedings of the National Academy of Sciences, USA* **87**: 1968–72.

Carlomagno, F., Devita, G., Berlingieri, T. et al. 1996. Molecular heterogeneity of *RET* loss of function in Hirschsprung's disease. *EMBO* **15**: 2717–25.

Carlomagno, F., Salvatore, G., Cirafici, A.M. et al. 1997. The different *RET*-activating capability of mutations of cysteine 620 or cysteine 634 correlates with the multiple endocrine neoplasia type 2 disease phenotype. *Cancer Research* **57**: 391–5.

Carlson, K.M., Dou, S., Chi, D. et al. 1994. Single missense mutation in the tyrosine kinase catalytic domain of the ret proto-oncogene is associated with multiple endocrine neoplasia type 2B. *Proceedings of the National Academy of Sciences, USA* **91**: 1579–83.

Carney, J.A. 1995. The Carney complex (myxomas, spotty pigmentation, endocrine overactivity, and schwannomas). *Dermatologic Clinics* **13**: 19–26.

Carney, J.A. and Stratakis, C.A. 1996. Ductal adenoma of the breast and the Carney complex. *Journal of Surgical Pathology* **20**: 1154–5.

Chakravarti, A. 1996. Endothelin receptor-mediated signaling in Hirschsprung disease. *Human Molecular Genetics* **5**: 303–7.

Chandrasekharappa, S.C., Guru, C., Manickam, P. et al. 1997. Positional cloning of the gene for multiple endocrine neoplasia-type 1. *Science* **276**, 404–6.

Cote, G.J., Wohllk, N., Evans, D., Goepfert, H. and Gagel, R.F. 1995. RET proto-oncogene mutations in multiple endocrine neoplasia type 2 and medullary thyroid carcinoma. *Ballieres Clinical Endocrinology and Metabolism* **9**: 609–30.

Creedon, D.J., Tansey, M.G., Baloh, R.H. et al. 1997. Neurturin shares receptors and signal tranduction pathways with glial cell line-derived neurotrophic factor in sympathetic neurons. *Proceedings of the National Academy of Sciences, USA* **94**: 7018–23.

Debelenko, L.V., Emmert-Buck, M.R., Manickam, P. et al. 1977. Haplotype analysis defines a minimal interval for the multiple endocrine neoplasia type 1 (*MEN1*) gene. *Cancer Research* **57**: 1039–42.

Ding, S.-F., Habib, N.A., Delhanty, J.D.A. et al. 1992. Loss of heterozygosity on chromosomes 1 and 11 in carcinoma of the pancreas. *British Journal of Cancer* **65**: 809–12.

Donis-Keller, H. 1995. The *RET* proto-oncogene and cancer. *Journal of Internal Medicine* **238**: 319–25.

Donis-Keller, H., Dou, S., Chi, D. et al. 1993. Mutations in the RET proto-oncogene are associated with MEN 2A and FMTC. *Human Molecular Genetics* **2**: 851–6.

Donow, C., Pipeleers-Marichal, M., Schröder, S., Stamm, B., Heitz, P.U. and Klöppel, G. 1991. Surgical pathology of gastrinoma: site, size, mulicentricity, association with multiple neoplasia type 1, and malignancy. *Cancer* **68**: 1329–34.

Durbec, P., Marcos-Gutierrez, C.V., Kilkenny, C. et al. 1996a. GDNF signalling through the Ret receptor tyrosine kinase. *Nature* **381**: 789–93.

Durbec, P.L., Larsson-Blomberg, L.B., Schuchardt, A., Costantini, F. and Pachnis, V. 1996b. Common origin and developmental dependence on *c-ret* of subsets of enteric and sympathetic neuroblasts. *Development* **122**: 349–58.

Easton, D.F., Ponder, M.A., Cummings, T. et al. 1989.The clinical and screening age-at-onset distribution for the MEN-2 syndrome. *American Journal of Human Genetics* **44**: 208–15.

Emmert-Beck, M.R., Lubensky, I.A., Dong, Q. et al. 1997. Localization of the multiple endocrine neoplasia type I (MEN1) gene based on tumor loss of heterozygosity analysis. *Cancer Research* **57**: 1855–8.

Eng, C., Clayton, D., Schuffenecker, I. et al. 1996a. The relationship between specific *RET* proto-oncogene mutations and disease phenotype in multiple endocrine neoplasia type 2: International *RET* Mutation Consortium. *JAMA* **276**: 1575–9.

Eng, C. and Mulligan, L.M. 1997. Mutations of the *RET* proto-oncogene in the multiple endocrine neoplasia type 2 syndromes, related sporadic tumours and Hirschsprung disease. *Human Mutation* **9**: 97–100.

Eng, C., Mulligan, L.M., Healey, C.S. et al. 1996b. Heterogeneous mutation of the *RET* proto-oncogene in subpopulations of medullary thyroid carcinoma. *Cancer Research* **56**: 2167–70.

Eng, C., Smith, D.P., Mulligan, L.M. et al. 1995. A novel point mutation in the tyrosine kinase domain of the *RET* proto-oncogene in sporadic medullary thyroid carcinoma and in a family with FMTC. *Oncogene* **10**: 509–13.

Eng, C., Smith, D.P., Mulligan, L.M. et al. 1994. Point mutation within the tyrosine kinase domain of the *RET* proto-oncogene in multiple endocrine neoplasia type 2B and related sporadic tumours. *Human Molecular Genetics* **3**: 237–41.

European Consortium on MEN1, The. 1997. Identification of the multiple endocrine neoplasia type 1 (MEN1) gene. *Human Molecular Genetics* **6**: 1177–83.

Falchetti, A., Bale, A.E., Amorosi, A. et al. 1993. Progression of uremic hyperparathyroidism involves allelic loss on chromosome 11. *Journal of Clinical Endocrinology and Metabolism* **76**: 139–44.

Farndon, J.R., Leight, G.S., Dilley, W.G., Baylin, S.B., Smallridge, R.C., Harrison, T.S. and Wells, S.A. 1986. Familial medullary thyroid carcinoma without associated endocrinopathies: a distinct clinical entity. *British Journal of Surgery* **73**: 278–81.

Frank-Raue, K., Höppner, W., Frillling, A. et al. 1996. Mutations of the *RET* proto-oncogene in German MEN families: relation between genotype and phenotype. *Journal of Clinical Endocrinology and Metabolism* **81**: 1780–3.

Friedman, E., De Marco, L., Gejman, P.V. et al. 1992. Allelic loss from chromosome 11 in parathyroid tumors. *Cancer Research* **52**: 6804–9.

Friedman, E., Sakaguchi, K., Bale, A.E. et al. 1989. Clonality of parathyroid tumors in familial multiple endocrine neoplasia type 1. *New England Journal of Medicine* **321**: 213–18.

Fujimori, M., Wells, S.A. and Nakamura, Y. 1992. Fine-scale mapping of the gene responsible for multiple endocrine neoplasia type 1 (*MEN 1*). *American Journal of Human Genetics* **50**: 399–403.

Gagel, R., C. Jackson, C., Block, M., Feldman, E., Reichlin, S., Hamilton, C. and Tashjian, A. 1982. Age-related probability of development of hereditary medullary thyroid carcinoma. *Journal of Pediatrics* **101**: 941–6.

Goldsmith, R.E., Sizemore, G.W., Chen, I.W., Zalme, E. and Altemeier, W.A. 1976. Familial hyperparathyroidism: description of a large kindred with physiologic observations and a review of the literature. *Annals of Internal Medicine* **84**: 36–43.

Heppner, C., Kester, M.B., Agarwal, S.K. et al. 1997. Somatic mutation of the *MEN1* gene in parathyroid tumours. *Nature* **16**: 375–8.

Heutink, P., van der Mey, A.G.L., Bardoel, A. et al. 1994. Further localization of the gene for hereditary paragangliomas (PGL), and evidence for linkage in unrelated families. *European Journal of Human Genetics* **2**: 148–58.

Heutink, P., van der Mey, A.G.L., Sandkuijl, L.A. et al. 1992. A gene subject to genomic imprinting and responsible for hereditary paragangliomas maps to chromosome 11q23-qter. *Human Molecular Genetics* **1**: 7–10.

Hofstra, R.M.W., Landsvater, R.M., Ceccherini, I. et al. 1994. A mutation in the *RET* proto-oncogene associated with multiple endocrine neoplasia type 2B and sporadic medullary thyroid carcinoma. *Nature* **367**: 375–6.

Howe, J.R., Norton, J.A. and Wells, S.A. 1993. Prevalence of pheochromocytoma and hyperparathyroidism in multiple endocrine neoplasia type 2A: Results of long-term follow-up. *Surgery* **114**: 1070–7.

Ikeda, I., Ishizaka, Y., Tahira, T., Suzuki, T., Onda, M., Sugimura, T. and Nagao, M. 1990. Specific expression of the *ret* proto-oncogene in human neuroblastoma cell lines. *Oncogene* **5**: 1291–6.

Ito, S., Iwashita, T., Asai, N., Murakami, H., Iwata, Y., Sobue, G. and Takahashi, M. 1997. Biological properties of Ret with cysteine mutations correlate with multiple endocrine neoplasia type 2A, familial medullary thyroid carcinoma, and Hirschsprung's disease phenotype. *Cancer Research* **57**: 2870–2.

Ivanchuk, S.M., Myers, S.M., Eng, C. and Mulligan, L.M. 1996. *De novo* mutation of *GDNF*: ligand of the RET/GDNFR-α receptor complex in Hirschsprung disease. *Human Molecular Genetics* **5**: 2023–6.

Iwashita, T., Asai, N., Murakami, H., Matsuyama, M. and Takahashi, M. 1996. Identification of tyroisine residues that are essential for transforming activity of the *ret* proto-oncogene with MEN2A or MEN2B mutation. *Oncogene* **12**: 481–7.

Jackson, C.E., Norum, R.A., Boyd, S.B., Talpos, G.B., Wilson, S.D., Taggart, T. and Mallette, L.E. 1990. Hereditary hyperparathyroidism and multiple ossifying jaw fibromas: a clinically and genetically distinct syndrome. *Surgery* **108**: 1006–13.

Jing, S., Wen, D., Yu, Y. et al. 1996. GDNF-induced activation of the Ret protein tyrosine kinase is mediated by GDNFR-α, novel receptor for GDNF. *Cell* **85**: 1113–24.

Kakinuma, A., Morimoto, I., Nakano, Y. et al. 1994. Familial primary hyperparathyroidism complicated with Wilms' tumor. *Internal Medicine* **33**: 123–6.

Klein, R.D., Sherman, D., Ho, W.-H. et al. 1997. A GPI-linked protein that interacts with Ret to form a candidate neurturin receptor. *Nature* **387**: 717–21.

Klöppel, G., Willemer, S., Stamm, B., Häcki, W.H. and Heitz, P.U. 1986. Pancreatic lesions and hormonal profile of pancreatic tumors in multiple endocrine neoplasia type 1: an immunocytochemical study of nine patients. *Cancer* **57**: 1824–32.

Komminoth, P., Kunz, E., Hiort, O. et al. 1994. Detection of *RET* proto-oncogene point mutations in paraffin-embedded pheochromocytoma specimens by nonradioactive single-strand conformation polymorphism analysis and direct sequencing. *American Journal of Pathology* **145**: 922–9.

Kotzbauer, Lampe, P.A., Heuckeroth, R.O., Golden, J.P., Creedon, D.J., Johnson, E.M. and Milbrandt, J. 1996. Neurturin, a relative of glial-cell-line derived neurotrophic factor. *Nature* **384**: 467–70.

Kytölä, S., Leisti, J., Winqvist, R. and Salmela, P. 1995. Improved carrier testing for multiple endocrine neoplasia, type 1, using new microsatellite-type DNA markers. *Human Genetics* **96**: 449–53.

Landsvater, R.M., Jansen, R.P., Hofstra, R.M., Buys, C.H.C., Lips, C.J. and Ploos van Amstel, H.K. 1996. Mutation analysis of the *RET* proto-oncogene in Dutch families with MEN 2A, MEN 2B and FMTC: two novel mutations and one *de novo* mutation for MEN 2A. *Human Genetics* **97**: 11–14.

Landsvater, R.M., Rombouts, A.G., te Meerman, G.J. et al. 1993. The clinical implications of a positive calcitonin test for C-cell hyperplasia in genetically unaffected members of an MEN2A kindred. *American Journal of Human Genetics* **52**: 335–42.

Larsson, C., Calender, A., Grimmond, S., Giraud, S., Hayward, N.K., Teh, B. and Farnebo, F. 1995. Molecular tools for presymptomatic testing in multiple endocrine neoplasia type 1. *Journal of Internal Medicine* **238**: 239–44.

Larsson, C., Shepherd, J., Nakamura, Y. et al. 1992b. Predictive testing for multiple endocrine neoplasia type 1 using DNA polymorphisms. *Journal of Clinical Investigation* **89**: 1344–9.

Larsson, C., Skogseid, B., Öberg, K., Nakamura, Y. and Nordenskjöld, M. 1988. Multiple endocrine neoplasia type 1 gene maps to chromosome 11 and is lost in insulinoma. *Nature* **332**: 85–7.

Larsson, C., Weber, G., Kvanta, E. et al. 1992a. Isolation and mapping of polymorphic cosmid clones used for sublocalization of the multiple endocrine neoplasia type 1 (*MEN1*) locus. *Human Genetics* **89**: 187–93.

Lin, L.-F.H., Doherty, D.H., Lile, J.D., Bektesh, S. and Collins, F. 1993. GDNF: a glial cell line-derived neurotrophic factor for midbrain dopaminergic neurons. *Science* **260**: 1130–2.

Lubensky, I.A., Debelenko, L.V., Zhuang, Z. et al. 1996. Allelic deletions on chromosome 11q13 in multiple tumors from individual MEN1 patients. *Cancer Research* **56**: 5272–8.

Mallette, L.E. 1994. Management of hyperparathyroidism in the multiple endocrine neoplasia syndromes and other familial endocrinopathies. *Endocrinology and Metabolism Clinics of North America* **23**: 19–36.

Mariman, E.C.M., van Beersum, S.E.C., Cremers, C.W.R.J., Struycken, P.M. and Ropers, H.H. 1995. Fine mapping of a putatively imprinted gene for familial non-chromaffin paragangliomas to chromosome 11q13.1: evidence for genetic heterogeneity. *Human Genetics* **95**: 56–62.

Mariman, E.C.M., van Beersum, S.E.C., Cremers, C.W.R.J., van Baars, F.M. and Ropers, H.H. 1993. Analysis of a second family with hereditary non-chromaffin paragangliomas locates the underlying gene at the proximal region of chromosome 11q. *Human Genetics* **91**: 357–61.

Marsh, D.J., Andrew, S.D., Eng, C. et al. 1996. Germline and somatic mutations in an oncogene: *RET* mutations in inherited medullary thyroid carcinoma. *Cancer Research* **56**: 1241–3.

Marsh, D.J., Andrew, S.D., Learoyd, D.L., Pojer, R., Eng, C. and Robinson, B.G. 1997. Deletion-insertion mutation encompassing *RET* codon 634 is associated with medullary thyroid carcinoma. *Human Mutation.* (In press.)

Matsuo, K., Tang, S.H. and Fagin, J.A. 1991. Allelotype of human thyroid tumours: loss of chromosome 11q13 sequences in follicular neoplasms. *Journal of Molecular Endocrinology* **5**: 1873–9.

McCutcheon, I.E. 1994. Management of individual tumor syndromes. Pituitary neoplasia. *Endocrinology and Metabolism Clinics of North America* **23**: 37–51.

Morelli, A., Falchetti, A., Weinstein, L. et al. 1995. RFLP analysis of human chromosome 11 region q13 in multiple symmetric lipomatosis and multiple endocrine neoplasia type 1-associated lipomas. *Biochemical and Biophysical Research Communications* **207**: 363–8.

Mount, H.T.J., Dean, D.O., Alberch, J., Dreyfus, C.F. and Black, I.B. 1995. Glial cell line-derived neurotrophic factor promotes the survival and morphologic differentiation of Purkinje cells. *Proceedings of the National Academy of Sciences, USA* **92**: 9092–6.

Mulligan, L.M., Eng, C., Attié, T. et al. 1994a. Diverse phenotypes associated with exon 10 mutations of the *RET* proto-oncogene. *Human Molecular Genetics* **3**: 2163–7.

Mulligan, L.M., Eng, C., Healey, C.S. et al. 1994b. Specific mutations of the *RET* proto-oncogene are related to disease phenotype in MEN 2A and FMTC. *Nature Genetics* **6**: 70–74.

Mulligan, L.M., Kwok, J.B.J., Healey, C.S. et al. 1993. Germ-line mutations of the *RET* proto-oncogene in multiple endocrine neoplasia type 2A. *Nature* **363**: 458–60.

Mulligan, L.M., Marsh, D.J., Robinson, B.G. et al. 1995. Genotype-phenotype correlation in multiple endocrine neoplasia type 2: report of the International *RET* Mutation Consortium. *Journal of Internal Medicine* **238**: 343–6.

Nakamura, T., Ishizaka, Y., Nagao, M., Hara, M. and Ishikawa, T. 1994. Expression of the *ret* proto-oncogene product in human normal and neoplastic tissues of neural crest origin. *Journal of Pathology* **172**: 255–60.

Öberg, K., Wälinder, O., Bostrom, H., Lundqvist, G. and Wide, L. 1982. Peptide hormone markers in screening for endocrine tumors in multiple endocrine adenomatosis type 1. *American Journal of Medicine* **73**: 619–30.

Pachnis, V., Mankoo, B. and Costantini, F. 1993. Expression of the *c-ret* proto-oncogene during mouse embryogenesis. *Development* **119**: 1005–17.

Pasini, B., Borrello, M.G., Greco, A. et al. 1995. Loss of function effect of *RET* mutations causing Hirschsprung disease. *Nature Genetics* **10**: 35–40.

352   H. Feilotter and L. Mulligan

Radford, D.M., Ashley, S.W., Wells, S.A. and Gerhard, D.S. 1990. Loss of heterozygosity of markers on chromosome 11 in tumors from patients with multiple endocrine neoplasia syndrome type 1. *Cancer Research* **50**: 6529–33.
Romei, C., Elisei, R., Pinchera, A. et al. 1996. Somatic mutations of the *RET* proto-oncogene in sporadic medullary thyroid carcinoma are not restricted to exon 16 and are associated with tumor recurrence. *Journal of Clinical Endocrinology and Metabolism* 81, 1619–22.
Salomon, R., Attié, T., Pelet, A. et al. 1996. Germline mutations of the *RET* ligand, *GDNF*, are not sufficient to cause Hirschsprung disease. *Nature Genetics.* **14**: 345–7.
Sanicola, M., Hession, C., Worley, D. et al. 1997. Glial cell line-derived neurotrophic factor dependent RET activation can be mediated by two different cell-surface accessory proteins. *Proceedings of National Academy of Sciences, USA* **94**: 6238–43.
Santoro, M., Carlomagno, F., Romano, A. et al. 1995. Activation of *RET* as a dominant transforming gene by germline mutations of MEN2A and MEN2B. *Science* **267**: 381–3.
Santoro, M., Rosati, R., Grieco, M., Berlingieri, M.T., D'Amato, G.L.C., deFranciscis, V. and Fusco, A. 1990. The RET proto-oncogene is consistently expressed in human pheochromocytomas and thyroid medullary carcinomas. *Oncogene* **5**: 1595–8.
Schimke, R.N. 1984. Genetic aspects of multiple endocrine neoplasia. *Annual Review of Medicine* **35**: 25–31.
Schneider, R. 1992. The human protooncogene *ret*: a communicative cadherin? *TIBS* **17**: 468–9.
Schuchardt, A., D'Agati, V., Larsson-Blomberg, L., Costantini, F. and Pachnis, V. 1994. Defects in the kidney and enteric nervous system of mice lacking the tyrosine kinase receptor Ret. *Nature* **367**: 380–3.
Schuchardt, A., Agati, V., Larsson-Blomberg, L., Costantini, F. and Pachnis, V. 1995. RET-deficient mice: an animal model for Hirschsprung's disease and renal agenesis. *Journal of Internal Medicine* **238**: 327–32.
Schuffenecker, I., Billaud, M., Calender, A. et al. 1994. *RET* proto-oncogene mutations in French MEN 2A and FMTC families. *Human Molecular Genetics* **3**: 1939–43.
Skogseid, B., Eriksson, B., Lundqvist, G. et al. 1991. Multiple endocrine neoplasia type 1: a 10-year prospective screening study in four kindreds. *Journal of Clinical Endocrinology and Metabolism* **73**: 281–7.
Skogseid, B., Larsson, C., Lindgren, P.-G. et al. 1992. Clinical and genetic features of adrenocortical lesions in multiple endocrine neoplasia type 1. *Journal of Clinical Endocrinology and Metabolism* **75**: 76–81.
Skogseid, B. and Öberg, K. 1995. Experience with multiple endocrine neoplasia type 1 screening. *Journal of Internal Medicine* **238**: 255–61.
Skogseid, B., Rastad, J. and Öberg, K. 1994. Multiple endocrine neoplasia type 1: clinical features and screening. *Endocrinology and Metabolism Clinics of North America* **23**: 1–18.
Songyang, Z., Carraway, K.L., Eck, M.J. et al. 1995. Catalytic specificity of protein-tyrosine kinases is critical for selective signalling. *Nature* **373**: 536–9.
Stratakis, C.A., Carney, J.A., Lin, J.P. et al. 1996. Carney complex, a familial multiple neoplasia and lentiginosis syndrome: analysis of 11 kindreds and linkage to the short arm of chromosome 2. *Journal of Clinical Investigation* **97**: 699–705.

Suvanto, P., Wartiovaara, K., Lindahl, M. et al. 1997. Cloning, mRNA distribution and chromosomal localisation of the gene for glial cell line-derived neurotrophic factor receptor β, a homologue of GDNFR-α. *Human Molecular Genetics* **6**: 1267–73.

Szabó, J., Heath, B., Hill, V.M. et al. 1995. Hereditary hyperparathyroidism-jaw tumor syndrome: the endocrine tumor gene HRPT2 maps to chromosome 1q21-q31. *American Journal of Human Genetics* **56**: 944–50.

Tahira, T., Ishizaka, Y., Itoh, F., Nakayasu, M., Sugimura, T. and Nagao, M. 1991. Expression of the *ret* proto-oncogene in human neuroblastoma cell lines and its increase during neuronal differentiation induced by retinoic acid. *Oncogene* **6**: 2333–8.

Tahira, T., Ishizaka, Y., Sugimura, T. and Nagao, M. 1988. Expression of proto-ret mRNA in embryonic and adult rat tissues. *Biochemical and Biophysical Research Communications* **153**: 1290–5.

Takahashi, M., Buma, Y. and Hiai, H. 1989. Isolation of *ret* proto-oncogene cDNA with an amino-terminal signal sequence. *Oncogene* **4**: 805–6.

Takahashi, M., Buma, T., Iwamoto, T., Inaguma, Y., Ikeda, H. and Hiai, H. 1988. Cloning and expression of the *ret* proto-oncogene encoding a tyrosine kinase with two potential transmembrane domains. *Oncogene* **3**: 571–8.

Thakker, R.V., Bouloux, P., Wooding, C. et al. 1989. Association of parathyroid tumours in multiple endocrine neoplasia type 1 with loss of alleles on chromosome 11. *New England Journal of Medicine* **321**: 218–24.

Thakker, R.V., Pook, M.A., Wooding, C., Boscaro, M., Scanarini, M. and Clayton, R.N. 1993a. Association of somatotrophinomas with loss of alleles on chromosome 11 and with *gsp* mutations. *Journal of Clinical Investigation* **91**: 2815–21.

Thakker, R.V., Wood, C., Pang, J.T. et al. 1993b. Linkage analysis of 7 polymorphic markers at chromosome 11p11.2-11q13 in 27 multiple endocrine neoplasia type 1 families. *Annals of Human Genetics* **57**: 17–25.

Thompson, N.W. 1995. The surgical management of hyperparathyroidism and endocrine disease of the pancreas in the multiple endocrine neoplasia type 1 patient. *Journal of Internal Medicine* **238**: 269–80.

Treanor J.J.S, Goodman, L., de Sauvage, F. et al. 1996. Characterization of a multicomponent receptor for GDNF. *Nature* **382**: 80–3.

Trupp, M., Rydén, M., Jörnvall, H., Funakoshi, H., Timmusk, T., Arenas, E. and Ibáñez, C. 1995. Peripheral expression and biological activities of GDNF, a new neurotrophic factor for avian and mammalian peripheral neurons. *Journal of Cell Biology* **130**: 137–48.

Trupp, M., Arenas, E., Fainzilber, M. et al. 1996. Functional receptor for GDNF encoded by the *c-ret* proto-oncogene. *Nature* **381**: 785–9.

van der Mey, A.G.L., Maaswinkel-Mooy, P.D., Cornelisse, C.J., Schmidt, P.H., and Kamp, J.J.P. 1989. Genomic imprinting in hereditary glomus tumors: evidence for new genetic theory. *Lancet* **II**: 1291–4.

Vasen, H.F., van de Feltz, M., Raue, F. et al. 1992. The natural course of multiple endocrine neoplasia type IIb. A study of 18 cases. *Archives of Internal Medicine* **152**: 1250–2.

Wassif, W.S., Moniz, C.F., Friedman, E. et al. 1993. Familial isolated hyperparathyroidism: a distinct genetic entity with an increased risk of parathyroid cancer. *Journal of Clinical Endocrinology and Metabolism* **77**: 1485–9.

Wilkinson, S., Teh, B.T., Davey, K.R., McArdle, J.P., Young, M. and Shepherd, J.J. 1993. Cause of death in multiple endocrine neoplasia type 1. *Archives of Surgery* **128**: 683–90.
Yuasa, H., Tokito, S., Nakagaki, H. and Kitamura, K. 1990. Familial pituitary adenoma: report of 4 cases from two unrelated families. *Neurologica Medico-Chirurgica* **30**: 1016–19.

17

Tobacco-related cancers of the respiratory and upper digestive tract

ZOLTAN TRIZNA and STIMSON SCHANTZ

Summary

Many enzymes are implicated in the metabolism of external carcinogens. Genetic polymorphisms in the genes that encode these enzymes have been described. This chapter reviews the possible relevance of some of the candidate enzymes that are involved with the metabolism of tobacco products. The role of polymorphisms in these enzymes in susceptibility to squamous cell carcinoma of the head and neck and lung is discussed. Mutagen sensitivity, as measured by bleomycin-induced chromosomal breakage, appears to be a marker for individuals' sensitivity to environmental carcinogens. The relevance of mutagen sensitivity to susceptibility to head and neck cancer is considered.

Introduction

Tobacco consumption is an epidemiologically well-established risk factor for cancer at a number of organ sites including the oral cavity, oesophagus, nasopharynx, lung, larynx, pancreas, bladder and kidney (susceptibility to the latter two cancers is discussed in Chapter 11). However, hereditary factors are probably involved in tobacco-related carcinogenesis. Some genetic traits show marked interactions with the environment in the carcinogenetic process. Others may influence the numbers of target cells, the proliferation of once-hit stem cells, the rates at which first and second events occur, or the occurrence of events critical for progression and metastasis, such as vascularization of a tumour.

Genetic polymorphisms

Genetic polymorphisms are mutations that are not incompatible with life, and by convention have a population frequency of at least 1%. However,

356   Z. Trizna and S. Schantz

such mutations may result in marked interindividual phenotypic differences. An example of this is the case of the metabolism of ingested and/or
inhaled foreign agents (xenobiotics). Several enzymatic systems act upon
these compounds, either by detoxifying reactive compounds or by con-
verting them into carcinogens. Genetically determined polymorphisms
have been found to be associated with increased susceptibility to cancers
of the lung, bladder, and gastrointestinal tract.

Glutathione S-transferases

Glutathione S-transferases (GSTs) catalyze the conjugation of glutathione to several electrophilic compounds, including carcinogenic polycyclic aromatic hydrocarbons and cytotoxic drugs. Such conjugated
xenobiotics are rendered harmless and their excretion is enhanced. The
human GST supergene family is divided into classes of alpha, mu, theta
and pi on the basis of chromosomal location and sequence homology.

Glutathione transferase mu 1-1 (GSTM1)

The GSTM1 gene is a part of a cluster of five genes on chromosome 1
and the products of this gene cluster are detectable in various organ
systems of the body (Seidegård et al., 1987, 1988, 1990). The presence
or absence of the GSTM1 gene constitutes the polymorphism and the
lack of GSTM1 (the GSTM1 null genotype) affects approximately 50%
of the population (Seidegård et al., 1988). A 98–100% correlation was
described between phenotyping and genotyping for GSTM1 (Zhong et
al., 1991). Studies employing more than 100 subjects mostly showed the
GSTM1 null genotype prevalence being between 0.31 and 0.58 (Bell et al.,
1993; Heckbert et al., 1992).

In phenotypic studies the activity of GSTM1 was determined toward
one of its substrates, trans-stilbene oxide, and it was suggested that the
lack of GSTM1 is a host determinant to lung cancer in smokers
(Seidegård et al., 1987, 1988, 1990). Smokers with GSTM1 deficiency
had a significantly elevated risk for developing laryngeal cancer
(Lafuente et al., 1993). The GSTM1 null genotype was positively associated with high DNA adduct levels in lung cancer, suggesting its role in
carcinogenesis (Shields et al., 1993). Another mechanistic explanation of
the GSTM1 null genotype comes from the in vivo observation that the
mutagenicity of urine from smokers with the GSTM1 null genotype was
significantly higher than urine from smokers in whom the GSTM1 gene

was present (Hirvonen et al., 1994). The *GSTM1* null genotype-associated lung cancer risk also appears to be dependent on the extent of tobacco smoke exposure (Kihara and Noda, 1994).

A positive correlation was found between the *GSTM1* null genotype and lung cancer (Seidegård et al., 1988), but contradictory findings have also been published (Brockmöller et al., 1993). The *GSTM1* null genotype was associated with higher risk for other environmentally-related cancers, e.g. cancers of the bladder (Brockmöller et al., 1993) and stomach (Harada et al., 1992).

In a case-control study of patients (167 blacks and 189 whites) with incident lung cancer and population control subjects (258 blacks and 473 whites), for patients with all lung cancers combined, the *GSTM1* null genotype was associated with an OR (odds ratio) of 1.29 (95% CI (confidence interval) = 0.94–1.77). The OR was similar among blacks (OR: 1.20; 95% CI: 0.72–2.00) and whites (OR: 1.37; 95% CI: 0.91–2.06). An OR of 1.77 (95% CI: 1.11–2.82) was detected for the *GSTM1* null genotype in relation to lung cancer risk among lighter smokers (< 40 pack-years), but no association was found among heavier smokers (London et al., 1995).

In a population of 42 patients with head and neck squamous cell cancers (HNSCCs) and their matched 42 controls the absence of the *GSTM1* genotype conferred OR of 2.56 ($p < 0.05$). Even though the study size is small, these preliminary data suggest an association between genetically determined factors of carcinogen metabolism and risk for HNSCC (Trizna et al., 1995).

Combined effects of GSTM1 and CYP1A1 polymorphisms

The combined effects of *GSTM1* and *CYP1A1* polymorphisms (see later) have also been investigated (Nakachi et al., 1993; Anttila et al., 1994; Hayashi et al., 1992). The combination of the *GSTM1* null genotype and the rare homozygous allele (G/G) of the *CYP1A1* gene resulted in a significantly higher relative risk for lung cancer than the relative risks calculated for either of these genotypes separately (Hayashi et al., 1992). A subsequent case-control study showed that individuals with the susceptible MspI or *G/G* genotype combined with the *GSTM1* null genotype had significantly elevated OR for lung cancer at a low dose level of cigarette smoking (Nakachi et al., 1993). Similarly, a European case-control study showed that expression of the *GSTM1* enzyme had a protective effect against contracting bronchial cancer in patients with inducible *CYP1A1* (Anttila et al., 1994).

In Sweden the *m1/m2* and *m2/m2* genotypes of the MspI site and the *Ile/Val* genotype of the *CYP1A1* gene were slightly over-represented in patients with squamous cell carcinoma of the lung in Sweden (Alexandrie et al., 1994). Among patients diagnosed before 66 years of age the *m1/m2* genotype was found in 28%, whereas the same genotype was observed in 16% of healthy controls. A combined risk of pulmonary squamous cell carcinoma was indicated for patients, diagnosed before 66 years of age, carrying both the *GSTM1* null genotype and the m2 alleles (OR: 3.0; 95% CI: 1.2–7.2).

Glutathione S-transferase theta (GSTT1)

GSTT1 differs from other GSTs in that it has no activity toward the model substrate 1-chloro-2,4-dinitrobenzene but has relatively high activity toward epoxy and peroxide compounds. GSTT1 is important in the detoxification of naturally occurring monohalomethanes, as well as the industrial compounds dichloromethane and ethylene oxide (Pemble et al., 1994).

Approximately 60–70% of the human population are able to carry out this conjugative reaction ('conjugators') whereas the remaining 30–40% are 'non-conjugators' because they are unable to do so. The conjugation is detoxifying with regard to monohalomethanes and ethylene oxide but conjugation of dichloromethane yields a mutagenic metabolite (Pemble et al., 1994). Because the agents mentioned above are widely used in industry as methylating agents, fumigants, pesticides and solvents, any polymorphism involved in their metabolism is of epidemiological interest in aerodigestive cancers.

The human *GSTT1* gene has been isolated. The product of the gene is the GST theta enzyme, and the null ('non-conjugator') phenotype results from homozygous deletion of the *GSTT1* gene (Pemble et al., 1994). The lack of this gene may be associated with elevated risk of head and neck cancer.

In a population of 42 patients with HNSCC and their matched 42 controls, the absence of the GSTT1 genotype conferred OR of 2.18 ($p = 0.06$). Despite the small study size, these data suggest that genetically determined factors of carcinogen metabolism may be associated with increased risk for HNSCC (Trizna et al., 1995).

Glutathione S-transferase pi (GSTP1)

GSTP1 isoenzyme is overexpressed in some models of malignant transformation and antineoplastic drug resistance, as well as in several chemically induced human neoplasms and tumour cell lines (Morrow et al.,
1989; Xia et al., 1993). In addition, the expression of the isoenzyme was
higher in the malignant tissue itself than in normal tissue (Morrow et al.,
1989), including a 2.5-fold increase in head and neck cancers (Toffoli et
al., 1992). Elevated plasma GSTP1 levels were found in patients with oral
cancer and were considered to be useful in early diagnosis, prognosis, and
determining treatment efficacy (Hirata et al., 1992).

However, a study of oesophageal cancer found that GSTP1 levels in
the tumour and adjacent tissue were markers of carcinogenic exposure
but not of the tumour itself (Sasano et al., 1993). Another study of several
metabolic enzymes did not show any difference of enzymatic activities
between tumourous and adjacent non-tumourous mucosa (Janot et al.,
1993). In the light of the theory of field cancerization these findings are
not surprising, because these tissues were subjected to similar environmental exposures. The gene sequence is known (Morrow et al., 1989), and
a polymorphic region has been described at the AT-rich 5'-flanking
region of the gene (Harada et al., 1992).

The cytochrome P450 system

The cytochrome P450-dependent mono-oxygenases represent a major
line of defense against toxic chemicals. The oxidation of the substrate
increases the hydrophilic nature of the molecule and facilitates further
metabolic processing and excretion. However, certain chemicals are not
detoxified but are activated into a carcinogenic form.

Cytochrome P450IA1 (CYP1A1)

Encoded by the *CYP1A1* gene, aryl hydrocarbon hydroxylase (AHH) is
involved in the biotransformation of tobacco-derived polycyclic aromatic
hydrocarbons (PAHs) into reactive diolepoxide metabolites with carcinogenic potential. The genetic polymorphism for AHH in humans is
reflected in the existence of populations sensitive and resistant to inducers
such as tobacco smoke (Petersen et al., 1991).

A statistically significant increase of AHH activity in neoplastic versus
normal lung tissues was found in smokers, and AHH activity in the
neoplastic tissues of smokers was higher than in those of non-smokers

(Pasquini et al., 1988). Significant correlations between high AHH inducibility and bronchogenic carcinoma (Anttila et al., 1994) and peripheral adenocarcinomas of the lung (Anttila et al., 1991) have also been described in smokers. Lower crude mortality rates were related to lower enzyme levels in surgically treated lung cancer patients (Bartsch et al., 1990). Smokers with a high AHH level had a four-fold higher risk of developing laryngeal cancer than non-smokers with low AHH levels; they also developed cancer earlier in their lives and had recurrences and secondary malignancies more frequently (Andreasson et al., 1987).

The tissue concentration of 10 CYP mRNA expression levels was quantitated in 19 human lung tumours and matched normal adjacent tissues. CYP expression was generally higher in the tumours than in normal adjacent tissue, for example, CYP1A1 mRNA levels were elevated 25-fold compared to normal adjacent tissue. A positive correlation between CYP1A1 expression in tumours and smoking was observed (Romkes-Sparks et al., 1995).

The sequencing of the *CYP1A1* gene allowed investigation of the genetic background of the findings described above (Petersen et al., 1991). Two polymorphisms seem to be important.

The frequency of restriction fragment length polymorphism (RFLP) after MspI or DraI digestion was correlated with tobacco-related lung cancer risk in Japanese populations (Kawajiri et al., 1990; Hayashi et al., 1991b) and with PAH-related colorectal cancer in Hawaiians (Sivaraman et al., 1994). Individuals with the susceptible *CYP1A1* genotype contracted smoking-induced pulmonary cancers at lower cigarette smoking levels than those with other *CYP1A1* genotypes (Nakachi et al., 1993). Similar RFLP studies of European and South American populations did not show clear associations between the *CYP1A1* genotype and susceptibility to lung cancer (Sugimura et al., 1990; Tefre et al., 1991; Hirvonen et al., 1992). This may be explained by insufficient study sizes for detecting an association between cancer and a putative risk factor whose prevalence is between 0.05 (Hirvonen et al., 1992b) and 0.08 (Sugimura et al., 1994).

The A/G mutation in exon 7 determines an Ile→Val amino acid change (Hayashi et al., 1992). The importance of this lies in the observation that the activity of the CYP1A1 enzyme, as determined with the ethoxyresorufin assay, was elevated in individuals with such mutations of the coding region of the *CYP1A1* gene (Cosma et al., 1993). The risk factor seems to be the *G/G* homozygous genotype, which has a prevalence between 0.02 (Hirvonen et al., 1992b) and 0.05 (Hayashi et al., 1992) in healthy controls. Whereas there was a significant association between this genotype and lung cancer in a Japanese study (Hayashi et al., 1992), a Finnish study did not demonstrate similar findings (Hirvonen et al., 1992b). The functional significance of these polymorphisms was further emphasized in a recent study, in which *CYP1A1* genotypes, gene expression levels and enzymatic activity levels were measured in mitogen-stimulated lymphocytes (Crofts et al., 1994). Genotypes were determined at two sites previously associated with lung cancer – a point mutation in exon 7 near the catalytic region of the enzyme and an Mspl RFLP in the 3′ non-coding region of the gene. There was a threefold elevation in CYP1A1 enzymatic activity in exon 7 variant genotypes. When Mspl and exon 7 genotypes were combined, there was an increased CYP1A1 inducibility and enzymatic activity in subjects with the exon 7 polymorphism, and in subjects with both polymorphisms.

In a recent publication (Hamada et al., 1995) an association between the exon 7 mutation and lung cancer risk was described in a patient population in which previously no associations were detected between lung cancer risk and the CYP1A1 MspI polymorphism or RsaI polymorphism of the CYP2ED (Sugimura et al., 1994).

Cytochrome P450 IIE1 (CYP2E1)

CYP2E1 metabolizes more than 75 substrates, including potentially important carcinogens such as benzene, dimethylnitrosoamine, vinylchloride and diethyldithiocarbamate (Persson et al., 1993). The region for either PstI or RsaI restriction sites is located in the transcriptional regulation region of CYP2E1 (Hayashi et al., 1991). Another polymorphism has been described which is located in intron 6 (Watanabe et al., 1990). Marked inter-ethnic differences have been described with regard to these RFLPs but there was no significant association with risk for lung cancer (Persson et al., 1993; Watanabe et al., 1990). In a recent study, CYP2E1 was the second most highly expressed CYP in lung tumours and the activity of this enzyme was also higher in vivo in lung cancer patients than young controls (Romkes-Sparks et al., 1995).

Cytochrome P450IID6 (CYP2D6)

The significance of the *CYP2D6* gene is that in metabolizes the tobacco-specific nitrosoamine, 4-(methylnitrosamino)-1-(3-pyridyl)-1-butanone (NNK), to mutagenic products. The genetic basis of the extensive metabolizer and poor metabolizer phenotypes is well understood, and PCR-based methodologies are available for their detection (Heim and Meyer, et al., 1991). The PCR-based methods are superior to the phenotypic assessment of metabolic status, as the latter may be influenced by previous drug therapy and the presence of the tumour itself (Idle and Daly, 1993). The correlation between phenotype and PCR-based genotyping is 95.0–97.5% (Heim and Meyer, 1991).

A polymorphism of the cytochrome P450 debrisoquine hydroxylase (*CYP2D6*) gene affects 5–10% of the Caucasian population and is responsible for the compromised metabolism and side-effects of several therapeutic drugs such as debrisoquine, dextrometorphan, propranolol. and bufuralol (Sugimura et al., 1990; Heim and Meyer, 1991; Wolf et al., 1992). The phenotypically determined debrisoquine metabolism shows a bimodal distribution. The defective metabolism, designated as the poor metabolizer genotype, was found to be associated with reduced susceptibility to lung cancer and other types of cancer (Heim and Meyer, 1991; Wolf et al., 1992). Several epidemiological studies initially indicated that lung cancer risk is increased in extensive metabolizers of debrisoquine (Hirvonen et al., 1992b, 1993; Idle and Daly, 1993). The *CYP2D6(C)* allelic variant was significantly overrepresented in patients with lung cancer (Agundez et al.,1994).

A case-control study of 335 white lung cancer patients and 373 matched controls investigated the debrisoquine metabolic phenotype. No increased risk was found among extensive or intermediate metabolizers or among either heavy smokers or light and non-smokers (Shaw et al., 1995). These initial findings are still to be confirmed. However, the value of some of these observations is limited because of their sample sizes. For instance, selection of an unmatched group of controls may explain the lack of association (Wolf et al., 1992). Another negative study used phenotyping with RFLP-based genotyping but because only 45 cases, 42 controls, and 38 healthy volunteers were included, the observations can be challenged on a statistical basis (Sugimura et al., 1990).

Genetic polymorphisms and DNA adducts

A large body of evidence shows that the carcinogenic process is a multi-stage process driven by the interaction of exogenous carcinogenic exposures, genetic traits, and other endogenous factors. Levels of carcinogen-DNA adducts reflect the net effect of exposure, absorption, metabolic activation, detoxification, and DNA repair. These effects are genetically predetermined, inducibility notwithstanding. The combination of adduct and genotyping assays provide an assessment of risk that reflects recent exogenous exposure as well as one's lifetime ability to activate and detoxify carcinogens.

There are several possible interactions between different genetic variables. For instance, activated carcinogen metabolites may bind to DNA and form DNA adducts, many of which can induce genetic mutations. Thus, if individuals have an increased capacity to activate carcinogens, they might form more carcinogen–DNA adducts and subsequently have an increased risk of cancer. In a study of autopsy specimens from 90 noncancerous lungs it was found that the levels of two different carcinogen-DNA adducts varied in lung tissue in association with three separate genetic polymorphisms (*CYP2D6*, *CYP2E1*, and *GSTM1*). These findings suggest that genetic polymorphisms are predictive of carcinogen-DNA adduct levels and would thus be predictive of an individual's lifetime response to carcinogen exposure (Kato et al., 1995).

In a recent study, leukocytes from 119 non-small cell carcinoma lung cancer cases and from 98 non-cancer controls were analyzed for PAH-DNA adducts by ELISA and for *GSTM1* genotype by PCR. When the subjects were classified by adducts (high/low) and *GSTM1* genotype (0/0 versus 0/+ or +/+), the risk was 12-fold higher for those individuals with both high adducts and *GSTM1* 0/0 compared to those with neither factor (Tang et al., 1995). A combination of genetic factors was found to be related to differences in DNA adduct levels and was consistent with higher relative risk of lung cancer in 95 Finnish iron foundry workers with *GSTM1* null and MspI RFLP in *CYP1A1* (Dickey et al., 1995).

The levels of DNA adducts were analyzed in normal lung tissue from 63 lung cancer patients and examined in relation to exposure and genetic factors (Ryberg et al., 1994). An excess of individuals with GSTM1 deficiency was found among male patients with high adduct levels. Among females, the DNA adduct levels were higher than in males when adjusted for smoking dose.

The association between the *GSTM1* null genotype and PAH-DNA adduct levels in peripheral white blood cells (WBCs) was investigated among 47 non-smoking wildland fire-fighters who were frequently consuming charbroiled food. The results suggested that neither the *GSTM1* null genotype nor the *CYP1A1* exon 7 polymorphism were associated with increased susceptibility for PAH–DNA adduct formation in peripheral WBCs (Rothman et al., 1995).

Mutagen-sensitivity and cancer risk

Chromosomal fragility is an indicator of genetic instability and is associated with an increased risk of cancer in syndromes such as Fanconi anaemia, xeroderma pigmentosum, ataxia-telangiectasia, and Bloom syndrome (Trizna and Schnantz, 1992). The genetic defects underlying these conditions are discussed in Chapter 18. An area of mutagen sensitivity that is particularly relevant to tobacco-related cancers is bleomycin-induced chromosomal breakage, which has been used as a potential measure of the individual's sensitivity to environmental carcinogens (Hsu et al., 1989; Schantz and Hsu, 1989; Schantz et al., 1990). It was also suggested that mutagen sensitivity is a constitutional factor which reflects the way in which genotoxic compounds are dealt with and is thereby directly related to cancer risk (Cloos et al., 1994).

One component of the enhanced mutagen sensitivity phenotype observed in cancer-prone individuals may involve an inherent chromatin alteration that allows a more efficient translation of DNA damage into chromosome damage following mutagen exposure. The degree of such an alteration might then be associated with an increased risk for second primary tumours in other carcinogen-exposed sites (Pandita et al., 1995).

The greatest sensitivity to bleomycin damage was found in patients with cancers developing in tissues directly exposed to the external environment, such as the upper aerodigestive tract (Hsu et al., 1989; Schantz and Hsu et al., 1989). Mutagen sensitivity has been shown to be an independent risk factor for tobacco-related malignancies, especially those of the upper aerodigestive tract (Spitz et al., 1989). Furthermore, within the head and neck cancer population, it was noted that field cancerization was more evident in those individuals with the highest degree of mutagen sensitivity; such patients demonstrated a greater frequency of second primary malignancies. This relationship was independent of age, sex, site, treatment of first primary cancer and tobacco or alcohol exposures (Schantz et al., 1990; Spitz et al., 1994).

In 108 previously untreated HNSCCs and 108 matched controls, 69% of the cases, compared with 44% of the controls, were classified as mutagen sensitive. On multivariate analysis, mutagen sensitivity (OR: 2.5), heavy cigarette smoking (OR: 4.8), and heavy alcohol consumption (OR: 3.1) were all associated with significantly increased risk. Stratified analyses showed that the combined effects of cigarette smoking (OR: 8.1) and mutagen sensitivity (OR: 3.2) were suggestive of a multiplicative effect, resulting in an OR of 23.0 (Spitz et al., 1993).

In a multicentre, case-control analysis of 313 patients with HNSCC and in 334 control subjects, it was found that non-sensitive, heavy smokers had an OR of 11.5 (95% CI: 5.0–26.6). This risk increased dramatically in mutagen-hypersensitive, heavy smokers to 44.5 (95% CI: 17.4–114.0). A significant trend was found for the dose-dependent increase in cancer risk by smoking. The consumption of alcohol potentiated the effects of smoking, resulting in an OR of 57.5 (95% CI: 17.5–188.0) in hypersensitive persons (Cloos et al., 1996).

In another study, lymphocytes from primary blood cultures of 78 controls and 75 cases with four histopathological types of lung cancer were subjected to the bleomycin assay, and the frequency of induced chromatid breakage and the locations of the breaks were determined in Q-banded preparations. Lung cancer risk had a dose-response relationship with breaks on chromosomes 4 and 5, and cigarette smoking had a strong interaction with breaks on chromosomes 2, 4, and 5. These findings suggest that the susceptibility of particular chromosome loci to mutagenic damage may be a risk factor for specific types of lung cancer (Wu et al., 1995).

In a study of black individuals (90 lung cancer cases and 119 controls), 55.3% of the cases were mutagen sensitive (defined as $\geq$ break/cell), compared with 24.6% of the controls, with an age-, sex-, and smoking-adjusted OR of 3.7 (95% CI: 1.4–9.4). Of interest, higher risks were noted for former smokers (OR: 5.4) compared with current smokers (OR: 3.1) and especially for younger former smokers (< 55 years). By histologic-specific analysis, mutagen sensitivity was significantly associated with risk for adenocarcinoma (OR: 4.8) and squamous cell carcinoma (OR: 8.5) by histologic-specific analysis (Spitz et al., 1995).

Another study evaluated the relationship between family history of cancer and bleomycin-induced mutagen sensitivity in 108 patients with squamous cell cancer of the upper aerodigestive tract. A significant OR was found (OR: 2.63; 95% CI: 1.06–6.53) for patients who were mutagen sensitive and had one first-degree relative affected with cancer. For mutagen-sensitive patients with two or more first-degree relatives affected with cancer, the OR increased to 6.59 (95% CI: 1.69–25.72). These findings suggested that patients with defective DNA repair capability as evidenced by the mutagen sensitivity assay are significantly more likely to report a family history of cancer than patients who are not mutagen sensitive (Bondy et al., 1993).

In a study of 25 patients with multiple malignant head and neck cancers, *TP53* expression in first primary and second primary cancers was compared to *TP53* expression in tumour tissues from 25 head and neck cancer patients with single cancer. In addition, bleomycin-induced chromosome fragility was investigated in both groups of patients and in 21 healthy controls. A higher sensitivity to bleomycin was demonstrated in patients with multiple tumours than of patients with a single cancer ($p < 0.01$). A significant correlation between chromosome fragility and *TP53* overexpression ($p < 0.01$) was found only in patients with multiple malignancies. Patients with *TP53*-positive staining of both first and second primaries showed a higher mutagen sensitivity than those with a single *p53* immunoreactive tumour or those in whom both cancers were *TP53* negative ($p < 0.01$). These data suggest that subjects with increased susceptibility to carcinogens after tobacco exposure are at higher risk for multiple cancers. In this process aberrant *TP53* expression may be one of the most common genetic events (Gallo et al., 1995).

The interaction between environmental factors and genotoxicity have also been studied in vitro. Several micronutrients, including ascorbic acid (Trizna et al., 1991), N-acetyl-L-cysteine (Trizna et al., 1991), tocopherols (Trizna et al., 1992a) and 13-cis-retinoic acid (Trizna et al., 1992a) have been found to exert a dose-dependent protective effect against mutagen-induced chromosomal damage in vitro.

A recent case-control study (Schantz et al., 1997) supported the concept that the risk of head and neck cancer is determined by a balance of factors that either enhance or protect against free radical oxygen damage, including innate capacities for DNA repair. In these investigations, mutagen hypersensitivity was strongly associated with increased risk of head and neck cancer (OR: 4.95; 95% CI: 2.67–9.17) after adjusting for age, sex, and race. Low intake of vitamins C and E was also associated with an increased risk of disease and was interactive with mutagen sensitivity in risk estimates. Individuals with both a low intake of various antioxidants and increased chromosomal sensitivity to oxidant-induced DNA damage were at greatest risk.

Head, neck and lung cancers in fragility/instability syndromes

Head and neck cancers in hereditary non-polyposis colorectal cancer (HNPCC)

Laryngeal carcinomas were described as a part of multiple cancers in HNPCC (Loury et al., 1987); it had been reported in a family in which the mother developed laryngeal cancer 26 years after she had cancer of the uterine cervix. Her son was diagnosed with laryngeal cancer at 31

(Lynch et al., 1988). Whether tobacco is also playing a role in those with mismatch repair gene mutations is unknown.

Head and neck cancers in Bloom and Fanconi syndrome

Bloom syndrome (BS) is an autosomal recessive disorder characterized by a high incidence of cancer at a young age (see Chapter 18). Twenty-eight of the first 103 identified BS patients developed cancers, and five of these were head and neck carcinomas (Berkower and Biller, 1988). Head and neck cancer is also reported in Fanconi anaemia (Snow et al., 1991). These cancers usually develop at an age when signficant tobacco consumption is unlikely.

Skin, head, and neck cancers in xeroderma pigmentosum

Xeroderma pigmentosum (XP), an autosomal recessive condition, is characterized by defective DNA repair of UV-induced damage (see Chapter 18). Ninety-seven percent of the reported basal and squamous cell carcinomas and 65% of the melanomas in XP were found on the face, head, or neck. Life expectancy for XP patients was reduced by 28 years compared with the general US population. Ocular abnormalities (including neoplasias), restricted to UV-exposed tissues, were reported in 40% of the patients (Kraemer et al., 1987).

In a review of reports of 726 XP patients (from 41 countries) published from 1874 to 1982, the XP patients under age 20 years had an estimated 2000-fold increase in frequency of basal cell and squamous cell carcinoma of the skin, of cutaneous melanoma, of cancer of the anterior eye, and of cancer of the anterior tongue, in comparison to the general population. In addition to these sites, which are all potentially exposed to UV radiation, XP patients under age 20 years also had an estimated 12-fold increase in occurrence of neoplasms in sites not exposed to UV radiation, such as the brain and oral cavity (Kraemer et al., 1984).

Conclusion

Tobacco-related cancers are among the commonest group of cancers in the world. They are not commonly part of inherited cancer syndromes, but it is quite likely that genetic variation in the population influences risk of cancer among tobacco users. The role of particular enzymes such as the glutathione *S*-transferases in cancer susceptibility is not fully established. Many methodological problems remain, but it is likely that in the coming years, this area of research will throw light on the role of low penetrance genes in cancer and other diseases.

References

Agundez, J.A., Martinez, C., Ladero, J.M. et al. 1994. Debrisoquine oxidation genotype and susceptibility to lung cancer. *Clinical Pharmacology and Therapeutics* **55**: 10–4.

Alexandrie, A.K., Sundberg, M.I., Seidegard, J., Tornling, G. and Rannug, A. 1994. Genetic susceptibility to lung cancer with special emphasis on CYP1A1 and GSTM1: a study on host factors in relation to age at onset, gender and histological cancer types. *Carcinogenesis* **15**: 1785–90.

Andreasson, L., Bjorlin, G., Hocherman, M., Korsgaard, R. and Trell, E. 1987. Laryngeal cancer, aryl hydrocarbon hydroxylase inducibility and smoking. A follow-up study. *Journal of Otorhinolargyngology Related Specialities* **49**: 187–92.

Anttila, S., Hietanen, E., Vainio, H. et al. 1991. Smoking and peripheral type of cancer are related to high levels of pulmonary cytochrome P450IA in lung cancer patients. *International Journal of Cancer* **47**: 681–5.

Anttila, S., Hirvonen, A., Husgavel-Pursiainen, K., Karjalainen, A., Nurminen, T. and Vainio, H. 1994. Combined effect of CYP1A1 inducibility and GSTM1 polymorphism on histological type of lung cancer. *Carcinogenesis* **15**: 1133–5.

Bartsch, H., Hietanen, E., Petruzzelli, S., Giuntini, C., Saracci, R., Mussi, A. and Angeletti, C.A. 1990. Possible prognostic value of pulmonary AH-locus-linked enzymes in patients with tobacco-related lung cancer. *International Journal of Cancer* **46**: 185–8.

Bell, D.A., Taylor, J.A., Paulson, D.F., Robertson, C.N., Mohler, J.L. and Lucier, G.W. 1993. Genetic risk and carcinogen exposure: a common inherited defect of the carcinogen-metabolism gene glutathione S-transferase M1 (*GSTM1*) that increases susceptibility to bladder cancer. *Journal of the National Cancer Institute* **85**: 1159–64.

Berkower, A.S. and Biller, H.F. 1988. Head and neck cancer associated with Bloom's syndrome. *Laryngoscope* **98**: 746–8.

Bondy, M.L., Spitz, M.R., Halabi, S., Fueger, J.J., Schantz, S.P., Sample, D. and Hsu, T.C. 1993. Association between family history of cancer and mutagen sensitivity in upper aerodigestive tract cancer patients. *Cancer Epidemiology, Biomarkers and Prevention* **2**: 103–6.

Brockmöller, J., Kerb, R., Drakoulis, N., Nitz, M. and Roots, I. 1993. Genotype and phenotype of glutathione S-transferase class mu isoenzymes mu and psi in lung cancer patients and controls. *Cancer Research* **53**: 1004–11.

Cloos, J., Braakhuis, B.J., Steen, I., Copper, M.P., de Vries, N., Nauta, J.J. and Snow, G.B. 1994. Increased mutagen sensitivity in head-and-neck squamous-cell carcinoma patients, particularly those with multiple primary tumours. *International Journal Cancer* **56**: 816–9.

Cloos, J., Spitz, M.R., Schantz, S.P., Hsu, T.C., Zhang, Z.F., Tobi, H., Braakhuis, B.J. and Snow, G.B. 1996. Genetic susceptibility to head and neck squamous cell carcinoma. *Journal of the National Cancer Institute* **88**: 530–5.

Cosma, G., Crofts, F., Taioli, E., Toniolo, P. and Garte, S. 1993. Relationship between genotype and function of the human CYP1A1 gene. *Journal of Toxicology and Environmental Health* **40**: 309–16.

Crofts, F., Taioli, E., Trachman, J., Cosma, G.N., Currie, D., Toniolo, P. and Garte, S.J. 1994. Functional significance of different human CYP1A1 genotypes. *Carcinogenesis* **15**: 2961–3.

Dickey, C.P., Bell, D.A., Santella, R. et al. 1995. *GSTM1*, CYP1A1 MspI and DNA adducts in workers exposed to PAH (Meeting abstract). *Proceedings of the Annual Meeting of the American Association for Cancer Research* **36**: A712.

Gallo, O., Bianchi, S., Giovannucci-Uzzielli, M.L. et al. 1995. p53 oncoprotein overexpression correlates with mutagen-induced chromosome fragility in head and neck cancer patients with multiple malignancies. *British Journal of Cancer* **71**: 1008–12.

Hamada, G.S., Sugimura, H., Suzuki, I. et al. 1995. The heme-binding region polymorphism of cytochrome P450IA1 (CypIA1), rather than the RsaI polymorphism of IIE1 (CypIIE1), is associated with lung cancer in Rio De Janeiro. *Cancer Epidemiology, Biomarkers and Prevention* **4**: 63–7.

Harada, S., Misawa, S., Nakamura, T., Tanaka, N., Ueno, E. and Nozoe, M. 1992. Detection of GST1 gene deletion by the polymerase chain reaction and its possible correlation with stomach cancer in Japanese. *Human Genetics* **90**: 62–4.

Hayashi, S., Watanabe, J. and Kawajiri, K. 1991a. Genetic polymorphisms in the 5'-flanking region change transcriptional regulation of the human cytochrome P450IIE1 gene. *Journal of Biochemistry* **110**: 559–65.

Hayashi, S., Watanabe, J. and Kawajiri, K. 1992. High susceptibility to lung cancer analyzed in terms of combined genotypes of P450IA1 and Mu-class glutathione S-transferase genes. *Japanese Journal of Cancer Research* **83**: 866–70.

Hayashi, S., Watanabe, J., Nakachi, K. and Kawajiri, K. 1991. Genetic linkage of lung cancer-associated MspI polymorphisms with amino acid replacement in the heme binding region of the human cytochrome P450IA1 gene. *Journal of Biochemistry* **110**: 407–11.

Heckbert, S.R., Weiss, N.S., Hornung, S.K., Eaton, D.L. and Motulsky, A.G. 1992. Glutathione S-transferase and epoxide hydrolase activity in human leukocytes in relation to risk of lung cancer and other smoking-related cancers. *Journal of the National Cancer Institute* **84**: 414–22.

Heim, M.H. and Meyer, U.A. 1991. Genetic polymorphism of debrisoquine oxidation: restriction fragment analysis and allele-specific amplification of mutant alleles of CYP2D6. *Methods of Enzymology* **206**: 173–83.

Hirata, S., Odajima, T., Kohama, G., Ishigaki, S. and Niitsu, Y. 1992. Significance of glutathione S-transferase-pi as a tumour marker in patients with oral cancer. *Cancer* **70**: 2381–7.

Hirvonen, A., Husgafvel Pursiainen, K., Anttila, S., Karjalainen, A., Pelkonen, O. and Vainio, H. 1993. PCR-based CYP2D6 genotyping for Finnish lung cancer patients. *Pharmacogenetics* **3**: 19–27.

Hirvonen, A., Husgafvel Pursiainen, K., Anttila, S., Karjalainen, A., Sorsa, M. and Vainio, H. 1992a. Metabolic cytochrome P450 genotypes and assessment of individual susceptibility to lung cancer. *Pharmacogenetics* **2**: 259–63.

Hirvonen, A., Husgafvel Pursiainen, K., Karjalainen, A., Anttila, S., Vainio, H. 1992b. Point-mutational MspI and Ile-Val polymorphisms closely linked in the CYP1A1 gene: lack of association with susceptibility to lung cancer in a Finnish study population. *Cancer Epidemiology, Biomarkers and Prevention* 1: 485–9.

Hirvonen, A., Nylund, L., Kociba, P., Husgafvel-Pursiainen, K. and Vainio, H. 1994. Modulation of urinary mutagenicity by genetically determined carcinogen metabolism in smokers. *Carcinogenesis* 15: 813–5.

Hsu, T.C., Johnston, D.A., Cherry, L.M. et al. 1989. Sensitivity to genotoxic effects of bleomycin in humans: Possible relationship to environmental carcinogenesis. *International Journal of Cancer* 43: 403–9.

Idle, J.R. and Daly, A.K. 1993. New opportunities in cancer risk evaluation using PCR-based DNA analysis for CYP2D6. *Environmental Health Perspectives* 101 (Suppl 3): 117–20.

Janot, F., Massaad, L., Ribrag, V. et al. 1993. Principal xenobiotic-metabolizing enzyme systems in human head and neck squamous cell carcinoma. *Carcinogenesis* 14: 1279–83.

Kato, S., Bowman, E.D., Harrington, A.M., Blomeke, B. and Shields, P.G. 1995. Human lung carcinogen-DNA adduct levels mediated by genetic polymorphisms in vivo. *Journal of the National Cancer Institute* 87: 902–7.

Kawajiri, K., Nakachi, K., Imai, K., Yoshii, A., Shinoda, N. and Watanabe, J. 1990. Identification of genetically high risk individuals to lung cancer by DNA polymorphisms of the cytochrome P450IA1 gene. *FEBS Letters* 263: 131–3.

Kihara, M. and Noda, K. 1994. Lung cancer risk of GSTM1 null genotype is dependent on the extent of tobacco smoke exposure. *Carcinogenesis* 15: 415–8.

Kraemer, K.H., Lee, M.M. and Scotto, J. 1984. DNA repair protects against cutaneous and internal neoplasia: evidence from xeroderma pigmentosum. *Carcinogenesis* 5: 511–14.

Kraemer, K.H., Lee, M.M. and Scotto, J. 1987. Xeroderma pigmentosum. Cutaneous, ocular, and neurologic abnormalities in 830 published cases. *Archives of Dermatology* 123: 241–50.

Lafuente, A., Pujol, F., Carretero, P., Villa, J.P. and Cuchi, A. 1993. Human glutathione S-transferase mu (GST mu) deficiency as a marker for the susceptibility to bladder and larynx cancer among smokers. *Cancer Letters* 68: 49–54.

London, S.J., Daly, A.K., Cooper, J., Navidi, W.C., Carpenter, C.L. and Idle, J.R. 1995. Polymorphism of glutathione S-transferase M1 and lung cancer risk among African-Americans and Caucasians in Los Angeles County, California. *Journal of the National Cancer Institute* 87: 1246–53.

Loury, M.C., Johns, M.E. and Danes, B.S. 1987. In vitro hyperdiploidy in head and neck cancer. A genetic predisposition? *Archives of Otolaryngology – Head and Neck Surgery* 113: 1230–3.

Lynch, H.T., Kriegler, M., Christiansen, T.A., Smyrk, T., Lynch, J.F. and Watson, P. 1988. Laryngeal carcinoma in a Lynch syndrome ii kindred. *Cancer* 62: 1007–13.

Morrow, C.S., Cowan, K.H. and Goldsmith, M.E. 1989. Structure of the human genomic glutathione S-transferase-pi gene. *Gene* 75: 3–11.

Nakachi, K., Imai, K., Hayashi, S. and Kawajiri, K. 1993. Polymorphisms of the CYP1A1 and glutathione S-transferase genes associated with susceptibility to lung cancer in relation to cigarette dose in a Japanese population. *Cancer Research* 53: 2994–9.

Tobacco-related cancers   371

Pandita, T.K. and Hittelman, W.N. 1995. Evidence of a chromatin basis for increased mutagen sensitivity associated with multiple primary malignancies of the head and neck. *International Journal of Cancer* **61**: 738–43.

Pasquini, R., Sforzolini, G.S., Cavaliere, A. et al. 1988. Enzymatic activities of human lung tissue: relationship with smoking habits. *Carcinogenesis* **9**: 1411–16.

Pemble, S., Schroeder, K.R., Spencer, S.R. et al. 1994. Human glutathione S-transferase theta (GSTT1): cDNA cloning and the characterization of a genetic polymorphism. *Biochemistry Journal* **300**: 271–6.

Persson, I., Johansson, I., Bergling, H. et al. 1993. Genetic polymorphism of cytochrome P4502E1 in a Swedish population: Relationship to incidence of lung cancer. *FEBS Letters* **319**: 207–11.

Petersen, D.D., McKinney, C.E., Ikeya, K., Smith, H.H., Bale, A.E., McBride, O.W. and Nebert, D.W. 1991. Human CYP1A1 gene: cosegregation of the enzyme inducibility phenotype and an RFLP. *American Journal Human Genetics* **48**: 720–5.

Romkes-Sparks, M., Parise, R., Adedoyin, A., Stiff, D., Landreneau, R. and Branch, R.A. 1995. Expression of cytochrome P450 mRNA in human lung tumours and normal adjacent tissue (Meeting abstract). *Proceedings of the Annual Meeting of the American Association for Cancer Research* **36**: A715.

Rothman, N., Shields, P.G., Poirier, M.C., Harrington, A.M., Ford, D.P. and Strickland, P.T. 1995. The impact of glutathione S-transferase M1 and cytochrome P450 1A1 genotypes on white-blood-cell polycyclic aromatic hydrocarbon-DNA adduct levels in humans. *Molecular Carcinogenesis* **14**: 63–8.

Ryberg, D., Hewer, A., Phillips, D.H. and Haugen, A. 1994. Different susceptibility to smoking-induced DNA damage among male and female lung cancer patients. *Cancer Research* **54**: 5801–3.

Sasano, H., Miuazaki, S., Shiga, K., Goukon, Y., Nishihira, T., and Nagura, H. 1993. Glutathione S-transferase in human esophageal carcinoma. *Anticancer Research* **13**: 363–8.

Schantz, S.P. and Hsu, T.C. 1989. Mutagen-induced chromosome fragility within peripheral blood lymphocytes of head and neck cancer patients. *Head and Neck* **11**: 337–42.

Schantz, S.P., Spitz, M.R. and Hsu, T.C. 1990. Mutagen sensitivity in patients with head and neck cancers: a biologic marker for risk of multiple primary malignancies. *Journal of the National Cancer Institute* **82**: 1773–5.

Schantz, S.P., Zhang, Z.F., Spitz, M.S., Sun, M. and Hsu, T.C. 1997. Genetic suceptibility to head and neck cancer – interaction between nutrition and mutagen sensitivity. *Laryngoscope* **107**: 765–81.

Seidegård, J., Guthenberg, C., Pero, R.W. and Mannervik, B. 1987. The trans-stilbene oxide-active glutathione transferase in human mononuclear leucocytes is identical with the hepatic glutathione transferase mu. *Biochemistry Journal* **246**: 783–5.

Seidegård, J., Pero, R.W., Markowitz, M.M., Roush, G., Miller, D.G. and Beattie, E.J. 1990. Isoenzyme(s) of glutathione transferase (class Mu) as a marker for the susceptibility to lung cancer: a follow-up study. *Carcinogenesis* **11**: 33–6.

Seidegård, J., Vorachek, W.R., Pero, R.W. and Pearson, W.R. 1988. Hereditary differences in the expression of the human glutathione transferase active on trans-stilbene oxide are due to a gene deletion. *Proceedings of the National Academy of Sciences, USA.* **85**: 7293–7.

372   Z. Trizna and S. Schantz

Shaw, G.L., Falk, R.T., Deslauriers, J. et al. 1995. Debrisoquine metabolism and lung cancer risk. *Cancer Epidemiology, Biomarkers and Prevention* **4**: 41–8.

Shields, P.G., Bowman, E.D., Harrington, A.M., Doan, V.T. and Weston, A. 1993. Polycyclic aromatic hydrocarbon-DNA adducts in human lung and cancer susceptibility genes. *Cancer Research* **53**: 3486–92.

Sivaraman, L., Leatham, M.P., Yee, J., Wilkens, L.R., Lau, A.F. and LeMarchand, L. 1994. CYP1A1 genetic polymorphisms and in situ colorectal cancer. *Cancer Research* **54**: 3692–5.

Snow, D.G., Campbell, J.B. and Smallman, L.A. 1991. Fanconi's anemia and post-cricoid carcinoma. *Journal of Laryngology and Otology* **105**: 125–7.

Spitz, M.R., Fueger, J.J., Beddingfield, N.A., Annegers, J.F., Hsu, T.C., Newell, G.R. and Schantz, S.P. 1989. Chromosome sensitivity to bleomycin-induced mutagenesis, an independent risk factor for upper aerodigestive tract cancers. *Cancer Research* **49**: 4626–8.

Spitz, M.R., Fueger, J.J., Halabi, S., Schantz, S.P., Sample, D. and Hsu, T.C. 1993. Mutagen sensitivity in upper aerodigestive tract cancer: a case-control analysis. *Cancer Epidemiology, Biomarkers and Prevention* **2**: 329–33.

Spitz, M.R., Hoque, A., Trizna, Z. et al. 1994. Mutagen sensitivity as a risk factor for second malignant tumours following malignancies of the upper aerodigestive tract. *Journal of the National Cancer Institute* **86**: 1681–4.

Spitz, M.R., Hsu, T.C., Wu, X., Fueger, J.J., Amos, C.I. and Roth, J.A. 1995. Mutagen sensitivity as a biological marker of lung cancer risk in African Americans. *Cancer Epidemiology, Biomarkers and Prevention* **4**: 99–103.

Sugimura, H., Caporaso, N.E., Shaw, G.L. et al. 1990. Human debrisoquine hydroxylase gene polymorphisms in cancer patients and controls. *Carcinogenesis* **11**: 1527–30.

Sugimura, H., Suzuki, I., Hamada, G.S. et al. 1994. Cytochrome P-450IA1 genotype in lung cancer patients and controls in Rio de Janeiro, Brazil. *Cancer Epidemiology, Biomarkers and Prevention* **3**: 145–8.

Tang, D.L., Chiamprasert, S., Santella, R.M. and Perera, F.P. 1995. Molecular epidemiology of lung cancer: carcinogen-DNA adducts, *GSTM1* and risk (Meeting abstract). *Proceedings of the Annual Meeting of the American Association for Cancer Research* **36**: A1689.

Tefre, T., Ryberg, D., Haugen, A., Nebert, D.W., Skaug, V., Brogger, A. and Borresen, A.L. 1991. Human CYP1A1 cytochrome P(1)450) gene: lack of association between the Msp I restriction fragment length polymorphism and incidence of lung cancer in a Norwegian population. *Pharmacogenetics* **1**: 20–5.

Toffoli, G., Viel, A., Tumiotto, L., Giannini, F., Volpe, R., Quaia, M. and Boiocchi, M. 1992. Expression of glutathione-S-transferase-pi in human tumours. *European Journal of Cancer* **28A**: 1441–6.

Trizna, Z., Clayman, G.L., Spitz, M.R., Briggs, K.L. and Goepfert, H. 1995. Glutathione S-transferase genotypes as risk factors for head and neck cancer. *American Journal of Surgery* **170**: 499–501.

Trizna, Z., Hsu, T.C. and Schantz, S.P. 1992a. Protective effects of vitamin E against bleomycin-induced genotoxicity in head and neck cancer patients in vitro. *Anticancer Research* **12**: 325–7.

Trizna, Z., Hsu, T.C., Schantz, S.P., Lee, J.J. and Hong, W.K. 1992b. Anticlastogenic effects of 13-cis-retinoic acid in vitro. *European Journal of Cancer* **29A**: 137–40.

Trizna, Z. and Schantz, S.P. 1992. Hereditary and environmental factors associated with risk and progression of head and neck cancer. *Otolaryngology Clinics of North America* **25**: 1089–103.

Trizna, Z., Schantz, S.P. and Hsu, T.C. 1991. Effects of N-acetyl-L-cysteine and ascorbic acid on mutagen-induced chromosomal sensitivity in patients with head and neck cancers. *American Journal of Surgery* **162**: 294–8.

Watanabe, J., Hayashi, S.I., Nakachi, K., Imai, K., Suda, Y., Sekine, T. and Kawajiri, K. 1990. PstI and RsaI RFLPs in complete linkage disequilibrum at the CYP2E gene. *Nucleic Acids Research* **18**: 7194.

Wolf, C.R., Dale Smith, C.A., Gough, A.C. et al. 1992. Relationship between the debrisoquine hydroxylase polymorphism and cancer susceptibility. *Carcinogenesis* **13**: 1035–8.

Wu, X., Hsu, T.C., Annegers, J.F., Amos, C.I., Fueger, J.J. and Spitz, M.R. 1995. A case-control study of nonrandom distribution of bleomycin-induced chromatid breaks in lymphocytes of lung cancer cases. *Cancer Research* **55**: 557–61.

Xia, C., Taylor, J.B., Spencer, S.R. and Ketterer, B. 1993. The human glutathione S-transferase P1-1 gene: modulation of expression by retinoic acid and insulin. *Biochemistry Journal* **292**: 845–50.

Zhong, S., Howie, A.F., Ketterer, B. et al. 1991. Glutathione S-transferase mu locus: use of genotyping and phenotyping assays to assess association with lung cancer susceptibility. *Carcinogenesis* **12**: 1533–7.

18

Inherited abnormalities of DNA processing and predisposition to cancer

A. MALCOLM TAYLOR

Summary

This chapter deals sequentially with the well-recognized conditions that, although phenotypically quite distinct, have in common an underlying abnormality of some aspect of DNA processing. The clinical features of such disorders as ataxia telangiectasia, xeroderma pigmentosum and Fanconi anaemia are discussed. There follows a detailed analysis of the biochemical abnormalities that feature as a result of mutations in the relevant genes whose products are implicated in DNA repair mechanisms. These mutations are also discussed where they are known. The disorders, the cancers seen, the chromosomal location, and function of the genes are tabulated.

Introduction

Defects of DNA repair, DNA replication, transcription and recombination are now well established steps in the development of some cancers. There have been enormous advances recently in the studies of patients with xeroderma pigmentosum (XP) Cockayne syndrome (CS), trichothiodystrophy (TTD), Fanconi anaemia (FA), Bloom syndrome (BS), ataxia-telangiectasia (A-T), and Nijmegen breakage syndrome (NBS) which make up this group. A rather different phenotype results from mutations in certain mismatch repair genes: hereditary non-polyposis colorectal cancer, which has been discussed in Chapter 9. There is an increased predisposition to cancer in all of these disorders with the apparent exception of Cockayne syndrome and trichthiodystrophy. Some of these disorders have previously been grouped together as chromosome instability syndromes or DNA repair disorders. They should, perhaps, now better be considered as all having a defect in the processing of DNA. Defective genes may include those whose products normally control replicative DNA synthesis, DNA repair synthesis, recombination, transcription, or combinations of these functions. The disorders are considered in turn below, including a clinical description, a description of the relationship of the DNA processing defect to cancer development and the range of mutations in these individuals and their relationship to the clinical phenotype.

Ataxia-telangiectasia and Nijmegen breakage syndrome

Although the clinical phenotypes of these two disorders are quite different their cellular features are remarkably similar.

Ataxia-telangiectasia

This is a recessively inherited neurological disorder in which the most striking clinical features are the effects of a progressive cerebellar degeneration, limb and truncal ataxia, dysarthria, and abnormal eye movements (Sedgwick and Boder, 1991). Other features of this pleiotropic disorder include chromosomal abnormalities, immunodeficiency, thymic hypoplasia, hypogonadism, high levels of serum AFP, growth retardation, evidence for premature aging, telangiectasia and increased incidence of leukaemia and lymphoma. (See Table 18.1.)

Cancer in A-T

Penetrance of the leukaemia or lymphoma phenotype is about 10–15% in A-T by early adulthood (Taylor et al., 1996). Childhood T cell tumours are seen at a greatly increased frequency compared with non-A-T

Table 18.1 *Ataxia-telangiectasia and Nijmegen breakage syndrome*

Disorder/group	Predisposition to cancer	Chromosome location	Function
Ataxia-teleangiectasia	Lymphoma/ leukaemia	11q22-23	Protein/lipid kinase? phosphatidylinositol-3 kinase domain
Nijmegen breakage syndrome	Lymphoma	?	?

patients, and myeloid tumours are apparently absent. In contrast with children, it is clear that young adult A-T patients have a particular predisposition to T cell prolymphocytic leukaemia (T-PLL). Little is known about the underlying mechanism by which T-ALL and T cell lymphoma develop in A-T children, but more is known about the development of T-PLL which appears in large translocation, t(14;14), inv(14;14) and t(X;14), containing clones in A-T patients (Taylor et al., 1996). With respect to the increased risk of developing epithelial cell tumours, again, little is known about the mechanism of this or the underlying cause of the breast cancers for which carriers (i.e. heterozygotes) of the gene are reported to be at increased risk (Swift et al., 1991).

The cellular phenotype

These features of A-T include an increased sensitivity to both ionizing radiation and a range of radiomimetic drugs all of which also cause cultured cells to die by apoptosis (Taylor et al., 1975; Taylor et al., 1994; Meyn, 1995). There is good evidence for a defective G_1/S checkpoint involving abnormal kinetics of TP53 accumulation following exposure of A-T cells to ionizing radiation (Kastan et al., 1992; Lu and Lane, 1993), a defective S phase checkpoint as shown by the failure to inhibit DNA synthesis following exposure to either gamma rays or radiomimetic drugs (Painter and Young, 1980) and a G_2/M checkpoint abnormality (Beamish and Lavin, 1994). There is an abnormality of immune system gene rearrangement (Lipkowitz et al., 1990) and A-T patients also show an increased rate of loss of telomere sequences compared with non-affected individuals (Metcalfe et al., 1996).

Nijmegen breakage syndrome

Patients with NBS show microcephaly, short stature, a bird-like face, both humoral and T cell mediated immunodeficiency, which appears to be more severe than in A-T (Weemaes et al., 1994), *café au lait* spots, and a predisposition to lymphoid tumours. There appears to be some clinical heterogeneity but cerebellar degeneration is not part of the disorder. Translocations occur in T lymphocytes between chromosomes 7 and 14 at the same breakpoints as seen in A-T. Inv(14)(q11q32) inversions and t(14;14)(q11;q32) translocations are rare but there are reports of clonal expansions of cells containing t(14;14)(q11;q32) and t(X;14)(q28;q11) in NBS patients (see Weemaes et al., 1994). Both of these chromosomal rearrangements in large clones are associated with the development of T cell leukaemia in A-T patients but leukaemia has, so far, not been diagnosed in NBS. Overall the proportion of chromosome 7 and 14 translocations is higher in NBS patients compared with A-T. Similarly the proportion of NBS patients developing lymphoma is higher than the proportion of A-T patients developing leukaemia or lymphoma (Weemaes et al., 1994).

The cellular phenotype

Cells from NBS patients show the same unusual sensitivity to the killing effects of ionizing radiation and chromosomally radiomimetic drugs (Taalman et al., 1983). An increased chromosomal radiosensitivity is also observed as seen in A-T. In addition, like A-T, there is a lack of inhibition of DNA synthesis in NBS cells following exposure of cells to either gamma rays or radiomimetic drugs. The gene for NBS has not yet been cloned. (See Table 18.1.)

ATM, *the A-T gene*

The gene for ataxia-telangiectasia has been cloned and encodes a large cDNA of 9,168kb and protein estimated to be about 350kDa (Savitsky et al., 1995a; Byrd et al., 1996a,b; Uziel et al., 1996). The function of the A-T protein is unknown with only a part of the C-terminal region showing homology to other proteins. This homology suggests that the ATM protein belongs to a conserved phosphatidylinositol kinase (PIK)-like family of proteins which contain the PI-3 kinase motif at their C-terminus and which are involved variously in checkpoint functions, DNA repair (Savitsky et al., 1995b), and maintenance of telomere length in yeast (Greenwell et al., 1995). Mouse models showed growth retardation, infertility, increased sensitivity to irradiation, a G_1 checkpoint abnormality, and, unlike A-T patients, the occurrence of thymic lymphomas (immature T cell) in all homozygotes at an early age (4.5 months) (Barlow et al., 1996; Xu et al., 1996; Xu and Baltimore, 1996). At four to five months there was no histological abnormality detected in the cerebellum of mice. Using an antibody against the Cor1 protein in the synaptonemal complex it could be shown that there was a general delay in synapsis in spermatocytes from homozygous *ATM* deficient mice (Xu et al., 1996). Antibody localization studies have shown that ATM associates with mouse spermatocyte chromosomes during meiosis (Keegan et al., 1996). B lymphocyes in the A-T knockout mice were functionally normal, but there was a defect in T cell immunity. ATM is suggested to have protein kinase activity by virtue of autophosphorylation and together with the Atr (ataxia-telangiectasia and rad3-related protein) is reported to associate, normally, with meiotic chromosomes; Atr at sites of unpaired or unsynapsed regions and ATM in synapsed regions (Keegan et al., 1996).

What is the role of the *ATM* gene in the cell? In considering this, both the cellular and clinical features of A-T have to be taken into account. A model for the function of the *ATM* gene has been put forward based on the suggestion that A-T patients lack DNA damage activated responses: (1) cell cycle checkpoints; (2) lack of damage activated DNA repair; and (3) a low threshold for triggering programmed cell death (Meyn, 1995). It has been suggested that the absence of both damage-sensitive cell cycle checkpoints and damage-induced DNA repair lead to abnormal levels of immune system gene rearrangements, genetic instability, and cancer, and that the triggering of apoptosis by normally non-lethal levels of DNA damage leads to increased radiation sensitivity and the major clinical features of A-T such as cerebellar degeneration (Meyn, 1995).

Do the components of this model adequately account for the clinical and cellular features of A-T? With respect to the defect in cell cycle checkpoints, it is not known how or if this contributes to the clinical features of A-T. Abnormalities of cell cycle checkpoints cannot, however, be responsible for cerebellar degeneration of non-cycling cells in G_0 in A-T patients. Patients with NBS show the same cellular features as A-T including the S phase checkpoint abnormality, but have no neurological abnormality (Taalman et al., 1989). In addition $p53-/-$ mice do not show degenerative neurological defects. Both of these observations tend to separate the role of the checkpoint abnormalities from degenerative features.

There is a 10- to 100-fold increased frequency of T cell cluster region (TCR) hybrid genes formed by interlocus recombination in A-T lymphocytes compared with normal (Lipkowitz et al, 1990). This increase has been explained as a result of failure to activate checkpoints in response to double-strand breaks in DNA and cells enter mitosis before resolving the rearrangements correctly, leading to hybrid molecules (translocations). In response to this argument it is seen that mice with no funtional p53 protein as a result of gene knockout ($p53-/-$) do not show aberrant gene rearrangements which suggests that the G_1/S cell cycle checkpoint, the basis for which is an absence or abnormality of p53 accumulation, is irrelevant to this process of constitutive abnormal translocation production. Normally, TCRγ, β and α genes rearrange in order and there is a developmental checkpoint or delay until the lymphocyte has undertaken particular rearrangements (Rajewsky, 1996). There is no evidence that this recombination is regulated by the cell cycle but there is evidence that accessibility, the availability of the locus in the chromatin, determines targeting of the recombinase (Stanhope-Baker et al., 1996). The increased number of inter-locus translocations in A-T patients is possibly the result of disordered rearrangement of TCRβ and α chain gene breaks.

In the absence of a demonstrated importance of the G_1/S checkpoint in gene rearrangements the argument has been put forward that S and G_2/M checkpoints contribute to genetic instability leading to cancer (Meyn, 1995) in both A-T and in p53−/− mice, but there is no direct evidence for this. In A-T patients, shorter telomeres are also argued to be the result of absent cell cycle checkpoints.

It is generally agreed that the role of the cell cycle in the causation of increased radiosensitivity in A-T cells is minimal (Thacker, 1994; Meyn, 1995). A-T cells are unusually radiosensitive even when not proliferating. The key evidence for this is the absence of 'liquid holding' recovery (holding cells in a non-dividing state following irradiation) in A-T cells (Cox et al., 1982). Other evidence suggesting that a defect in the G_1/S checkpoint is not important for cell killing comes from observations on p53−/− mice which do not show increased radiosensitivity (Donehower et al., 1992). For both the increased X-ray induced cell killing and the decreased level of chromosome restitution, an alternative mechanism may involve a defect in some form of DNA repair.

Since there is sequence homology between Mec1 and ATM proteins it is possible that at least part of the function of ATM is involvement in signalling, although ATM is predominantly a nuclear protein. There are, however, differences between ATM and its various homologues e.g. rad3 and *MEC1* which caution against any close comparison. Overall the biochemical mechanisms of checkpoint controls are not well understood but several protein products are involved which include DNA repair functions (Lydall and Weinert, 1995; Lehmann and Carr, 1995).

Another response to damage is constitutive DNA repair. A-T cells are unusually sensitive to irradiation even when not proliferating (liquid holding) when the cell cycle is not operating, which itself is some indirect evidence for a DNA repair defect. The unusual radiosensitivity may be due to a subtle defect in repair of some DNA double strand breaks (Thacker, 1994). It is important to note that in yeast the extra radio-sensitivity of checkpoint *rad* mutants cannot be accounted for entirely by checkpoint defects and the rad proteins are postulated also to be directly involved in DNA repair processes (Lehmann and Carr, 1995).

A third response of damaged cells, however, is to undergo apoptosis. In addition to cerebellar degeneration many of the clinical features of A-T, thymic and gonadal dysplasia, and liver abnormalities leading to high levels of serum AFP are consistent with a defect in the regulation of apoptosis. It has been suggested that the primary cause of the spontaneous loss of dividing and non-dividing cells in A-T patients is a lower threshold of DNA damage for activation of programmed cell death. A-T cells treated with streptonigrin or X-rays have been reported to show a higher level of apoptosis than normal cells (Meyn et al., 1994) although there is also contrary evidence (Duchaud et al., 1996) suggesting that the hypersensitivity of A-T cells to irradiation is not due to an increased apoptotic response.

The roles of checkpoint abnormalities, repair, and apoptosis in the development of the A-T phenotype are far from clear. Another model for *ATM* gene function is that the ATM protein operates in dividing cells as part of a complex common to various forms of DNA processing. The substrates for such DNA processing would include any form of DNA strand breakage whether it occurred during normal cellular processes or after exposure to DNA damaging agents. The DNA processing itself would include recombination, repair, telomeric replication, and recognition of damaged DNA prior to inhibition of DNA synthesis. In this way the ATM protein is likely to influence control over several different cellular processes and have different effects in different cell types. For example, A-T patients appear to develop T cell tumours more frequently than B cell tumours suggesting some preferential abnormality in T cells possibly as a result of being unusually prone to translocations rather than as the result of a cell cycle checkpoint abnormality. One possibility underlying these observations is that there is an abnormality in chromatin 'accessibility' (Stanhope-Baker et al., 1996) in A-T cells. The abnormal ATM protein could also affect regulation of apoptosis in both dividing and non-dividing cells again by affecting chromatin structure. Sensitivity to radiation and neuronal degeneration appear to vary independently in A-T patients, suggesting quite different interactions of the ATM protein in different cell types. Another possibility is that the ATM protein is a component of a transcription complex or controls such a factor.

ATM belongs to a growing number of high molecular weight phosphatidylinositol 3-kinase (PIK) related kinases including Tor1p, Tor2p, FRAP, rad3/Mec1. They are related more to the lipid kinases than protein kinases by virtue of containing the PI-3 kinase domain. Although Tor2p has PI-4 kinase activity (Cardenas et al., 1995), there is no evidence that DNA-PK, or other PIK related kinases, functions as a lipid kinase. Some PIK related kinases and possibly ATM may act as protein kinases with a role in DNA damage recognition and repair (Hartley et al., 1995). The major questions to be answered are: (1)) what are the substrates for the ATM protein in different cell types?; (2) is it acting solely as a protein kinase with different effects in different cells or differentiated states?; (3) does ATM act in a fundamentally different way in dividing and non-dividing (including neuronal) cells?; and (4) is there a single fundamental role which underlies all the cellular and clinical features?

Mutations in ATM

More than 100 different mutations have been identified in A-T patients, (Savitsky et al., 1995a; Byrd et al., 1996a; Gilad et al., 1996; McConville et al., 1996; Teletar et al, 1996; Wright et al., 1996). Most of these are predicted to be null mutations, consisting of exon skipping, small out of frame insertions or deletions and a small proportion of missense mutations. It is possible to study genotype–phenotype correlations in A-T and we have examined a distinct group of A-T patients in which the clinical and cellular phenotype was less severe. About 15% of all UK patients fall into this subgroup. All the patients had a 137 bp insertion in their cDNA, caused by a point mutation in a sequence resembling a splice donor site. Although the insertion causes truncation of the protein, the less severe phenotype probably results from the small degree of normal splicing which occurs as an alternative product from the insertion containing allele (McConville et al., 1996). It is possible that this normal splicing also protects these patients from the same risk of leukaemia and lymphoma seen in other A-T patients.

The clinical and cellular phenotype is also less severe in A-T patients with missense mutations. We have described a family with A-T patients homozygous for a missense mutation in which the cerebellar degeneration is much less marked, life expectancy appears to be no different from normal and where there is fertility.

The vast majority of A-T patients are compound heterozygotes for *ATM* mutations. Patients with two truncating mutations are likely to show the most severe phenotype – those with two missense mutations show the least severe phenotype. The range of phenotypes is clearly very wide and in A-T patients native to the British Isles about 20% of cases are predicted to have a milder phenotype.

Table 18.2. *Fanconi anaemia (FA)*

Disorder/group	Predisposition to cancer	Chromosome location	Function
FA-A	AML	16q24.3	?
FA-B		?	?
FA-C		9q22.3	?
FA-D		3p	?
FA-E		?	?

Fanconi anaemia

Fanconi anaemia (FA) is a recessively inherited disorder in which patients present with short stature, a pancytopaenia which develops between the ages of 5 and 10 years of age, and the presence of some dysmorphic features the most prominent of which are dysplastic or absent thumbs and/or radii. In addition there may be skin hyperpigmentation, growth retardation, deafness, and genital, ocular, renal and cardiac defects (Taylor et al., 1992). There is, however, considerable clinical heterogeneity in presentation of the disorder and it may not always be readily recognized since some patients may show a minimal number of these features (Taylor et al., 1992). Most but not all patients show an elevated level of chromosome breakage, which is quite different from the specific translocations observed in A-T patients. They also have a predisposition to the development of acute myeloblastic leukaemia.

FA cells are characterized by an increased sensitivity to bifunctional cross-linking agents such as nitrogen mustard, mitomycin C, and diepoxybutane as shown by colony forming assays on cultured skin fibroblasts or on lymphocyte chromosomes (Taylor et al., 1992). A defect in DNA–DNA cross-link repair has been suggested for FA but the precise gene defect remains unknown. The presence of clinical heterogeneity is consistent with the finding of genetic complementation in FA and there is evidence for at least five groups, designated FA-A to FA-E (Joenje et al., 1995; Table 18.2) which would account for the clinical heterogeneity seen in the disorder. At present group FA-A is believed to be the major gene causing the disorder in 66% of cases, with FA-B in 4%, FA-C in 13%, FA-D in 4%, and FA-E in 13% of cases (Buchwald, 1995). The FA-A group has been localized to chromosome 16q24.3 by both linkage analysis and homozygosity mapping (Pronk et al., 1995; Gschwend et al., 1996). Recently the *FA-A* gene has been cloned and found to encode a

1455 amino acid protein of approximately 160 kDa. The presence of two nuclear localization signals suggests that, unlike the FA-C protein, FA-A is a nuclear protein. No significant homologies to the base or amino acid sequence have been found, including to FA-C (Lo Ten Foe et al., 1996; The Fanconi Anaemia/Breast Cancer Consortium, 1996). The gene for FA-D was mapped to chromosome 3p using microcell mediated chromosome transfer into an TFA-D cell line (Whitney et al., 1995). Most is known, however, about group FA-C. The *FAC-C* gene was been localized to chromosome 9q22.3 (Strathdee et al., 1992a). The gene has been cloned and complements the increased cellular sensitivity to diepoxybutane and mitomycin C in the group C cells (Strathdee et al, 1992b). The coding region is a 1674 bp long encoding 14 exons. No homology to known proteins has been reported and no functional domains have been recognized. The FA-C protein is widely expressed. Work with antibodies has shown it to be a 60 kDa protein. FA-C cell lines expressed full length, truncated, or absent protein. Cell fractionation studies indicated that FA-C protein is localized to the cytoplasm (Yamashita et al., 1994).

Homozygous FA-C null (FA−/FA−) mice developed normally and did not show any developmental or haematological problems before the age of nine months. Their spleen cells showed a much higher level of mitomycin C and diepoxybutane-induced chromosome damage compared with wild type cells. Both male and female mice also showed impaired fertility (Chen et al., 1996). The mouse model does show some of the features of FA, but as with the A-T knockout mouse, the correspondence between the mouse model and the human disorder is not complete.

Mutations in FA

Verlander et al. (1994) found mutations in 25 of 174 racially and ethnically diverse FA families screaned for mutations in *FAC-C*. The most frequent muations were IVS4 + 4A→T in 12 families and 322delG in exon 1 in 9 families. The IVS + 4A→T mutation is responsible for most Fanconi anaemia in Ashkenazi Jewish patients (Verlander *et al* 1995) and in the 12 families reported by Verlander et al., (1994) all the affected patients were homozygous for this mutation. Patients with the IVS + 4A→T mutation are all severely affected with multiple congenital malformations. Jewish patients without this mutation may have mutations in other FA genes. All but one of the patients with 322delG had a mild phenotype. One patient was homozygous for the 322delG mutation suggesting this does confer a milder phenotype. The Q13X mutation in exon 1 also appears to be mild. Other mutations found include R185X and D195V in exon 6 and L554P in exon 14. Both R185X and L554P can give severe phenotypes. Six different intragenic deletions (five leading to truncation of the protein) have been identified in the *FA-A* gene in FA patients. At least three of these mutations also give exon skipping. A seventh mutation present in two families was a large insertion resulting from a splice site mutation. It appears that a founder mutation in this gene has contributed to the high incidence of FA in the Afrikaner population of South Africa (Pronk et al., 1995) although no mutations have so far been published.

Xeroderma pigmentosum, Cockayne syndrome, trichothiodystrophy

Patients who show an unusual sensitivity to UV (ultraviolet) light have been diagnosed as having one of the three disorders: xeroderma pigmentosum (XP); Cockayne syndrome (CS); or trichothiodystrophy (TTD).

Xeroderma pigmentosum

XP patients clearly have an increased sensitivity to sunlight although the degree depends on the level of exposure and also on their particular mutation. They also show an increased likelihood of developing tumours early in life on sun exposed areas of the skin. Tumour types include basal and squamous cell carcinomas and malignant melanomas. Some patients also show neurological abnormalities. Skin fibroblast cultures from most XP patients show an increased sensitivity to killing by UV light resulting from a defect in nucleotide excision repair (NER), which can repair a broad spectrum of DNA damage including UV-induced thymine dimers and other adducts. The repair defect is in a process that, in most groups, affects the whole of the genome irrespective of transcriptional state. At least seven different complementation groups, designated XPA-XPG (Vermeulen et al., 1993) which are deficient in NER, have been identified by cell fusion studies and the genes are located in different parts of the genome (Table 18.3). The level of measurable repair varies between complementation groups. Cells from groups A, B and G have very little residual repair capacity, repair in groups C and F is 10–20% and in D and E, 25–50% of normal levels. One additional group (XP variant), has normal levels of NER but a less well defined defect in daughter strand

Table 18.3. *Xeroderma pigmentosum (XP)*

Disorder/group/ cloned gene	Predisposition to cancer	Chromosome location	Function
XPA	Skin	9q34	?DNA binding
XPB (ERCC3)		2q21	3' → 5' helicase (TFIIH)
XPC	Skin	3p25.1	ssDNA binding
XPD (ERCC2)	Skin	19q13.3	3' → 5' helicase (TFIIH)
XPE		11	?DNA binding
XPF (ERCC4/ ERCC11)		16p13	5' endonuclease
XPG (ERCC5)		13q32-33	3' endonuclease
XPV	Skin	?	?

gap repair. Most XP patients fall into complementation groups A and C, groups B, E, F and G are rare. Group D patients are of intermediate frequency. Proneness to skin cancer appears to be more associated with the common XP groups A and C. All XP-A patients develop neurological abnormalities, e.g. gait ataxia, possibly as a result of the accumulation of unrepaired DNA damage in the neurons.

Cockayne syndrome

Whereas the major clinical features of XP are associated with the skin, CS patients show a quite different clinical phenotype. Interestingly, cancer is not a feature of CS (Table 18.4) but it has been included in this chapter for comparison and completeness (see below). Although there is also sun sensitivity, the major features are dwarfism, mental retardation, microcephaly, retinal and skeletal abnormalities. There is also progressive neurological degeneration caused by dysmyelination rather than the neuronal changes seen in XP. A readily measurable result of the defect in CS cells is the failure of the rapid recovery of RNA synthesis following UV exposure (Mayne and Lehmann, 1982). Using an assay based on this observation most CS patients can be assigned to one of two complementation groups (CKN1 and CKN2). In classical CS patients in complementation group 2 (formerly CSB) the excision defect has been reported to preferentially affect the ability of their cells to repair damage in actively transcribing genes (Venema et al., 1990). This is the so-called

Table 18.4. *Cockayne syndrome (CKN)*

Disorder/group	Predisposition to cancer	Chromosome location	Function
CKN1	Nil	5	WD repeat helicase
CKN2 (ERCC6)	Nil	10q11-21	
XPB (ERCC3)	Nil	2q21	$3' \to 5'$ helicase TFIIH
XPD (ERCC2)	Nil	19q13	$5' \to 3'$ helicase TFIIH
XPG (ERCC5)	Nil	13q32-33	3' endonuclease ?interacting with TFIIH

Note: XP: xeroderma pigmentosum.

transcription coupled repair pathway. This repair occurs only on the transcribed strand of transcriptionally active genes and is dependent on transcription. This contrasts with the defect in repair across the whole genome (global genome repair) in most XP patients. Since repair of actively transcribing regions makes a small contribution to total repair in the cell, overall repair rates appear to be normal in CS.

Trichothiodystrophy

Some patients with TTD also show unusual sun sensitivity, but the major features of this disorder are mental and physical retardation, sulphur-deficient brittle hair and ichthyotic skin (The term PIBIDS, an acronym for Photosensitivity, Ichthyosis, Brittle hair, Impaired intelligence, Decreased fertility, and Short stature is sometimes used for these patients) (Stefanini et al., 1992). In TTD there is heterogeneity in the biochemical defect. Some patients have no defects in excision repair but others have a severe defect in this repair pathway. Some TTD patients may show a deficiency in the repair of 6–4 photoproducts. In most TTD patients showing increased photosensitivity the defect has been assigned to XP complementation group D (Stefanini et al., 1992). It is clear, therefore, that mutations in the *XPD* gene can be found in patients with XP or TTD. A second excision repair complementation group (TTDA) has been described in TTD (Stefanini et al., 1993). There is no evidence for the same predisposition to skin cancer in CS and TTD that is seen in XP patients. Comparing Table 18.3 with Tables 18.4 and 18.5, it can be seen that mutations in the same *ERCC* genes can

Table 18.5. *Trichothiodystrophy (TTD)*

Disorder/Group	Predisposition to cancer	Chromosome location	Function
XPD (ERCC2)	Nil	19q13	5′ → 3′ helicase (TFIIH)
TTDA	Nil	?	TFIIH component
XPB (ERCC3)	Nil	2q21	3′ → 5′ helicase (TFIIH)

Note: XP: xeroderma pigmentosum.

cause very different phenotypes, with and without cancer predisposition, see section 'The XP gene family' below.

Complementation studies

In addition to the human genes identified by complementation analysis of cells from XP, CS and TTD patients, another approach has also identified human repair genes. Rodent cells mutated to be hypersensitive to the killing effects of UV can be corrected to normal UV sensitivity by transfection of normal human DNA (Hoeijmakers, 1993). The cloned human genes conferring this normal phenotype are designated *ERCC* genes (Excision Repair Chinese hamster Complementing). *ERCC2, 3, 4, 5* and *6* have now been found to correct the defects in XPD, XPB, XPF, XBG and CKN2 respectively (Fletjer et al., 1992; Weeda et al., 1990; O'Donovan et al., 1993; Troelstra et al., 1992, Sijbers et al., 1996). In addition, *ERCC11* and *ERCC4* are equivalent genes to XPF and *ERCC1* forms a heterodimer with the XPF gene product. Most of these genes also have identified yeast homologues (Jaspers and Hoeijmakers, 1995).

The XP gene family

All the known XP genes, *XPA, XPB, XPC, XPD, XPF,* and *XPG* have now been cloned and a factor defective in some XPE cells has also been identified (Hoeijmakers, 1994). A total of about 25–30 proteins are required to reconstitute the complex NER reaction in vitro (Aboussekhra et al., 1995). The first stage in NER is lesion recognition and incision of the damaged strand on each side of the lesion after which a 27-29-mer oligonucleotide is removed (Sancar 1996). The single strand region is protected by a single strand binding protein (HSSB) and the gap is filled in by DNA polymerase δ or ε PCNA and ligase. The XPB and XPD products are $3' \rightarrow 5'$ and $5' \rightarrow 3'$ helicases, respectively, causing unwinding of DNA at the site of the damage. The XPA protein acts as a binding site for the endonuclease XPG that cuts $3'$ to the dimer and the heterodimer XPF/ERCC1 that cuts $5'$ to the dimer. The product of the *XPE* gene may help cleavage by the XPG protein as it creates a DNase I hypersensitive site at the XPG cleavage point. The XPC product forms a heterodimer with RAD23B protein – its function is still unclear. Residual repair in these cells (10–20%) and presumably also the skin cancer, in XPC patients, results from a deficiency in repair of non-transcribed regions of the genome (deficiency in the global genome repair pathway). This contrasts with CS where the global DNA repair pathway is normal and where there is no skin cancer. Cells from XP variants show normal NER but are deficient in repair of single stranded DNA during DNA replication (daughter strand gap repair).

NER is, therefore, a complex DNA metabolic process and interactions with transcription, replication and recombination have recently become apparent. In particular, the human multiprotein TFIIH basal transcription factor complex, which consists of nine or more subunits, has been shown to contain at least three known repair proteins, XPB (ERCC3), XPD (ERCC2) and TTDA, involved in NER (Hoeijmakers et al., 1996). The transcription factor TFIIH is therefore involved in both repair and basal transcription. This means that mutations in *XP-B* and *XPD* genes have to be thought of as causing TFIIH related disorders. There is a clinical spectrum associated with defects in TFIIH (mutations in *XPB*, *XPD* and *TTDA*). Consequently, it is possible that different mutations in *XPB* or *XPD* could produce a clinical phenotype resulting principally from either loss of repair function or, alternatively, defective transcription or possibly both. Three patients in two families who simultaneously displayed features of both XP and CS carried a mutation in *XPB*. A TTD patient also showed a mutation in *XPB*. Similarly, different *XPD* mutations gave rise to XP, XP with CS and TTD. The XPB helicase appears to be more important for NER and transcription than XPD since complete inactivation of XPD helicase function still allows some repair and is not essential for transcription, but loss of XPB function completely prevents both repair and transcription. Two of the seven NER genes which can cause XP alone (*XPD* and *XPG*) can also result in partial or complete CS. In contrast, the *XPA*, *XPC*, *XPF* and *XPE* genes are associated only with a DNA repair disorder, XP. Mutations in the *XPG* gene are associated with patients showing features of both XP and CS (Vermeulen et al., 1993) which suggests that the XPG protein is also likely to interact with TFIIH (Hoeijmakers et al., 1996).

Loss of complete NER function in XPA gives the typical repair deficient phenotype. In contrast, inactivation of transcription is lethal but some deficiency in transcription may lead to the clinical features associated with some patients with CS or TTD; hence the association of different phenotypes with different mutations in *XPD* and *XPB* which are involved in both repair and transcription. Repair is also coupled with transcription through another set of genes, the CS genes *CKN1* and *CKN2*. The CKN1 and CKN2 proteins do not appear to be essential for trancription, but, nevertheless, mutations in these genes give rise to CS suggesting some role for these genes in the transcription process. Recently it has been suggested that the sensitivity of CS cells to UV and other DNA damaging agents is not due to defective transcription coupled repair of active genes. This was shown by measuring the rate of removal of of DNA adducts produced by NA-AAF in the *ADA* gene of normal human cells and CKN1 and CKN2 cells. Repair of the adducts in the *ADA* gene occurred at similar rates in the normal and CS cells. It was postulated that the undoubted increased sensitivity of CS cell to the killing effects of NA-AAF and the failure of recovery of RNA synthesis is due to a defect in transcription (van Oosterwijk et al., 1996). Following exposure of cells to UV light or NA-AAF, there is recruitment of the TFIIH transcription factor for nucleotide excision repair. It was suggested that the CS proteins uncouple repair from transcription. If the uncoupling process is defective then RNA synthesis will not recover.

Studies in mice

Mice homozygous for mutations in the *XPA* and *XPC* genes have been generated (Sands et al., 1995; Nakane et al., 1995; de Vries et al., 1995). Cultured cells from all three homozygous deficient mice were unusually sensitive to the killing effects of UV light and the mice were also unusually senitive to UV light induced skin cancer. Cells from the XPC mice were not unusually sensitive to the chemical 4-NQO, compared with wild type cells. This is rather unusual as XP cells have been reported to be unusually sensitive to 4-NQO. Homozygous mutations in the murine *XPA* gene also caused more DMBA-induced papillomas compared with wild type although these did not progress to carcinomas. Interestingly the *XPA* mice did not show any of the neurological degeneration of *XPA* patients. The ERCC1-XPF complex makes the 5' incision during NER. Mice totally deficient in ERCC1 protein die of liver failure soon after birth and show elevated levels of p53 (McWhir et al., 1993), suggesting functions additional to those in NER which may be related to recombination (Sijbers et al., 1996).

Mutations in XP, TTD, and CS

Mutations have been described in XP patients from groups XPA (Maeda et al., 1995; Kondoh et al., 1995; Satakata et al., 1995), XPB, (Weeda et al., 1990), XPD (Frederick et al., 1994; Takayama et al., 1995), XPF (Sijbers et al., 1996) and XPG (Okinaka et al., 1995). In addition *XPD* gene mutations have been described in patients with TTD (Broughton et al., 1994, Takayama, et al., 1996) and in patients with features of both XP and CS (Broughton et al., 1995). Mutations in *CKN1*, *ERCC6* (*CKN2*) have also been described. Much of the recent work on these mutations is concerned with making genotype–phenotype correlations in order to understand the development of the different disorders and also the importance of different domains of the genes in defining the clinical conditions. The mutations in cells from XP-F patients occur in the region predicted to be involved in ERCC1 binding.

The *ERCC2* gene is perhaps one of the most interesting genes because of the relatively large number of mutations available for study and the association of mutations with XP, XP/CS and TTD. Mutations in the C-terminal region of *ERCC2* have been shown to be important in determining the clinical features of TTD and many of the mutations are in the region 713-760. Mutation Arg722→Trp correlated with high UV sensitivity in a TTD cell strain and Arg658→His or Lys with an intermediate level of UV sensitivity. *ERCC2* mutation Arg683→Trp in the likely nuclear localization signal was found in XPD strains but not in TTD or XPD/CS strains. The suggestion has been made that TTD is due to mutations that alter the transcriptional role of *ERCC2* and that XPD is due to mutations affecting the repair role of this protein (Takayama et al., 1996).

Bloom syndrome

BS patients are characterized by their small birth size, growth retardation, narrow face and telangiectasia in the butterfly area of the face. They are also immunodeficient. A major feature of the disorder is the high frequency of malignant disease with about a quarter of patients developing cancer early in life. Unlike the other disorders described above, BS is remarkable for the variety of histological types of tumour including acute leukaemia, lymphoma and various carcinomas (Table 18.6).

BS patients also show a spontaneous chromosome breakage similar to that in FA with the important difference that the characteristic interchanges tend to occur between homologous chromosomes. The most striking and unique chromosomal feature of BS is the large increased frequency of sister chromatid exchanges (SCE). Cells from patients with BS appear to be unusually sensitive to the killing effects of simple alkylating agents such as EMS and N-ethyl-N-nitrosourea.

Using microcell mediated chromosome transfer it was shown that introduction of normal chromosome 15 into BS cells led to a decrease in the number of SCE. Using homozygosity mapping the location of the gene was refined to 15q26 and the BS gene subsequently cloned revealing a 1417 amino acid protein homologous to the RecQ subfamily of DExH box-containing DNA and RNA helicases (Ellis et al., 1995; Ellis and German, 1996). Antibody to the N-terminal domain of the protein detected a 180 kDa nuclear protein absent from BS patients cells. It is interesting that two other members of this RecQ gene family are the Werner's syndrome gene, *WRN*, and the yeast gene product SGS1. The SGS1 gene protein interacts with the yeast topoisomerase products Top3p and Top2p. It has recently been shown that SGS1 has helicase activity (Lu et al., 1996). Site-directed mutagenesis experiments that remove helicase activity, however, can still complement some yeast SGS1 mutants. This suggests that SGS1 has another important function unrelated to helicase. This notion is consistent with the observation that Werner mutations truncate the protein beyond the helicase domain, and thereby may retain helicase activity.

The single patient 46BR showed dwarfism, a profound immunodeficiency resulting in recurrent serious chest infection, and a slow growing lymphomatous liver infiltration. She died at age 19 from acute pulmonary infection. Cultured cells from this patient showed an increased sensitivity to different alkylating agents, UV light, and ionizing radiation. The level of SCE in her cells was slightly higher than normal but much lower than levels seen in BS patients. Patient 46BR appeared, therefore, to be quite distinct from BS patients (Barnes et al., 1992; Table 18.6).

Cellular defects in BS cells include delayed joining of large DNA replication intermediates, a reduced rate of progression of replication forks. In contrast the major feature of 46BR cells was the retarded rate of

Table 18.6. *Bloom syndrome*

Disorder/group	Predisposition to cancer	Chromosome location	Function
Bloom syndrome	Lymphoma/leukaemia/ carcinoma	15q26	Rec Q helicase
46BR	Lymphoma	19q13	DNA ligase

rejoining of Okazaki fragments during DNA replication and the greatly reduced rate of DNA single strand rejoining following exposure of cells to DNA damaging agents (Barnes et al., 1992). No coding mutations were found in DNA ligase 1 in several BS lines in two studies (Petrini et al., 1991; Barnes et al., 1992,) but two missense mutations occurring in different alleles of the DNA ligase gene were found in patient 46BR (Barnes et al., 1992). At the biochemical level, in 46BR cells, there is a strongly reduced ability of DNA ligase 1 to form a labelled enzyme-adenylate intermediate. 46BR appears, therefore, to represent the phenotype caused by coding changes in the DNA ligase 1 gene.

Mutations in Bloom syndrome

BS is more common in the Ashkenazi Jewish population than in any other group with the estimate of about 1% of Ashkenazi Jews being carriers of the same mutation. As discussed above, the gene for BS, *BLM* has been identified (Ellis et al., 1995). Seven unique mutations have been identified. Four are predicted to result in truncated proteins, and three are missense mutations, with no effect on protein. Of particular note is the six base-pair insertion–seven base-pair deletion mutation that has only been observed in Ashkenazi Jewish individuals with BS.

Hereditary nonpolyposis colorectal cancer and mismatch repair genes

Over recent years it has been shown that hereditary nonpolyposis colorectal cancer (HNPCC) is due to an inherited defect in mismatch repair. As a result of this defect, tumour cells of HNPCC patients have a characteristic replication error (RER$^+$) phenotype. This consists first, of loss of the ability to maintain microsatellite length. In HNPCC tumours new microsatellite alleles not found in the patients normal cells are observed. New alleles for di- and trinucleotide repeats are seen across the genome suggesting an instability of the replication or repair of short repeat sequences. Secondly, RER$^+$ cancer cells exhibit an increased level of base substitutions, the so called 'mutator phenotype', which probably contributes to the development of cancer, and thirdly, there is a loss of mismatch repair capacity. HNPCC patients inherit one mismatch repair mutant allele and have to acquire a mutation in the second allele in order for a tumour to develop. Following the establishment of linkage of HNPCC to chromosome 2 it was shown that a human homologue, *hMSH2*, of the bacterial gene *MutS* was located on chromosome 2 and subsequently germline mutations in *hMSH2* were indeed identified in HNPCC families. The majority of HNPCC families have germline mutations in one of the two mismatch repair genes *hMSH2* and *hMLH1* (chromosome 3) and fewer than 10% of families in *hPMS2* (Kinzler and Vogelstein, 1996). Mutations in *hPMS1* are rarely seen. Sporadic colonic tumours with microsatellite instability resulting from mutations in *GTBP* (*S. cerevisiae* MSH6), *hMSH2* and *hMLH1* have been reported (see Eshleman and Markowitz, 1996). Recent work suggests a functional role for MSH3 in mismatch repair since mutations have been found in an endometrial tumour and an endometrial tumour cell line (Risinger et al., 1996).

All RER$^+$ phenotypes were reversed when a single copy of chromosome 3 containing wild type *hMLH1* is introduced into an *hMLH1* mutant cell line. Generally it is seen that defects associated with mutations in *hMSH2*, *hMLH1* or *hMSH6* are also corrected by introduction of the appropriate chromosome containing the wild-type copy of the gene (Umar et al., 1997).

The role of mismatch repair is to recognize and repair errors made by DNA polymerase during replication or to recognize mismatches resulting from strand slippage. The microsatellite instability in human cells is similar to that seen in bacteria carrying mismatch repair gene mutations such as *MutS* and *MutL*. In bacteria the MutS protein recognizes the mismatch and in human cells this is achieved by *MutS* homologues, *MSH2* and *GTBP* and *hMSH3*. In bacteria *MutL* (human homologues are *hMLH1*, *hPMS1* and *hPMS2*) and *MutH* form a complex with MutS and the mismatches are repaired using exonuclease, helicase II, DNA polymerase II single strand binding protein and DNA ligase (Kolodner, 1996).

Mice homozygous for mutations in the *msh2*, *pms2* and *mlh1* genes have been generated and all are mismatch repair-defective. Both male and female *mlh1* mice are sterile although in *pms2* null mice only the males are sterile, but this is due to a different mechanism. *mlh1* and *pms1* may have a function in meiosis, such as mismatch repair, for which *msh2* is not required. A proportion of the *msh2* and *pms2* mice develop lymphomas but so far the *mlh1* mice have not yet developed such tumours (Edelmann et al., 1996). The clinical features of the HNPCC syndrome are described in Chapter 9.

Conclusion

The different genetic complementation groups described in XP, CS, TTD and FA have each proved to be a consequence of the involvement of several different genes. Little is known at present about the function of the FA genes and indeed not all the putative genes have been cloned. In contrast, work over the past few years, on XP, CS and TTD, and in parallel work on both NER and transcription factors has illuminated the relationships between these disorders and these aspects of DNA processing. In addition, recent work suggests that XPB and XPD helicases may be components of the TP53 mediated apoptotic pathway (Wang et al., 1996). There was also evidence for genetic complementation in A-T cell lines but the cloning of the A-T gene showed that patients homozygous for the same mutation had been assigned to different complementation groups and, at present, there is no evidence for more than one A-T gene. It is possible, of course, that the A-T gene and NBS gene (and possibly other genes) are involved in the same pathway or protein complex, bearing in mind their very similar cellular phenotypes. There is still, however, considerable clinical and cellular heterogeneity in A-T caused by the large number of mutations. Biochemical analyses of the various products of these genes and analysis of the effects of different mutations in the disorders will eventually lead to an understanding of the functions of these genes.

The gene knockout mouse models do not usually provide a carbon copy of the human disorder, but the similarities will allow a further understanding of the human disorders. In some instances, breeding to give double knockouts will also be informative, e.g. whether or not *p53* and *ATM*, or *DNA-PK* and *ATM* or *ATM* and *scid* have any overlapping roles. Mice with knockouts of the *TTD* and *CS* genes are still awaited.

The dramatic improvements in our understanding of these DNA processing disorders over the past few years is set to continue for a while yet.

Acknowledgements

I thank the Cancer Research Campaign, the Wellcome Trust, Medical Research Council, the Kay Kendall Leukaemia Fund, the A-T Society, and the A-T Research and Support Trust for their support.

References

Aboussekhra, A., Biggersaff, M., Shivji, M.K.K. et al. 1995. Mammalian DNA nucleotide excision repair reconstituted with purified components. *Cell* **80**: 859–68.

Barlow, C., Hirotsune, S., Paylor, R., et al. 1996. *Atm*-deficient mice: a paradigm of ataxia telangiectasia. *Cell* **86**: 159–71.

Barnes, D.E,. Tomkinson, A.E., Lehmann, A.R., Webster, A.D.B. and Lindahl T. 1992. Mutations in the DNA ligase 1 gene of an individual with immunodeficiencies and cellular hypersensitivity to DNA-damaging agents. *Cell* **69**: 495–503.

Beamish, H. and Lavin, M.F. 1994. Radiosensitivity in ataxia telangiectasia: anomalies in radiation induced cell cycle delay. *International Journal of Radiation Biology* **65**: 175–84.

Broughton, B.C., Steinsgrimsdottir, H., Weber, C.A. and Lehmann, A.R. 1994. Mutations in the xeroderma pigmentosum group D DNA repair/ transcription gene in patients with trichothiodystrophy. *Nature Genetics.* **7**: 189-94

Broughton, B.C., Thompson, A.F., Harcourt, S.A., Vermeulen, W., Hoeijmakers, J.H.J., Botta, E., Stefanini M. et al., 1995. Molecular analysis of the DNA repair defect in a patient in xereoderma pigmentosum complementation group D who has the clinical features of xeroderma pigmentosum and Cockayne syndrome. *American Journal of Human Genetics* **56**: 167-74.

Buchwald, M. (1995). Complementation groups: one or more per gene. *Nature Genetics* **11**: 228–30.

Byrd, P.J., McConville, C.M., Cooper, P. et al. 1996a. Mutations revealed by sequencing the 5′ half of the gene for ataxia telangiectasia *Human Molecular Genetics* **5**: 145–9.

Byrd, P.J,. Cooper, P.R., Stankovic, T., Kullar, H.S., Watts, G.D.J., Robinson, P.J. and Taylor, A.M.R. 1996b. A gene transcribed from the bidirectional ATM promoter coding for a serine rich protein; amino acid sequence, structure and expression studies. *Human Molecular Genetics* **5**: 1785–91.

Cardenas, M.E. and Heitman, J. 1995. FKBP12-rapamycin target TOR2 is a vacuolar protein with an associated phosphatidylinositol-4 kinase activity. *EMBO Journal* **14**: 5892–907.

Chen, M., Tompkins, D.J., Auerbach W. et al. 1996. Inactivation of *Fac* in mice produces inducible chromosomal instability and reduced fertility reminiscent of Fanconi anaemia. *Nature Genetics* **12**: 448–51.

Cox, R. 1982. A cellular description of the repair defect in ataxia telangiectasia. In *Ataxia Telangiectasia – A Cellular and Molecular Link Between Cancer, Neuropathology and Immune Deficiency*, ed. B.A.Bridges and D.G. Harnden, pp 141–53. Chichester: Wiley.

396   A.M. Taylor

de Vries, A., van Oostrom, C.Th. M., Hofhuls, F.M.A. et al. 1995. Increased susceptibility to ultraviolet-B and carcinogens of mice lacking the DNA excision repair gene XPA. Nature 377: 169–73.

Donehower, L.A., Harvey, M., Slagle, B.L., McArthur M.J., Montgomery, C.A., Butel, J.S. and Bradley, A. 1992. Mice deficient for p53 are developmentally normal but susceptible to spontaneous tumours. Nature 356: 215–21.

Duchaud, E., Ridet, A., Stoppa-Lyonnet, D., Janin, N,. Moustacchi, E. and Rosselli, F. 1996. Deregulated apoptosis in ataxia telangiectasia; association with clinical stigmata and radiosensitivity. Cancer Research 56: 1400–4.

Edelman, W., Cohen, P.E., Kane, M. et al. 1996. Meiotic pachytene arrest in MLH1-deficient mice. Cell 85: 1125–34

Ellis, N.A., Groden, J., Ye, T-Z. et al. 1995. The Bloom's syndrome gene product is homologous to RecQ helicases. Cell 83: 655–66.

Ellis, N.A. and German, J. 1996. Molecular genetics of Bloom's Syndrome. Human Molecular Genetics 5: 1457–63.

Eshleman, J.R. and Markowitz, S.D. 1996. Mismatch repair defects in human carcinogenesis. Human Molecular Genetics 5: 1489–94.

The Fanconi Anaemia/Breast Cancer Consortium. 1996. Positional cloning of the Fanconi anaemia group A gene. Nature Genetics 14: 324–8.

Fletjer, W.L., McDaniel, L.D., Johns, D., Friedberg, E.C. and Schultz, R.A. 1992. Correction of xeroderma pigmentosum complementation group D mutant cell phenotypes by chromosome and gene transfer: involvement of the human ERCC2 DNA repair gene. Proceedings of the National Academy of Sciences, USA 89: 261–5.

Gilad, S., Khosravi, R. and Shkedy, D. 1996. Predominance of null mutations in ataxia-telangiectasia. Human Molecular Genetics 5(4): 433–9.

Greenwell, P.W,. Kronmal, S.L., Porter, S.E., Gassenhuber, J., Obermaier, B. and Petes, T.D. 1995. TEL1, a gene involved in controlling telomere length in S. cerevisiae is homologous to the human ataxia telangiectasia gene. Cell 82: 823–9.

Frederick, G.D., Amirkan, R.H., Schultz, R.A. and Friedberg, E.C. 1994. Structural and mutational analysis of th xeroderma pigmentosum group D (XPD) gene. Human Molecular Genetics 3: 1783–8.

Gschwend, M., Levran, O., Kruglyak, L. et al. 1996 A locus for Fanconi anaemia on 16q determined by homozygosity mapping. American Journal of Human Genetics 59: 377–84.

Hartley, K.O., Gell, D. Smith, G.C.M. et al. 1995. DNA-dependent protein kinase catalytic subunit: a relative of phosphatidylinositol 3-kinase and the ataxia telangiectasia gene product. Cell 82: 849–56.

Hoeijmakers, J.H.J. 1993. Nucleotide excision repair II: from yeast to mammals. Trends in Genetics 9: 211–17.

Hoeijmakers, J.H.J. 1994. Human nucleotide excision repair syndromes: molecular clues to unexpected intricacies. European Journal of Cancer 30A: 1912–21.

Hoeijmakers, J.H.J., Egly, J-M. and Vermeulen, W. 1996. TFIIH: a key component in multiple DNA transactions. Current Opinion in Genes and Development 6: 36–3.

Jaspers, N.G.J. and Hoeijmakers, J.H.J. 1995. Nucleotide excision-repair in the test tube. Current Biology 5: 700–2.

Joenje, H., Lo Ten Foe, J.R., Oostra, A.B. et al. 1995. Classification of Fanconi anaemia patients by complementation analysis; evidence for a fifth genetic subtype. Blood 86: 2156–60.

Kastan, M.B., Zhan, Q.M., Eldeiry, W.S. et al. 1992. A mammalian cell cycle checkpoint pathway utilising p53 and GADD 45 is defective in ataxia telangiectasia. *Cell* **71**: 587–97.

Keegan, K.S., Holtzman, D.A., Plug, A.W. et al. 1996. The atr and atm protein kinases associate with different sites along meiotically pairing chromosomes. *Genes and Development* **10**: 2423–37.

Kinzler, K.W. and Vogelstein, B. 1996. Lessons from hereditary colorectal cancer. *Cell* **87**: 159–70.

Kolodner, R. 1996. Biochemistry and genetics of eukaryotic mismatch repair. *Genes and Development* **10**: 1433–42.

Kondoh, M., Ueda, M. and Ichihashi, M. 1995. Correlation of the clinical manifestations and gene mutations of Japanese xeroderma pigmentosum group A patients. *British Journal of Dermatology* **133**: 579–85.

Lehmann, A.R. and Carr, A.M. 1995. The ataxia-telangiectasia gene: a link between checkpoint controls, neurodegeneration and cancer. *Trends in Genetics* **11**: 375–7.

Lipkowitz, S., Stern, M-H. and Kirsch, I.R. 1990. Hybrid T cell receptor genes formed by interlocus recombination in normal and ataxia telangiectasia lymphocytes. *Journal of Experimental Medicine* **172**: 409–18.

Lo Ten Foe, J.R., Rooimans, M.A., Bosnoyan-Collins, L. et al. 1996. Expression cloning of a cDNA for the major Fanconi anaemia gene, FAA. *Nature Genetics* **14**: 320–3.

Lu, J., Mullen, J.R., Brill, S.J., Kleff, S., Romeo, A.M. and Sternglanz, R. 1996. Human homologues of yeast helicase. *Nature* **383**: 678–9.

Lu, X. and Lane, D.P. 1993. Differential induction of transcriptionally active p53 following UV or ionising radiation; defects in chromosome instability syndromes? *Cell* **75**: 765–78.

Lydall, D. and Weinert, T. 1995. Yeast checkpoint genes in DNA damage processing: implications for repair and arrest. *Science* **270**: 1488–91.

Maeda, T., Sato, K., Minami, H., Taguchi, H. and Yoshikawa, K. 1995. Chronological difference in walking impairment among Japanese group A xeroderma pigmentosum (XP-A) patients with various combinations of mutation sites. *Clinical Genetics* **48**: 225–31.

Mayne, L.V. and Lehmann, A.R. 1982. Failure of RNA synthesis to recover after UV irradiation: an early defect in cells from individuals with Cockayne's syndrome and xeroderma pigmentosum. *Cancer Research* **42**: 1473–8.

McConville, C.M., Stankovic, T., Byrd, P.J., McGuire, G.M., Yao, Q-Y., Lennox, G.G., and Taylor, A.M.R. 1996. Mutations associated with variant phenotypes in ataxia telangiectasia. *American Journal of Human Genetics* **59**: 320–30.

McWhir, J., Selfridge, J., Harrison, D.J., Squires, S. and Melton, D.W. 1993. Mice with DNA repair gene (*ERCC-1*) deficiency have elevated levels of p53, liver nuclear abnormalities and die before weaning. *Nature Genetics* **5**: 217–23.

Metcalfe, J.A., Parkhill, J., Byrd, P.J., Campbell, L., Stacey, M., Biggs, P. and Taylor, A.M.R. 1996. Accelerated telomere shortening in ataxia telangiectasia. *Nature Genetics* **13**: 350–3.

Meyn, M.S .1995. Ataxia telangiectasia and cellular responses to DNA damage. *Cancer Research* **55**: 5991–6001.

Meyn, M.S., Strasfeld, L. and Allen, C. 1994. Testing the role of p53 in the expression of genetic instability and apoptosis in ataxia telangiectasia. *International Journal of Radiation Biology* **66**: S141–S149.

Nakane, H., Takeuchi, S., Yuba, S. et al. 1995. High incidence of ultraviolet-B- or chemical-carcinogen-induced skin tumours in mice lacking the xeroderma pigmentosum group G gene. *Nature* 377: 165–8.

O'Donovan, A. and Wood, R.D. 1993. Identical defects in DNA repair in xeroderma pigmentosum group G and rodent ERCC group 5. *Nature* 363: 185–8.

Okinaka, R.T., Perez, A., Laubscher, K.H., Sena, A.P., Macinnes, M.A. and Kraemer, K.H. 1995. Identification of mutations within the *ERCC5* gene in a xeroderma pigmentosum group G pedigree. *Journal of Cellular Biochemistry* 285: S21A:SIA.

van Oosterwijk, M.F., Versteeg, A., Filon, R., van Zeeland, A.A. and Mullenders, L.H.F. 1996. The sensitivity of Cockayne's syndrome cells to DNA-damaging agents is not due to defective transcription-coupled repair of active genes. *Molecular Cellular Biology* 16: 4436–44.

Painter, R.B. and Young, B.R. 1980. Radiosensitivity in ataxia telangiectasia; a new explanation. *Proceedings of the National Academy of Sciences, USA* 77: 7315–17.

Petrini, J.M., Huwiler, K.G. and Weaver, D.T., 1991. A wild type DNA ligase 1 gene is expressed in Bloom's syndrome cells. *Proceedings of the National Academy of Sciences, USA* 88: 7615–19.

Pronk, J.C., Gibson, R.A., Savoia A. et al. 1995. Localisation of the Fanconi anaemia complementation group A gene to chromosome 16q24.3. *Nature Genetics* 11: 338–40.

Rajewsky, C. 1996. Clonal selection and learning in the antibody system. *Nature* 381: 751–8.

Risinger, J.I., Umar, A., Boyd, J., Berchuck, A., Kunkel, T.A. and Barrett, J.C. 1996, Mutation of MSH3 in endometrial cancer and evidence for its functional role in heteroduplex repair. *Nature Genetics* 14: 102–5.

Sancar, A. 1996. DNA excision repair. *Annual Review of Biochemistry* 65: 43–81.

Sands, A.T., Abuin, A., Sanchez, A., Conti, C. and Bradley, A. 1995. High susceptibility to ultraviolet-induced carcinogenesis in mice lacking XPC. *Nature* 377: 162–5.

Satakata, I., Uchiyama, M. and Tanaka, K. 1995. Two novel splicing mutations in the XPA gene in patients with group A xeroderma pigmentosum. *Human Molecular Genetics* 4: 1993–4.

Savitsky, K., Bar-Shira, A., Gilad, S. et al. 1995a A single ataxia telangiectasia gene with a product similar to PI-3 kinase. *Science* 268: 1749–53.

Savitsky, K., Sfez, S., Tagle, D.A. et al. 1995b. The complete sequence of the coding region of the ATM gene reveals similarity to cell cycle regulators in different species. *Human Molecular Genetics* 4: 2025–32.

Sedgwick, R.P. and Boder, E. 1991. Ataxia telangiectasia. In: *Handbook of Clinical Neurology. Hereditary Neuropathies and Spinocerebellar atrophies*, vol.16, ed. J.M.B.V. de Jong, pp. 347–423. Amsterdam: Elsevier.

Sijbers, A.M., de Laat, W.L., Ariza, R.R., et al. 1996. Xeroderma pigmentosum group F caused by a defect in a structure-specific DNA repair endonuclease. *Cell* 86: 811–22.

Stanhope-Baker, P., Hudson, K.M., Shaffer, A.L., Constatinescu, A. and Schlissel, M.S. 1996. Cell type-specific chromatin structure determines the targeting of V(D)J recombinase activity in vitro. *Cell* 85: 887–97.

Stefanini, M., Giliani, S., Nardo, T., Marinoni, S., Nazzaro, R., Rizzo, R. and Trevisan, G., 1992. DNA repair investigations in nine Italian patients affected by trichothiodystrophy. *Mutation Research* 273: 119–25.

Stefanini, M., Vermeulen,W., Weeda, G. et al. 1993. A new nucleotide-excision-repair gene associated with the disorder trichothiodystrophy. *American Journal of Human Genetics* **53**: 817–21.

Strathdee, C.A., Duncan, A.M.V., and Buchwald, M., 1992a. Evidence for at least four Fanconi anaemia genes including FACC on chromosome 9. *Nature Genetics*. 1: 196-8.

Strathdee, C.A., Gavish, H., Shannon, W.R. and Buchwald, M. 1992b. Cloning of cDNAs for Fanconi's anaemia by functional complementation. *Nature* **356**: 763–7.

Swift, M., Morellm D., Massey, R. and Chase, C.L. 1991. Cancer incidence in 161 ataxia telangiectasia families studied prospectively. *New England Journal of Medicine* **326**: 1831–6.

Taalman, R.D.F.M., Jaspers, N.G.J., Scheres, J.M.J.C., de Wit, J. and Hustinx, J.W.J. 1983. Hypersensitivity to ionising radiation *in vitro* in a new chromosome breakage disorder, the Nijmegen breakage syndrome. *Mutation Research* **112**: 23–32.

Takayama, K., Salazar, E.P., Lehmann, A.R., Stefanini, M., Thompson, L.H. and Weber, C.A. 1995. Defects in the DNA repair and transcription gene ERCC2 in the cancer prone disorder xeroderma pigmentosum group D. *Cancer Research* **55**: 5656–63.

Takayama, K., Salazar, E.P., Broughton, B.C., Lehmann, A.R., Sarasin, A., Thompson, L.H. and Weber, C.A. 1996. Defects in the DNA repair and transcription gene ERCC2 (XPD) in trichothiodystrophy. *American Journal of Human Genetics* **58**: 263–70.

Taylor, A.M.R., Harnden, D.G., Arlett, C.F., Harcourt, S.A., Lehmann, A.R., Stevens, S. and Bridges B.A. 1975. Ataxia telangiectasia: a human mutation with abnormal radiation sensitivity. *Nature* **258**: 427–8.

Taylor, A.M.R. and McConville, C.M. 1992. Chromosome breakage disorders. In *Prenatal Diagnosis and Screening,* ed. J.H. Brock, C.H. Rodeck and M.A. Ferguson-Smith, pp. 405–21. Edinburgh: Churchill Livingstone.

Taylor, A.M.R., Byrd, P.J., McConville, C.M. and Thacker, S. 1994. Genetic and cellular features of ataxia telangiectasia. *International Journal of Radiation Biology* **65**: 65–70.

Taylor, A.M.R., Metcalfe, J.A., Thick, J. and Mak, Y-F. 1996. Leukaemia and lymphoma in ataxia telangiectasia. *Blood* **87**: 423–38.

Teletar, M., Wang, Z., Udar, N. et al. (1996). Ataxia telangiectasia: mutations in ATM cDNA detected by protein truncation screening. *American Journal of Human Genetics* **59**: 40–4.

Thacker, J. 1994. Cellular radiosensitivity in ataxia telangiectasta. *International Journal of Radiation Biology* **66**: S87–S96.

Troelstra, C., van Gool, A., de Wit, J., Vermeulen, W., Bootsma, D. and Hoeijmakers, J.H.J. 1992. ERCC6, a member of a subfamily of putative helicases, is involved in Cockayne's syndrome and preferential repair of active genes. *Cell* **70**: 939–53.

Umar, A., Koi, M., Risinger, J.L., et al. 1997. Correction of hypermutability N-methyl-N'-nitro-N-nitrosoguanidine resistance, and defective DNA mismatch repair by introducing chromosome 2 into human tumor cells with mutations in MSH2 and MSH6. *Cancer Research* **57**: 3949–55.

Uziel, T., Savitsky, K., Platzer, M. et al. 1996. Genomic organisation of the ATM gene. *Genomics* **33**: 317–20.

Venema, J., Mullenders, L.H.F., Natarajan, A.T., Van Zeeland, A.A. and Mayne, L.V. 1990. The genetic defect in Cockayne syndrome is associated with a defect in repair of UV-induced DNA damage in transcriptionally active DNA. *Proceedings of the National Academy of Sciences, USA*. 87: 4707–11.

Verlander, P.C., Lin, J.D., Udono, M.U., Zhang, Q., Gibson, R.A., Mathew, C.G. and Auerbach, A.D. 1994. Mutation analysis of the Fanconi anaemia gene *FACC*. *American Journal of Human Genetics* 54: 595–601.

Verlander, P.C., Kaporis, A., Liu, Q., Zhang, Q., Seligsohn, U. and Auerbach, A.D. 1995. Carrier frequency of the IVS4+4A→T mutation of the Fanconi anaemia gene *FAC* in the Ashkenazi Jewish population. *Blood* 86: 4034–8.

Vermeulen, W., Jaeken, N.G., Jaspers, N.G.J., Bootsma, D. and Hoeijmakers, J.H.J. 1993. Xeroderma pigmentosum complementation group G associated with Cockayne syndrome. *American Journal of Human Genetics* 53: 185–92.

Wang, X.W., Vermeulen, W., Coursen, J.D. et al. 1996. The XPB and XPD DNA helicases are components of the p53 mediated apoptosis pathway. *Genes and Development* 10: 1219–32.

Weeda, G., van Ham, R.C.A,. Vermeulen, W., Bootsma, D., van der Eb, A.J. and Hoeijmakers, J.H. 1990. A presumed DNA helicase encoded by the excision repair gene ERCC-3 is involved in the human repair disorders xeroderma pigmentosum and Cockayne's syndrome. *Cell* 62: 777–91.

Weemaes, C.M.R., Smeets, D.F.C.M. and van der Burgt, C.J.A.M. 1994. Nijmegen Breakage Syndrome: a progress report. *International Journal of Radiation Biology* 66: S185–S188.

Whitney, M., Thayer, M., Reifstock, C. et al. 1995. Microcell mediated chromosome transfer maps the Fanconi anaemia group D gene to chromosome 3p. *Nature Genetics* 11: 341–3.

Wright, J., Teraoka, S., Onengut, S., Tolun, A., Gatti, R.A., Ochs, H.D. and Concannon, P. 1996. A high frequency of distinct ATM gene mutations in ataxia telangiectasia. *American Journal of Human Genetics* 59: 839–46.

Xu Y. and Baltimore, D. 1996. Dual roles of ATM in the cellular response to radiation and in cell growth control. *Genes and Development* 10: 2401–10.

Xu, Y., Ashley, T., Brainerd, E.E., Bronson, R.T., Meyn, M.S. and Baltimore, D. 1996. Targeted disruption of *ATM* leads to growth retardation, chromosomal fragmentation during meiosis, immune defects, and thymic lymphoma. *Genes and Development* 10: 2411–22.

Yamashita, T., Barber, D.L., Zhu, Y., Wu, N. and D'Andrea, A.D. 1994. The Fanconi anaemia polypeptide FACC is localized to the cytoplasm. *Proceedings of the National Academy of Sciences, USA* 91: 6712–16.

19
Childhood cancer
KATHY PRITCHARD-JONES

Summary

This chapter discusses the genetic contribution to childhood cancer. It might be expected that heredity plays a larger role in childhood cancer than in adult cancer, but in fact the hereditary fraction of childhood cancer is approximately 5%. The genetics of retinoblastoma and Wilms' tumour are discussed in detail. The hereditary contribution to neuroblastoma is outlined and the childhood component of Li–Fraumeni syndrome is considered. The genetic contributions to leukaemia and brain tumours are discussed in turn. The chapter concludes with a consideration of the role of adult cancer-predisposing genes in childhood cancer.

Introduction

Childhood cancer is fortunately uncommon, affecting approximately 1 in 500 children before the age of 15 years (Parkin et al., 1988). More than half such children can now expect to be long term survivors (Stiller, 1994a). Therefore it is of increasing importance to be able to identify those individuals who are genetically predisposed, as they will be at increased risk both of second tumours and of passing on this predisposition to their children, assuming their treatment has not impaired fertility. It is now ten years since the first cancer predisposition gene, that for retinoblastoma, was cloned on the basis of its involvement in a heritable form of the disease. (The *TP53* gene had been isolated several years earlier but was not realized to underlie a familial cancer syndrome until 1990.) Retinoblastoma laid down the paradigm for the localization and identification of cancer predisposition genes and showed that a single gene could underlie both heritable and sporadic forms of a cancer. It also proved at a molecular level Knudson's hypothesis that as few as two genetic events were sufficient for tumourigenesis in childhood. With the subsequent cloning of the Wilms' tumour gene, *WT1*, it became apparent that the genetics of childhood cancers could be more complex, with several different genes underlying the same tumour type and with multiple genetic events being necessary for tumour development in some cases, as in adult cancers.

Within the last decade, several more childhood cancer-predispostion genes have been cloned. Those involving DNA processing disorders (ataxia-telangiectasia, Bloom syndrome and Fanconi anaemia complementation group C genes) are reviewed in detail in Chapter 18. These types of disorder predispose mainly to leukaemias and lymphomas, a bias which may reflect the naturally high turnover of haematopoietic cells and hence their greater tendency to a rapid accumulation of mutations. However, even within this group of disorders, there is a preferred type of leukaemia or lymphoma associated with each disease category, showing that much more detailed structure–function analyses of these genes are required to dissect the pathways leading to cancer predisposition. Several other genes that predispose to both childhood and adult cancers have recently been cloned. These include the neurofibromatosis genes 1 and 2 (reviewed in Chapter 13) and the recognition that specific *RET* oncogene mutations may underlie either heritable forms of medullary thyroid cancer or the congenital malformation syndrome, Hirschsprung disease (reviewed in Chapter 16 and van Heyningen, 1994). This chapter will concentrate on genetic predisposition to the tumours specific to childhood, namely the embryonal tumours and certain leukaemias.

Retinoblastoma

Retinoblastoma (RB) is the only childhood cancer in which a significant proportion (10–15%) show a clear familial tendency and, including all sporadic bilateral cases, the total heritable fraction is over 40% (Draper et al., 1992). Predisposition to RB is transmitted as an autosomal dominant trait with a high degree of penetrance; over 90% of carriers develop the disease. In some families, ophthalmic examination of apparently unaffected adults reveals retinomas, which may represent either spontaneously regressed retinoblastomas or precusor lesions which never underwent full malignant conversion (Gallie et al., 1990). Survivors of the heritable form of retinoblastoma have a greatly increased risk of second primary tumours, particularly osteosarcoma and soft tissue sarcoma (Draper et al., 1986). These may occur at any site but show a predilection for previously irradiated tissue, emphasizing the interaction of enviromental insult with the genetic makeup of the cell.

The retinoblastoma gene, RB1

It was noted in the 1960s that a few patients with the sporadic form of RB had other congenital abnormalities and karyotypic analyses showed constitutional abnormalities of the long arm of chromosome 13. The familial cases also mapped to the same locus. Using the now classic approach of positional cloning or 'reverse genetics', the *RB1* gene was isolated from 13q14 (reviewed by Gallie et al., 1990). The gene is a large one, comprising 27 exons spanning more than 100 kb of genomic DNA. It encodes a ubiquitously expressed nuclear protein, pRB, which appears to act as a critical link between the cell cycle clock and the transcriptional machinery of the cell (Weinberg, 1995). The activity of pRB is regulated by phosphorylation and it seems to exert most of its effects during the first two-thirds of the G_1 phase of the cell cycle. The underphosphorylated form inhibits passage through the R (restriction) point, beyond which the cell becomes mitogen-independent and committed to undergoing mitosis (Pardee, 1989). A variety of physiological growth inhibitory signals are known to prevent pRB phosphorylation and thus block progression through the cell cycle. pRB is phosphorylated by the G_1 cyclins and their associated kinases. The underphosphorylated form normally binds to a family of transcription factors known as E2Fs but it can also bind to the transforming proteins of several tumour viruses, such as large T antigen of SV40 and the E7 protein of human papilloma virus. These viral proteins sequester pRB from performing its normal function and their binding sites are common sites for mutation of the *RB1* gene in tumours not associated with oncogenic DNA virus. Upon phosphorylation, pRB releases its hold on the E2Fs, which then presumably activate expression of other genes necessary for cell cycle progression. To date, few of the target genes of the E2Fs are known, although some of the cyclins appear to be activated, thus increasing the positive feedback on RB phosphorylation. RB is therefore truly a key regulator of the cell cycle.

At a molecular level, retinoblastoma has fulfilled all of the tenets of Knudson's two-hit hypothesis; both familial and sporadic forms of RB involve the same gene and both alleles are mutated in the tumours

404   K. Pritchard-Jones

(Gallie, 1990). The mutations usually cause loss of function, either through complete *RB1* gene deletion or production of a truncated protein. Some families with incomplete penetrance and mild expression of the RB phenotype have been shown to carry missense mutations in *RB1*, which may allow partial protein function (Onadim et al., 1992a). Thus, a degree of genotype–phenotype correlation exists. Mutations of the *RB1* gene have also been found in a variety of other tumour types, including sporadic osteosarcomas and soft tissue sarcomas and in sporadic adult breast cancer, which is not normally associated with RB predisposition. Relatives of RB patients have an excess risk of developing non-ocular cancers in adult life, particularly melanoma and lung, bladder, and brain tumours. This increased risk is mainly confined to relatives known to be carriers and who themselves were affected by retinoblastoma (Sanders et al., 1989).

Screening for mutations in **RB1**

Despite knowledge of the genomic structure of the *RB1* gene for almost a decade, screening for carriers can still be a laborious process due to the size of the gene. There is no common clustering of mutations and carrier detection is still often more efficiently performed by using linked markers rather than searching for the individual's mutation (Onadim et al., 1990). However, since only 10–15% of cases have a family history, direct mutational analysis is still required in almost a third of all cases. A functional screening test for the presence of the intact protein (as is possible for TP53) is still awaited. Molecular definition of carrier status is important as a negative result means avoidance of the three-monthly ophthalmoscopic examinations under general anaesthetic that comprise current clinical screening (Onadim et al., 1992b).

RB1 knockout as a clue to organ-specificity of cancer for **RB1** *mutations*

It is still not clear why a gene that is expressed in every cell and whose somatic mutation can contribute to a variety of tumour types, predisposes so specifically to retinoblastoma in early childhood and osteosarcoma and soft tissue sarcomas in adolescence. This tissue preference is not dictated by type of mutation, as germline and somatic mutational spectra are similar. Some answers (and more questions!) come from studies on *rb-1* deficient ('knockout') mouse models. Complete loss of rb-1 function is embryo-lethal just after midgestation with defects in neurogenesis and haematopoiesis. Heterozygous mice do not show the predisposition to RB seen in their human counterparts but develop pituitary adenocarcinoma and medullary thyroid carcinoma with high frequency, accompanied by mutation of the remaining wildtype *Rb* allele (Jacks et al., 1992). Remarkably, *rb-1* null cells can contribute to all adult tissues examined, including the retina, when they are injected into wild type blastocysts to generate chimaeric mice (Williams et al., 1994). These mice still do not develop retinoblastoma, suggesting that the relevant cell type in the mouse is refractory to loss of rb-1 function and requires additional genetic events before succumbing to tumourigenesis. Possible explanations may include the existence of Rb homologous proteins, which might compensate for loss of rb-1 function to a greater or lesser degree depending on cell type and species or a critical interaction of RB with cyclin D1 in the retina (Sicinski et al., 1995). Currently, there is no evidence for any gene other than *RB1* being responsible for retinoblastoma in humans.

Wilms' tumour

The genetics of Wilms' tumour

Wilms' tumour (WT) is an embryonal kidney cancer affecting 1 in 10,000 children worldwide. In large series from both the US and Europe, it is clear that familial WT is extremely rare, comprising only 1% of all cases (Breslow et al., 1988; Pastore et al., 1988). Direct parent–child transmission is uncommon and many of the pedigrees described have affected members only in second degree relatives and beyond (Bonaiti-Pellie et al., 1992). This has been interpreted as meaning that predisposition to WT is inherited as an autosomal dominant with a variable and much lower penetrance than for retinoblastoma. WT has been postulated to follow Knudson's two-hit model or Matsunaga's host resistance model, the latter perhaps explaining the variable expressivity (Knudson and Strong, 1972; Matsunaga, 1981). Although Knudson's original mathematical treatise of RB was based on the premise that familial cases occur earlier and are more likely to be bilateral, analysis of a large number of familial cases of WT now documented shows that they behave more like the sporadic cases in their median age of onset and frequency of bilaterality. The apparently sporadic bilateral cases (5–8%), which were assumed to all represent germline carriers of a WT-predisposition gene, also appear to be heterogeneous, with their age of onset showing a bimo-

406   K. Pritchard-Jones

dal peak, suggestive of early postzygotic initiation in a subgroup (Breslow
et al., 1993). Such somatic mosaicism may also explain the excess of
unilateral multicentric tumours over bilateral ones, assuming they represent independent primaries rather than intrarenal spread (Bonaiti-Pellie
et al., 1993).

The Wilms' tumour gene, WT1

WT1 encodes a zinc-finger protein which can function as a transcription
factor. The *WT1* mRNA is the subject of alternative splicing and RNA
editing to produce eight potential protein isoforms which differ in their
DNA binding specificity and their effect on transcription (reviewed by
Hastie, 1994). Unlike the *RB1* gene, *WT1* is expressed only in certain
tissues, particularly in the developing kidney and gonad, which is in
keeping with its role in both malformation and tumourigenesis of these
organs (reviewed by Pritchard-Jones and Hastie, 1990). Children with the
WAGR (Wilms', aniridia, genitourinary malformation and mental retardation) syndrome carry a germline complete deletion of one *WT1* allele
and, in the majority of their tumours, there is a second hit in the remaining *WT1* allele (Baird et al., 1992). Some cases of bilateral WT have also
been shown to be due to germline *WT1* mutation and again, the second
WT1 allele is usually but not always mutated in the tumours (Huff et al.,
1991). In several large studies of sporadic WTs, it is now clear that *WT1*
mutations are present in only 5–15% of tumours (Gessler et al., 1994;
Varansi et al., 1994). The majority produce a truncated protein and are
homozygous in the tumours, in accordance with WT1 functioning as a
tumour suppressor. However, a significant number of cases have been
described where the *WT1* mutation affects only one allele and produces
an abnormal protein that may have gained new properties or may interfere with the action of the remaining normal WT1 protein ('dominant-
negative').

   Intriguingly, *WT1* is highly expressed in the three cell types (metaneph-
ric blastema, renal podocytes, and developing gonad) which are abnormal in Denys–Drash syndrome (DDS) making *WT1* an ideal candidate
gene for this syndrome (Pritchard-Jones et al., 1990). This proved to be
the case and germline missense mutations have been found in most cases,
over half affecting a critical arginine residue in the third zinc finger
(reviewed by Coppes et al., 1993). A few cases of DDS have been
shown to carry either intronic *WT1* mutations that abolish the normal
splicing pattern or nonsense mutations which produce a truncated pro-

tein lacking the zinc finger region. This shows that the ratio of WT1 isoforms is essential for normal genitourinary development and suggests that the truncated protein may be acting in a dominant or dominant-negative fashion. A comparison of DDS with the WAGR syndrome emphasizes that complete absence of one allele of the *WT1* gene has less severe effects on development of the gonad and podocytes than does the presence of a mutated protein. WT1 is essential for development of the genitourinary system in the mouse. Mice homozygous for a *WT1* null mutation fail to form either kidneys or gonads and must have other more subtle abnormalities responsible for the intrauterine death at mid-gestation (Kreidberg, 1993).

Genetic heterogeneity in Wilms' tumour

Two loci on chromosome 11p are implicated in Wilms' tumour:WT1 at 11p13, and a more distal locus involved in Beckwith–Wiedemann syndrome (BWS – see below). A third locus involved in WT is suggested by allele loss studies in sporadic cases showing that 20% have LOH at chromosome 16q (Maw et al., 1992), but linkage to this region has been negative in several large pedigrees. Several affected individuals with con-stitutional abnormalities of chromosome 7p have been identified, suggest-ing a fourth WT locus. Familial WT, not attributable to loci on chromosome 11p or 16q has been linked to chromosome 17q, near *BRCA1*, in one large pedigree (Rahman et al., 1996). Preliminary analysis of other families, however, suggests that familial WT is genetically het-erogeneous.

Congenital abnormalities, genetic syndromes, and Wilms' tumour

Children with Wilms' tumour have an excess of congenital abnormalities, particularly cryptorchidism/hypospadias or hemihypertrophy, which occur in 2.5% and 3.5 % respectively (Breslow et al., 1988). A further 2% of cases of WT occur in children with a recognizable malformation syndrome, usually as a de novo event. The three best studied syndromes are the WAGR, DDS and Beckwith–Wiedemann (BWS) (Table 19.1). The first two result from different types of mutations in the same WT-predisposition gene, termed *WT1*, whereas BWS involves a second gene (or genes), as yet uncloned, on chromosome 11p15.5. Some other rare syndromes also carry an increased risk of Wilms' tumour including the gene for the hereditary hyperparathyroidism–jaw tumour syndrome,

Table 19.1. *Genetics of Wilms' tumour-associated syndromes.*

	WAGR syndrome	Denys–Drash syndrome	Beckwith–Wiedemann syndrome
Prevalence among Wilms' tumour cases	~ 1%	< 1%	~ 0.5%*
Risk of Wilms' tumour	30–50%	High (> 50%)	3–5%
Genetics and mode of inheritance	Sporadic *de novo* germline mutation	Sporadic *de novo* germline mutation	Sporadic *de novo* germline mutation 85%
	Rarely familial (AD)	Very rarely familial	Familial 15% (AD with variable expressivity)
Chromosomal locus	11p13	11p13	11p15.5
Disease gene(s)	*WT1* aniridia gene, *PAX6*	*WT1*	unknown
Types of mutation	Contiguous gene syndrome Complete deletion of one allele of *WT1* *PAX6*	Point mutation (mainly missense) Frameshift Aberrant mRNA splicing	

Note: WAGR: Wilms' tumour, aniridia, genitourinary malformation and mental retardation; AD: autosomal dominant.
*A further 2.5% of all cases have hemihypertrophy, which may represent a 'forme fruste' of Beckwith–Wiedemann syndrome.

which has been mapped to chromosome 1q21-q31 (Szabo et al., 1995) and the gene for the overgrowth syndrome of Simpson–Golabi–Behmel has recently been cloned (Pilia et al., 1996) but its contribution to sporadic WT has not yet been reported. Perlman syndrome, an autosomal recessive condition with fetal gigantism, nephroblastomatosis and genital abnormalities has been reported in fewer than 10 families worldwide (Greenberg et al., 1988). The risk of WT appears to be very high in this condition but the gene has not yet been localized. Sotos syndrome of cerebral gigantism has been associated with Wilms' and other embryonal tumours but the relative risk has not been quantified and again the disease locus is unknown (Hersh et al., 1992). An increased risk of WT is found in Turner syndrome, where the predisposition may be related to the renal malformation that frequently occurs (Olson, 1995). WT may also occur in neurofibromatosis type 1 and the breast–ovarian cancer syndrome (Stay and Vawter, 1977; Narod, 1994). Thus it appears several genes may be responsible for both heritable and sporadic forms of WT.

Wilms' tumour and aniridia

The association of WT with sporadic aniridia was recognized in the early 1960s and was termed the WAGR syndrome due the frequent occurrence of other characteristic abnormalities – i.e. Wilms' tumour, aniridia, genitourinary malformation and mental retardation. These children have a constitutional interstitial chromosomal deletion encompassing band 11p13. Aniridia is fully penetrant but WT develops only in 30–50%. Gonadal tumours are also occasionally seen in this syndrome. The 11p13 deletion can rarely be inherited, either by carriers of balanced translocations who transmit an unbalanced form or by carriers of submicroscopic deletions who have escaped the abnormal genital phenotype and therefore masquerade as familial aniridia, which does not normally carry an increased risk of WT (Fantes et al., 1992). By deletion mapping in individuals with varying phenotypes, the aniridia locus has been placed distal to the WT locus within 11p13 whereas the WT locus cannot be separated from that for genitourinary abnormalities, implying that tumourigenesis and malformation can be pleiotropic effects of mutations in the same WT-predisposition gene (van Heyningen et al., 1990). By positional cloning, both the aniridia gene, *PAX6* and the Wilms' tumour gene, *WT1* have now been isolated.

Beckwith–Wiedemann syndrome, Wilms' tumour and chromosome 11p15

BWS is usually sporadic but rarely may be familial (Koufos et al., 1989; Ping et al., 1989). Both forms involve changes at chromosome 11p15.5 and it appears that the phenomenon of genomic imprinting is important (Henry et al., 1991). Several imprinted genes lie in this area, including the fetal mitogen, insulin like growth factor 2 (IGF2), which is expressed from the paternal allele, and the *H19* gene, which is imprinted in the opposite direction and has tumour suppressor activity. BWS frequently involves constitutional duplication of the paternal 11p15.5 region, resulting in overexpression of *IGF2* and loss of *H19*. A preferential loss of the maternal 11p allele is seen in one-third of sporadic WTs, suggesting a similar mechanism may be operating. Loss of imprinting results in the same effect on IGF2 expression and is also found in sporadic WTs

(Ogawa et al., 1993; Steenman et al., 1994). However, proof that either *IGF2*, *H19* or any other gene actually *is* the BWS gene remains to be shown. Indeed, high resolution mapping of constitutional translocation breakpoints in BWS patients has defined two regions separated by over 4 Mb, neither of which encompasses the *IGF2* gene, although one is adjacent (Hoovers et al., 1995). It therefore seems that if IGF2 is the initiator of WT in these cases, then it is being disregulated by long range position effects. Since such effects have never been described to operate over 4Mb, it seems likely that there are at least two BWS genes in this region. Disturbances of IGF2 expression occur frequently in sporadic WTs which are not associated with BWS. It is therefore intriguing that the recently cloned glypican 3 gene, which underlies another overgrowth syndrome with an increased WT risk, the Simpson–Golabi–Behmel syndrome, appears to be an IGF binding protein.

Second primary cancers in children with Wilms' tumour

The *WT1* gene seems to predispose almost exclusively to specific cancers during childhood. There is no clear cut pattern of second primary tumours (SPTs) in survivors of Wilms' tumour but this may simply reflect the likelihood that only a small proportion carry a germline mutation in a WT-predisposition gene (Breslow et al., 1995). Acute lymphoblastic leukaemia and mesothelioma are unusual SPTs which have occurred after Wilms' tumour (Austin et al., 1986; Moss et al., 1989). Since somatic *WT1* mutations have been described in acute leukaemias in adults and in a single case of peritoneal mesothelioma, it is possible that this group represents children with germline *WT1* mutations (Park et al., 1993; King-Underwood et al., 1996).

Screening for Wilms' tumour

Children with certain congenital malformations should be considered at increased risk of developing Wilms' tumour and screened accordingly. Children with sporadic aniridia and a normal karyotype can be analysed for submicroscopic deletions of the *WT1* gene by FISH. Any child with early onset nephrotic syndrome even in the absence of genital abnormalities, should be evaluated to see if they have the DDS, including *WT1* gene analysis (Schmitt et al., 1995). The fetal overgrowth syndromes present greater difficulties, as many of the genes have not yet been isolated. Any child with a degree of hemihypertrophy as well as those with the full phenotype of BWS should be screened (Sotelo-Avila et al., 1980). Clinical screening for early WT can be done either by regular abdominal ultrasound examinations or by teaching the parents abdominal palpation. It is not clear which is most effective. Indeed, in a UK study, planned regular ultrasound did not decrease the stage of the tumour at time of diagnosis (Craft et al., 1995). The risk to siblings or children of survivors of unilateral sporadic Wilms' tumour seems to be extremely low and they do not require screening (Hawkins et al., 1995).

Neuroblastoma

Familial neuroblastoma is a recognized but very rare entity (reviewed by Brodeur 1995). Kushner et al. (1986) described a series of 55 such patients from a worldwide literature review. These comprised 45 siblings, of which eight were identical twins; only four cases had an affected parent. Familial cases were associated with an early age of onset, usually less than 12 months, and multiple primary sites. Familial neuroblastoma has been calculated to follow the two-hit hypothesis but, due to small numbers, the predicted 25% of sporadic patients who should represent heritable cases is probably an overestimate. The risk to a sibling of a neuroblastoma patient of developing the same cancer is only 1 in 1000 (Draper et al., 1996).

Li–Fraumeni syndrome in children

The association of early onset soft tissue sarcoma and breast cancer has been described in Chapter 10. In most families that fulfill the strict criteria for definition of the Li–Fraumeni syndrome (LFS), a germline mutation in the *TP53* gene has been found. However, such mutations are also found in approximately 10% of families that contain only two cases of LFS-spectrum cancers and are termed 'Li–Fraumeni-like' (Eeles, 1995). All such families are rare, and perhaps of more importance to the paediatric oncologist is the question 'how likely is it that a young patient with a sarcoma and no family history is a carrier of a *TP53* mutation?'. This question is particularly pertinent in paediatric practice as the close relatives of the proband are young and therefore may not yet have been diagnosed with cancer. In a study of 204 cases of soft tissue sarcomas in the Manchester children's tumour registry, 41 of 45 first degree relatives developing a cancer did so after the diagnosis of an apparently sporadic sarcoma in the child (Prof. J. Birch, pers. comm. 1996). An increased breast cancer risk has been documented in the mothers of children with soft tissue sarcomas, suggesting that some may belong to LFS families. The relative risk is highest when the index child is male with a diagnosis of embryonal rhabdomyosarcoma under the age of 3 years (Birch et al., 1990). Analyses for germline *TP53* mutations in children with apparently sporadic forms of tumours falling within the LFS-spectrum have shown that approximately 3–4% of osteosarcomas, up to 9% of rhabdomyosarcomas and over half of adrenocortical carcinomas are due to such a predisposing mutation (Sameshima et al., 1992, McKintyre et al., 1994, Diller et al., 1995). Children and young adults who develop a SPT are also more likely to be carriers of a germline *TP53* mutation, which has been found in 7% of such cases (Malkin et al., 1992). Germline *TP53* mutations only rarely contribute to childhood leukaemia (Felix et al., 1992). The issue of screening children with cancer for *TP53* mutations is fraught with ethical problems, as there is presently no reliable screening test available for early detection of SPTs. Knowledge of the *TP53* status prior to commencing therapy for the primary tumour could theoretically be used to modify treatment to reduce the risk of inducing a second cancer, for example by avoiding radiotherapy. Unfortunately, however, many of these children have very resistant tumours which require maximal therapy. In the future, if surveillance or preventive treatment became available to reduce cancer risk, both in the proband and their parent/ siblings, then such testing could be justified. At present, the main justification would be that if a carrier mother were to be identified, she could be offered screening for breast cancer, or prenatal testing for mutation carriers, if appropriate. Until screening for LFS-spectrum tumours is of proven benefit, routine testing of children with cancer is perhaps premature (see Chapter 3).

Genetic predisposition to leukaemia in childhood

Trisomy 21

Down syndrome accounts for over 90% of leukaemias associated with a known genetic condition, and was found in 1.7% of childhood acute lymphoblastic leukaemia (ALL) and 5.3% of childhood acute myeloid leukaemia (AML) in a large population-based survey (Narod et al., 1991). Children with Down syndrome have a 10-fold relative risk for ALL, which shows similar clinical features to sporadic ALL. By contrast, children with Down syndrome and AML have a significantly younger age of onset and an excess of the erythroid (M6) and megakaryocytic (M7)

Childhood cancer 413

subtypes (Levitt et al., 1990; Narod et al., 1991). The mechanism by which trisomy 21 imparts an increased risk of leukaemia is unclear. Certainly, this seems to be due to the genetic constitution of the cell rather than the overall phenotype of the patient, as leukaemia/transient leukaemoid reactions occur preferentially in trisomic cells in patients exhibiting mosaicism, and trisomy 21 is a common abnormality in sporadic leukaemias (Sacchi, 1992). In general, their leukaemias respond well to standard treatment but they require a high level of supportive care.

Neurofibromatosis type 1 (NF1)

Children with NF1 have only a fivefold relative risk of ALL but a 221-fold relative risk of juvenile chronic myeloid leukaemia, where they comprise 9% of the children with this diagnosis (Stiller et al., 1994b). They do not have an increased risk of AML or adult-type CML. Children with NF1 are more likely to develop a brain or spinal cord tumour than leukaemia.

Other genetic disorders associated with an increased risk of leukaemia
DNA processing disorders

The most diverse group of children predisposed to leukaemias/lymphomas comprises the DNA processing disorders, which have been discussed in Chapter 18. A component of many of these syndromes is immunodeficiency and it is unclear how much of the increased cancer risk is due to defective immunosurveillance rather than an increased accumulation of mutations. Their relative contributions should follow from a fuller characterization of the molecular defects in these syndromes, now that the genes for ataxia-telangiectasia, Bloom syndrome, and Fanconi anaemia group C have been cloned.

Fanconi anaemia (FA)

This group comprises a mixture of different autosomal recessive syndromes, which are all very rare and are characterized by progressive pancytopaenia, variable congenital abnormalities which often include defects of the thumb/radii and predisposition to malignancy. Most patients show increased chromosomal breakage, particularly in response to DNA cross-linking agents such as mitomycin C. The commonest malignancy is AML, which develops in almost 10% of patients (Auerbach and Allen, 1991). However FA was found in <0.5% of

1435 cases of childhood AML diagnosed in the UK between 1971 and 1990 (C. Stiller, pers. comm.). The cytogenetic abnormalities found in the leukaemic cells are diverse and include a high proportion of monosomy 7 and duplications of 1q. Cell fusion experiments have revealed the existence of at least four complementation groups in FA (Strathdee et al., 1992a). The gene for complementation group C, *FACC*, has been isolated from chromosome 9q22 but its function is as yet unknown (Strathdee et al., 1992b; Joenje et al., 1995).

Bone marrow failure syndromes

Blackfan–Diamond anaemia and Shwachman's syndrome of congenital neutropenia and pancreatic insufficiency are also considered to be pre-leukaemic states, although the absolute risk of leukaemia in these rare syndromes is not quantified (Woods et al., 1981; Mori et al., 1992; van Dijken and Verwijs, 1995). Kostmann's disease of severe congenital neutropaenia has been reported to progress to AML during treatment with G-CSF. It is probable that the G-CSF hastens the malignant transformation of an underlying preleukaemic state rather than being causative (Weinblatt et al., 1995).

Wiskott–Aldrich syndrome (WAS)

This syndrome is characterized by eczema, increased infections and risk of tumours, particularly leukaemias. The gene underlying this disorder, *WASP*, has recently been cloned (Derry et al., 1994). Although the normal function of the gene is as yet unknown, it is of great interest that different mutations within the same gene seem to determine whether or not there is a predisposition to cancer. X-linked thrombocytopenia (XLT) has been shown to be an allelic variant of WAS, which lacks both the increased risk of infections and of tumours (Villa et al., 1995). It is not yet clear whether the increased cancer susceptibility is a direct consequence of the effect of specific mutant WAS proteins on susceptibility of the cell to carcinogenic stimuli or whether it is a secondary phenomenon due to defective immunosurveillance. So far, there seems to be some overlap between the mutational spectra found in each condition, with both producing missense mutations or truncated proteins. Further studies are required before any firm genotype–phenotype correlations can be drawn.

Familial leukaemia

Outside the context of a cancer predisposition syndrome, familial clustering of leukaemia is extremely rare. Only nine sibling-pairs were diagnosed
with acute leukaemia in the UK over a 40 year period from 1952 to 1992
(Draper et al., 1996). Four of these pairs were identical twins, where the
increased risk of leukaemia is well recognized and is thought to be due to
intrauterine metastasis rather than an identical genetic predisposition
when the proband is an infant (Mahmoud et al., 1995).

Genetic predisposition to brain tumours in childhood

The commonest predisposing condition is NF1, which accounts for
1.5% of all childhood brain and spinal cord tumours, but a much
greater proportion of optic nerve glioma (23%) and meningioma
(5%) (Narod et al., 1991). The second largest genetic group is children
with tuberous sclerosis, who have a 70-fold relative risk and account for
0.5% of childhood brain tumours. Turcot syndrome of brain tumours
associated with familial polyposis accounts for < 1% of childhood
brain tumours (Narod et al., 1991). The familial naevoid basal cell
carcinoma (BCC) syndrome (Gorlin syndrome), an autosomal dominant disorder characterized by multiple BCCs and diverse structural
developmental abnormalities, carries an increased risk of medulloblastoma. In a population-based study from the Manchester Childhood
Tumour Registry, Gorlin syndrome was diagnosed in 3 of 173 consecutive cases of primitive neuroectodermal tumours (PNET) and
accounted for 5% of tumours diagnosed in children under the age of
five years (Evans et al., 1991). The characteristic appearance of BCCs,
at the edge of the radiation field could occur from three to nine years
post-radiotherapy. In the same series, the risk of developing childhood
medulloblastoma in Gorlin syndrome was 3.6% (3 of 84 cases). The
gene for Gorlin syndrome has been mapped to chromosome 9q22, the
same interval as the *FACC* gene (Farndon et al., 1994) and has recently
been isolated by a candidate gene approach (Hahn et al., 1996; Johnson
et al., 1996). The gene is the human homologue of the *Drosophila* segment polarity gene, *patched*, which encodes a transmembrane signalling
protein involved in precise determination of spatial patterns in developing flies. Mutations of the *PTC* gene have so far been found in a small
percentage of Gorlin syndrome carriers and sporadic BCCs. The predisposition to skin cancer associated with *PTC* mutations is discussed in

416   K. Pritchard-Jones

Chapter 15. As with the *WT1* gene, this reflects the intimate relationship of developmental control and tumour biology, and provides yet another molecular illustration of the classic two-hit model. Remarkably, homologues of two other *Drosophila* segment polarity genes have also been implicated in human cancer; *WNT1* in breast cancer and *GLI1* in glioblastoma. These latter genes seem to function as oncogenes and may be negatively regulated by PTC in the same pathway (Pennisi, 1996).

Adult cancer predisposition genes causing cancer in childhood

Familial adenomatous polyposis (FAP)

This is a dominantly inherited disorder characterized by the presence of hundreds of adenomatous large bowel polyps, which predisposes to colorectal cancer in young adults. It is discussed in more detail in Chapter 9. The causative *APC* gene on chromosome 5q is recessive for tumourigenesis and both functional copies are lost during the progression from benign adenoma to carcinoma. FAP is associated with a greatly increased relative risk of the rare childhood liver tumour–hepatoblastoma. However, due to the rarity of hepatoblastoma, the absolute risk to children of parents with FAP is less than 1% (Hughes and Michels, 1992). An analysis of apparently sporadic hepatoblastomas showed that mutations of the *APC* gene are uncommon and, when present, are due to an underlying germline mutation even in the absence of a family history of FAP (Kurahashi et al., 1995). FAP also carries a 10% risk of desmoid tumours which may occur in childhood. One such tumour in an FAP carrier has been shown to have homozygous inactivating mutations of the *APC* gene (de Silva et al., 1996).

Hereditary nonpolyposis colorectal carcinoma (HNPCC)

HNPCC has been shown to be due to germline mutations in a series of DNA mismatch repair genes, which cause errors in DNA replication (see Chapters 9 and 18). Although colon carcinoma is extremely rare in childhood, it appears that a significant proportion of apparently sporadic cases in adolescents are due to a germline mutation in one of these genes (Liu et al., 1995).

Thyroid cancer

Thyroid cancer is very rare in childhood and the commonest type is papillary carcinoma. Medullary thyroid carcinoma, a component of the hereditary multiple endocrine neoplasia (MEN) syndromes (see Chapter 16), accounts for less than one-fifth of childhood thyroid cancer but over half of these children belong to MEN2 families (Narod et al., 1991). The *RET* oncogene on chromosome 10 is the target for mutation in both types of thyroid cancer; germline mutations underlie the heritable medullary carcinomas whereas sporadic mutations, which can be radiation-induced, are seen in papillary carcinomas. Indeed, over 60% of the epidemic of childhood thyroid cancer seen after the Chernobyl nuclear fallout have translocations involving *RET* (Klugbauer et al., 1995). As discussed in Chapter 16, the type of *RET* mutation determines the associated phenotype, which can range from Hirschsprung disease to various types of thyroid cancer.

Conclusions

Rectinoblastoma and adrenocortical carcinoma are commonly hereditary. However, only a small fraction of all childhood cancer, probably less than 5%, is due to inherited predisposition (Narod et al., 1991). The commonest underlying genetic abnormalities are Down syndrome (0.8%), Li–Fraumeni syndrome (0.7%), neurofibromatosis (0.5%), and tuberous sclerosis (0.1%). The remainder of the diverse syndromes that include a predisposition to childhood cancer, while fascinating at a molecular level, contribute very little individually to the total childhood cancer incidence. Studies of cancer in the offspring of childhood cancer survivors suggests that the heritable fraction of non-syndrome associated cancers is very low (Hawkins, 1994). However, a note of caution is justified in that many of the now adult survivors were treated before the era of modern chemotherapy. The genotoxicity of current chemotherapy regimens remains to be established. Ongoing prospective studies of the risk of congenital malformation and cancer in offspring should establish whether current treatment regimens increase the risk of new germ cell mutations.

References

Auerbach., A.D. and Allen, R.G., 1991. Leukemia and preleukemia in Fanconi anemia patients. *Cancer Genetics and Cytogenetics* **51**: 1–12.

Austin, M.B., Fechner, R.E. and Roggli, V.L. 1986. Pleural malignant mesothelioma following Wilms' tumour. *American Journal of Clinical Pathology* **86**: 227–30.

Baird, PN., Groves, N., Haber, D.A., Housman, D.E. and Cowell, J.K. 1992. Identification of mutations in the WT1 gene in tumours from patients with the WAGR syndrome. *Oncogene* **7**: 2141–9.

Birch, J.M., Hartley, A.L., Blair, V. et al. 1990. Identification of factors associated with high breast cancer risk in the mothers of children with soft tissue sarcoma. *Journal of Clinical Oncology* **8**: 583–90.

Bonaiti-Pellie, C., Chompret, A., Tournade, M.F. et al. 1992. Genetic and epidemiology of Wilms' tumor: the French Wilms" tumor study. *Medical and Pediatric Oncology* **20**: 284–91.

Bonaiti-Pellie, C., Chompret, A., Tournade, M.F., Lemerle, J., Voute, P.A. and Delemarre, J.F.M. 1993. Excess of multifocal tumors in nephroblastoma: implications for mechanisms of tumor development and genetic counseling. *Human Genetics* **91**: 373–6.

Breslow, N., Beckwith, J.B., Ciol, M. and Sharples, K. 1988. Age distribution of Wilms' Tumor: Report from the National Wilms' Tumor Study. *Cancer Research* **48**: 1653–7.

Breslow, N., Olshan, A., Beckwith J.B. and Green, D.M. 1993. Epidemiology of Wilms' Tumor. *Medical and Pediatric Oncology* **21**: 172–81.

Breslow, N.E., Takashima, J.R., Whitton J.A., Moksness, J., D'Angio, G.J. and Green, D.M. 1995. Second malignant neoplasms following treatment for Wilms' tumor: a report from the National Wilms' Tumor Study Group. *Journal of Clinical Oncology* **13**: 1851–9.

Brodeur, G.M. 1995. Genetics of embryonal tumours of childhood: retinoblastoma, Wilms' tumour and neuroblastoma. *Cancer Survey* **25**: 67–99.

Coppes, M.J., Campbell, C.E. and Williams, B.R.G. 1993. The role of WT1 in Wilms' tumorigenesis. *FASEB Journal* **7**: 886–95.

Craft, A.W., Parker, L., Stiller, C. and Cole, M. 1995. Screening for Wilms' tumour in patients with aniridia, Beckwith syndrome, or hemihypertrophy. *Medical and Pediatric Oncology* **24**: 231–4.

De Silva, D.C., Wright, M.F., Stevenson, D.A.J. et al. 1996. Cranial desmoid tumour associated with homozygous inactivation of the APC gene in a 2-year old girl with familial adenomatous polyposis. *Cancer* **77**: 972–6.

Derry, J.M., Ochs, H.D. and Francke, U. 1994. Isolation of a novel gene mutated in Wiskott-Aldrich syndrome. *Cell* **78**: 635–44.

Diller, L., Sexsmith, E., Gottlieb, A., Li, F.P. and Malkin, D. 1995. Germline p53 mutations are frequently detected in young children with rhabdomyosarcoma. *Journal of Clinical Investigation* **95**: 1606–11.

Draper, G.J., Sanders, B.M. and Kingston, J.E. 1986. Second primary neoplasms in patients with retinoblastoma. *British Journal of Cancer* **53**: 661–71.

Draper, G.J., Sanders, B.M., Brownbill, P.A. and Hawkins, M.M. 1992. Patterns of risk of hereditary retinoblastoma and applications to genetic counselling. *British Journal of Cancer* **66**: 211–19.

Draper, G.M., Sanders, B.M., Lennox, E.L., and Brownbill, P.A. 1996. Patterns of childhood cancer among siblings. *British Journal of Cancer* **74**: 152–8.

Eeles, R.A. 1995. Germline mutation in the TP53 gene. *Cancer Survey* **25**: 101–24.

Evans, D.R.G., Farndon, P.A., Burnell, L.D., Gattamaneni, R. and Birch, J.M. 1991. The incidence of Gorlin syndrome in 173 consecutive cases of medulloblastoma. *British Journal of Cancer* **64**: 959.

Fantes, J.A., Bickmore, W.A., Fletcher, J.M., Ballesta, F., Hanson, I.M. and Van-Heyningen, V. 1992. Submicroscropic deletions at the WAGR locus, revealed by nonradioactive in situ hybridization. *American Journal of Human Genetics* **51**: 1286–94.

Farndon, P.A., Morris, D.J., Hardy, C., McConville, C.M., Weisenbach, J., Kilpatric, M. and Reis, A. 1994. Analysis of 133 meioses places the genes for nevoid basal cell carcinoma (Gorlin) syndrome and Fanconi anemia group C in a 2.6-cM interval and contributes to the fine map of 9q22.3. *Genomics* **23**: 486–9

Felix, C.A., Nau, M.M., Takahashi, T. et al. 1992. Hereditary and acquired p53 gene mutations in childhood acute lymphoblastic leukemia. *Journal of Clinical Investigation* **89**: 640–7.

Gallie, B.L., Squire, J.A., Goddard, A. et al. 1990. Mechanism of oncogenesis in retinoblastoma. *Laboratory Investigation* **62**: 394–408.

Gessler, M., Koing, A., Arden, K. et al. 1994. Infrequent mutation of the WT1 gene in 77 Wilms' tumours. *Human Mutations* **3**: 212–22.

Greenberg, F., Copeland, K. and Gresik, M.V. 1988. Expanding the spectrum of the Perlman syndrome. *American Journal of Medical Genetics* **29**: 773–6.

Hahn, H., Wicking, C., Zaphiropoulos, P.G. et al. 1996. Mutations of the human homolog of Drosophila *patched* in the nevoid basal cell carcinoma syndrome. *Cell* **85**: 841–51.

Hastie, N.D. 1994. The genetics of Wilms' tumour. A case of disrupted development. *Annual Review of Genetics* **28**: 523–58.

Hawkins, M.M. 1994. Pregnancy outcome and offspring after childhood cancer. *British Medical Journal* **309**: 1034.

Hawkins, M.M., Winter, D.L., Burton, H.S. and Potok, M.H., 1995. Heritability of Wilms' tumor. *Journal of the National Cancer Institute* **87**: 1323–4.

Henry, I. Bonaiti-Pelie, C., Chehensse, V., Beldjord, C., Schwartz, C., Utermann, G. and Junien, C. 1991. Uniparental paternal disomy in a genetic cancer-predisposing syndrome. *Nature* **351**: 665–7.

Hersh, J.H., Cole, T.R., Blom, A.S., Bertolone, S.J., Huges, H.E. 1992. Risk of malignancy in Sotos syndrome. *Journal of Pediatrics* **120**: 572–4.

Hoovers, J.M.N., Kalikin, L.M., Johnson, L.A. et al. 1995. *Proceedings of the National Academy of Sciences, USA* **92**: 12456–60.

Huff, V., Miwa, H., Haber, D.A., Call, K.M., Housman, D., Strong, L.C. and Saunders, G.F. 1991. Evidence for WT1 as a Wilms' tumour (WT) gene: intragenic germinal deletion in bilateral WT. *American Journal of Medical Genetics* **48**: 997–1003.

Hughes, L.J. and Michels, V.V. 1992. Rick of hepatoblastoma in familial adenomatous polyposis. *American Journal of Medical Genetics* **43**: 1023–5.

Jacks, T., Fazeli, A., Schmitt, E.M., Bronson, R.T., Goodell, M.A. and Weinberg, R.A. 1992. Effects of an *Rb* mutation in the mouse. *Nature* **359**: 295–300.

Joenje, H., Mathew, C. and Gluckman, E. 1995. Fanconi Anaemia research : current status and prospects. *European Journal of Cancer* **31A**: 268–72.

Johnson, R.L., Rothman, A.L., Xie, J. et al. 1996. Human homolog of *patched*, a candidate gene for the basal cell nevus syndrome. *Science* **272**: 1668–71.

King-Underwood L., Renshaw, J. and Pritchard-Jones, K. 1996. Mutations in the Wilms' tumour gene WT1 in leukaemias. *Blood* **87**: 2171–9.

Klugbauer, S., Lengfelder, E., Demidchik, E.P. and Rabes, H.M. 1995. High prevalence of RET rearrangement in thyroid tumors of children from Belarus after the Chernobyl reactor accident. *Oncogene* **11**: 2459–67.

Knudson, A.G. Jr. and Strong, L.C. 1972. Mutation and cancer: a model for Wilms' tumour of the kidney. *Journal of the National Cancer Institute* **40**: 313–24.

Koufos, A., Grundy, P., Morgan, K. et al. 1989. Familial Wiedemann–Beckwith syndrome and a second Wilms' tumor locus both map to 11p15.5. *American Journal of Human Genetics* **44**: 711–19.

Kreidberg, J.A., Sariola, H., Loring, J.M., Maeda, M., Pelletier, J., Housman, D. and Jaenisch, R. 1993. WT1 is required for early kidney development. *Cell* **74**: 679–91.

Kurahashi, H.,Takami, K., Oue, T. et al. 1995. Biallelic inactivation of the APC gene in hepatoblastoma. *Cancer Research* **55**: 5007–11.

Kushner, B.H., Gilbert, F. and Helson, L. 1986. Familial neurobalstoma. *Cancer* **57**: 1887–93.

Levitt, G.A., Stiller, C.A. and Chessells, J.M. 1990. Prognosis of Down's Syndrome with acute leukaemia. *Archives of Disease in Childhood* **65**: 212–16.

Liu, B., Farrington, S.M., Petersen, G.M. et al. 1995. Genetic instability occurs in the majority of young patients with colorectal cancer. *Nature Medicine* **1**: 348–52.

Mahmoud, H.H., Ridge, S.A., Behm, F.G., Pui, C.H., Ford, A.M., Raimondi, S.C. and Greaves, M.F. 1995. Intrauterine monoclonal origin of neonatal concordant acute lymphoblastic leukemia in monozygotic twins. *Medical Pediatric Oncology* **24**: 77–81.

Malkin, D., Jolly, K.W., Barbier, N. et al. 1992. Germline mutations of the p53 tumor suppressor gene in children and young adults with second malignant neoplasms. *New England Journal of Medicine* **326**: 1309–15.

Matsunaga, E. 1981. Genetics of Wilms' Tumour. *Human Genetics* **57**: 231–46.

Maw, M.A., Grundy, P.E., Millow, L.J., et al. 1992. A third Wilms' tumor locus on chromosome 16q. *Cancer Research* **52**: 3094–8.

McIntyre, J.F., Smith-Sorensen, B., Friend, S.H. et al. 1994. Germline mutations of the p53 tumor suppressor gene in children with osteosarcoma. *Journal of Clinical Oncology* **12**: 925–30.

Mori, P.G., Haupt, R., Fugazza, G., Sessarego, A.,C., Strigini, P. and Sansone, R. 1992. Pentasomy 21 in leukemia complicating Diamond–Blackfan anemia. *Cancer Genetics and Cytogenetics* **63**: 70–2.

Moss, T.J., Strauss, L.C., Das, L. and Feig, S.A. 1989. Secondary leukaemia following successful treatment of Wilms' tumour. *American Journal of Pediatric Hematology and Oncology* **11**: 158–61.

Narod, S.A. 1994. Genetics of breast and ovarian cancer. *British Medical Bulletin* **50**: 656–76.

Narod, S.A., Stiller, C. and Lenoir, G.M., 1991. An estimate of the heritable fraction of childhood cancer. *British Journal of Cancer* **63**: 993–9.

Ogawa, O., Eccles, M.R., Szeto, J. et al. (1993). Relaxation of insulin-like growth factor II gene imprinting implicated in Wilms' tumour. *Nature* **362**: 749–51.

Olson, J.M., Hamilton, A. and Breslow, N.E. 1995. Non-11p constitutional chromosome abnormalities in Wilms' tumor patients. *Medical and Pediatric Oncology* **24**: 305–9.

Onadim, Z., Mitchell, C.D., Rutland, P.C. et al. 1990. Application of intragenic DNA probes in prenatal screening for retinoblastoma gene carriers in the United Kingdom. *Archives of Disease in Childhood* **65**: 651–6

Onadim, Z., Hogg, A., Baird, P.N. and Cowell, J.K. 1992a. Oncogenic point mutations in exon 20 of the RB1 gene in families showing incomplete penetrance and mild expression of the retinoblastoma phenotype. *Proceedings of the National Academy of Sciences, USA* **89**: 6177–81.

Onadim, Z., Hungerford, J. and Cowell, J.K. 1992b. Follow-up of retinoblastoma patients having prenatal and perinatal predictions for mutant gene carrier status using intragenic polymorphic probes from the RB1 gene. *British Journal of Cancer* **65**: 711–16.

Pardee, A.B. 1989. G1 events and regulation of cell proliferation. *Science* **246**: 603–8.

Park, S., Schalling, M., Bernard, A. et al. 1993. The Wilms' tumour gene WT1 is expressed in murine mesoderm-derived tissues and mutated in a human mesothelioma. *Nature Genetics* **4**: 415–20.

Parkin, D.M., Stiller, C.A., Draper, G.J., Bieber, C.A., Terracini, B. and Young, J.L. (Eds.). 1988. *International Incidence of Childhood Cancer*. IARC Scientific Publications No.87.

Pastore, G., Carli, M., Lemerle, J. et al. 1988. Epidemiological features of Wilms' tumor: results of studies by the international society of pediatric oncology (SIOP). *Medical and Pediatric Oncology* **16**: 7–11.

Pennisi, E. 1996. Gene linked to commonest cancer. *Science* **272**: 1583–4.

Pilia, G., Hughes-Benzie, R. M., MacKenzie, A. et al. 1996. Mutations in GPC3, a glypican gene, cause the Simpson–Golabi–Behmel overgrowth syndrome. *Nature Genetics* **12**: 241–7.

Ping, A.J., Reeve, A.E., Law, D.J.,Young, M.R., Boehnke, M. and Feinberg, A.P. 1989. Genetic linkage of Beckwith–Wiedemann syndrome to 11p15. *American Journal of Human Genetics* **44**: 720–3.

Pritchard-Jones, K. and Hastie, N.D. 1990. Wilms' tumour as a paradigm for the relationship of cancer to development. *Cancer Surveys* **9**: 555–78.

Pritchard-Jones, K., Fleming, S., Davidson, D. et al. 1990. The candidate Wilms' tumour gene is involved in genitourinary development. *Nature* **346**: 194–7.

Rahman, N., Arbour, L., Tonin, P. et al. 1996. Evidence for a familial Wilms' tumour gene (FWT1) on chromosome 17q12-q21. *Nature Genetics* **13**: 461–3.

Sacchi, N. 1992. Down syndrome and chromosome 21 abnormalities in leukaemia. *Baillieres Clinics in Haematology* **5**: 815–31.

Sameshima, Y., Tsunematsu, Y., Watanabe, S. et al. 1992. Detection of novel germ-line p53 mutations in diverse cancer prone families identified by selecting patients with childhood adrenocortical carcinoma. *Journal of the National Cancer Institute* **84**: 703–7.

Sanders, B.M., Jay, M., Draper, G.J., and Roberts, E.M. 1989. Non-ocular cancer in relatives of retinoblastoma patients. *British Journal of Cancer* **60**: 358–65.

Schmitt, K., Zabel, B., Tulzer, G., Eitelberger, F. and Pelletier, J. 1995. Nephropathy with Wilms' tumour or gonadal dysgenesis: incomplete Denys–Drash syndrome or separate diseases? *European Journal of Pediatrics* **154**: 577–81.

Sicinski, P., Donaher, J.L., Parker, S.B. et al. 1995. Cyclin D1 provides a link between development and oncogenesis in the retina and breast. *Cell* **82**: 621–30.

Sotelo-Avila, C., Gonzalez-Crussi, F. and Fowler, J.W. 1980. Complete and incomplete forms of Beckwith–Wiedemann syndrome: their oncogenic potential. *Journal of Pediatrics* **96**: 47–50.

Stay, E.J. and Vawter, G. 1977. The relationship between nephroblastoma and neurofibromatosis (Von Recklinghausen's disease). *Cancer* **39**: 2550–5.

Steenman, M.J.C., Rainier, S., Dobry, C.J. et al. 1994. Loss of imprinting of 1GF2 is linked to reduced expression and abnormal methylation of H19 in Wilms' tumour. *Nature Genetics* 7: 433–9.

Stiller, C., 1994a. Population based survival rates for childhood cancer in Britain 1980–91. *British Medical Journal* 309: 1612–16.

Stiller, C.A., Chessells, J.M. and Fitchett, M. 1994b. Neurofibromatosis and childhood leukaemia/lymphoma: A population-based UKCCSG study. *British Journal of Cancer* 5: 969–72.

Strathdee, C.A., Duncan, A.M.V. and Buchwald, M., 1992a. Evidence for at least four Fanconi anaemia genes including FACC on chromosome 9. *Nature Genetics* 1: 196–8.

Strathdee, C.A., Gavish, H., Shannon WR. and Buchwald, M. 1992b. Cloning of cDNAs for Fanconi's anaemia by functional complementation. *Nature* 356: 763-767. (Correction 358: p. 434.)

Szabo, J., Heath, B., Hill, V.M. et al. 1995. Hereditary hyperparthyroidism-jaw tumor sundrome: The endocrine tumor gene HRPT2 maps to chromsosome 1q21-q31. *American Journal of Human Genetics* 56: 944–50.

van Dijken, P.J. and Verwijs, W. 1995. Diamond-Blackfan anemia and malignancy. *Cancer* 76: 517–19.

Van Heyningen, V., Bickmore, W.A., Seawright, A. et al. 1990. Role for the Wilms' tumour gene in genital development? *Proceedings of the National Academy of Sciences, USA* 87: 5383–6.

Van Heyningen, V. 1994. Genetics. One gene – four syndromes. *Nature* 27: 319–20.

Varanasi, R., Bardeesy, N., Ghahremani, M. et al. 1994. Fine structure analysis of the WT1 gene in sporadic Wilms' tumour. *Proceedings of the National Academy of Sciences, USA* 91: 3554–8.

Villa, A., Notarangelo, L., Macchi, P. et al. 1995. X-Linked thrombocytopenia and Wiskott-Aldrich syndrome are allelic diseases with mutations in the WASP gene. *Nature Genetics* 9: 414–17.

Weinberg, R.A. 1995. The retinoblastoma protein and cell cycle control. *Cell* 81: 323–30.

Weinblatt, M.E., Scimeca, P., James-Herry, A., Sahdev, I. and Kochen, J. 1995. Transformation of congenital neutropenia into monosomy 7 and acute nonlymphoblastic leukemia in child treated with granulocyte colony-stimulating factor. *Journal of Pediatrics* 126: 263–5.

Williams, B.O., Schmitt, E.M., Remington, L., Bronson, R.T., Albert, D.M., Weinberg R.A. and Jack, T. 1994. Extensive contribution of *Rb*-deficient cells to adult chimeric mice with limited histopathological consequences. *EMBO Journal* 13: 4251–9.

Woods, W.G., Roloff, J.S., Lukens, J.N. and Krivit, W. 1981. The occurrence of leukemia in patients with the Shwachman syndrome. *Journal of Pediatrics* 99: 425–8.

20

Late-breaking developments

WILLIAM FOULKES AND SHIRLEY HODGSON

Summary

In this chapter we detail some advances that have occurred since the individual chapter authors submitted their manuscripts. We hope to convey details of some of the extraordinary discoveries that have taken place within the last year (i.e. 1997/8) or so by discussing the most notable findings. We stress that there have been important developments in the ethical and legal issues as well as in molecular genetics.

Chapter 2: Screening for cancer in high risk individuals – difficult problems to solve

In the past few years there has been increasing interest in developing 'consensus statements' pertaining to the management of hereditary cancer (Burke et al., 1977a,b). With regard to screening, one statement recommends that full colonoscopy should be offered to all unaffected family members from HNPCC (hereditary nonpolyposis colorectal cancer) kindreds, commencing at age 20 to 25 years, and that this should be repeated every one to three years (Burke et al., 1977b). The authors recommend this intervention on the basis of studies in HNPCC families (Järvinen et al., 1995), studies in the general population (Selby et al., 1992) and on expert opinion. However, many of the recommendations end with the comment that no randomized trials exist to answer these questions. It seems quite unlikely that randomized controlled trials of sufficient size will ever be conducted to answer all hereditary cancer management questions, and we may have to rely upon retrospective studies. For example, in answering the question of whether mammography is capable of detecting early breast cancers in *BRCA1* mutation carriers, existing national mammography data could be useful if it were possible to collect mutation and survival data on participants who, for example, developed interval cancers. However, a randomized trial, in high risk women, of clinical genetics referral with tailored mammographic surveillance and possible genetic testing versus standard care is underway in Wales. As this trial would be impossible in North America, its findings are awaited with great interest.

Chapters 3 to 6: Ethical, legal, social and genetic counselling issues – protecting the individual at risk

The extraordinary increases in knowledge of the inherited basis of a fraction of common cancers has naturally and properly led to concern that this information could be accessed and used by third parties, against the interests of those at increased risk. Indeed, the phrase 'genetic underclass' has become a well-worn cliché only a year or two after its first use. In the past two years, health agencies have increased research activity in these areas, now collectively referred to as ELSI (ethical, legal, social issues). Much of the research has been prompted by the discovery of 'cancer genes', since several highly-penetrant cancer susceptibility genes have been identified and in some populations, certain disease-associated mutations are particularly prevalent (Struewing et al., 1995; Oddoux et al., 1996; Roa et al., 1996).

In the US, over the past few years, 19 states have passed legislation protecting individuals against genetic discrimination, but the word 'genetic' is often interpreted somewhat narrowly. Now, the Kennedy–Kassebaum Law (the Health Insurance Portability and Accountability Act) prohibits insurance companies from denying health coverage based on an individual's medical history, including any genetic information. This law does not protect individuals working for an increasingly large group of 'self-insuring' employers (i.e. they pay directly for the medical costs resulting from illnesses arising in the workforce). Moreover, denial of insurance *per se* may be less of a problem than grossly elevated premiums, applied by insurance companies 'across the board' to those at high risk. In order to increase protection. Congresswoman Louise Slaughter (Democrat, New York) has introduced a bill, HR 306, that would extend protection by prohibiting health plans from insurance discrimination on the basis of current or future genetic information. President Clinton is proposing legislation of his own that would extend both HR 306 and the Kennedy–Kassebaum Law by banning the disclosure of genetic information unless the Secretary of Health and Human

Services deemed that disclosure might be necessary for biomedical research. President Clinton believes that the problem of increased premiums has also to be addressed. Differences in health insurance policies between Canada and the US might be expected to result in different uptake rates of genetic tests in otherwise rather comparable populations (Beardsley, 1996; Rosenblatt et al., 1996).

In the UK, the main issue is life, rather than medical insurance. The Association of British Insurers decided that genetic information likely to be detrimental to an applicant would not be taken into account if the life insurance policy was associated with a household mortgage of less than £100,000. For sums greater than this, the information could be used by the insurance companies if they so wished (Association of British Insurers, 1997). Clearly, if insurance companies are going to be permitted to use molecular genetic information at all, both positive and negative test results must be made available to them. Perhaps the best outcome from the debate would be an assurance payment based on income, rather than risk.

The Ashkenazi Jewish population has recently been intensively studied regarding breast, ovary and colorectal cancer genes (see below). This has occurred almost entirely because of the relative reproductive isolation of the population and the presence of founder effects, rather than for any nefarious reason. Many of the leading researchers in the field are themselves Ashkenazi Jewish. However, given the extraordinarily poor record of geneticists and scientists in protecting the interests of their research subjects and patients (Kelves, 1985; Muller-Hill, 1988), it is entirely understandable that real concerns as to the wisdom of co-operating in genetic research have now been raised (Lehrman, 1997). It is likely that dialogue between community representatives and officials and scientists at the National Human Genome Research Institute (NHGRI) will now take place.

The more general issue of the information that a person should receive and understand before undergoing a cancer genetic test was recently the topic of a 'consensus statement' produced by the Cancer Genetics Studies Consortium (Geller et al., 1997). In essence, the consortium felt that there are significant barriers to truly informed consent to adult-onset cancer gene susceptibility testing and that consent should be a multi-step process. This aim is laudable, but at present it is difficult to see how it can be met within existing resources. Many more resources (manpower, educational aids, etc.) will be required to ensure that the decision-making process is as informed as possible. Nevertheless, it is clear that informed consent issues have come increasingly to the forefront of clinicians' and researchers' minds over the last two years, and this document outlines the process and content of informed consent in a detailed manner. A more practical approach was set out in a 'position paper' from the National Society of Genetic Counselors (USA), which was published after two years of deliberation. It provides a series of recommendations for professionals considering offering clinical genetic testing for late-onset adult disorders. The document does not state that genetic testing should only be carried out in the context of an IRB-approved research protocol (McKinnon et al., 1997).

There has been a huge debate about the topic of informed consent in the pages of the *British Medical Journal* (see for example, the issues of 12 April and 26 July 1997). One of the issues raised by the *British Medical Journal* is whether they should publish research that does not include fully informed consent as part of the research protocol. The whole debate on informed consent, from the perspective of cancer genetics research is very important, as pathology departments around the world have thousands of tissue blocks that could be used to study the presence or absence of cancer gene mutations, and correlate these findings with clinicopathological findings and vital status, providing much sought-after information. Obtaining informed consent for all individuals may be neither possible nor desirable. However, the interests of the research subjects must be paramount. One relevant question is whether a person is harmed by having a research test unknowingly performed on tissue removed at operation in such a fashion that the result is not directly linked to the patient's name. Historically, the collective answer has been 'No'. Now, the answer is less certain.

Chapters 7 and 8: Finding genes and mutations

Technical and statistical advances now make it easier than ever to locate cancer genes and identify mutations in them. For example, a possible way of speeding up the identification of new genes is suggested by the recent application of comparative genomic hybridization (CGH) in sporadic breast cancer (Tirkkonen et al., 1997). The findings led the investigators to speculate the *BRCA2* might have been identified by the high frequency of loss of heterozygosity at this locus seen in breast cancers occurring in women carrying *BRCA2* mutations. By mapping CGH patterns seen in *BRCA1*- and BRCA2-related tumours, it may be possible to compare the patterns seen in other, apparently unlinked families.

Elevated, but discordant regions of loss of heterozygosity in these latter breast cancer families might point to the position of a new locus. This could then be tested in a panel of families. This approach was successfully used to locate the Peutz–Jeghers gene (see Chapter 9).

Chapter 9: Cancers of the digestive tract – new genes, mutations and modifiers

In the January 1997 issue of *Nature Genetics*, a susceptibility locus for Peutz–Jeghers syndrome (PJS) was localized to chromosome 19 using comparative genomic hybridization and subsequent linkage analysis in PJS families (see above). With a pleasing symmetry, one year later, *Nature* and *Nature Genetics* have published papers identifying mutations in PJS families in the same gene (Hemminki et al., 1998; Jenne et al., 1998). Unusually, the two papers are derived from work carried out by a single consortium based in Helsinki. The PJS gene is a serine–threonine kinase, which had been previously identified and named *LKB1* but had not been mapped. The segregating mutations identified were deletions predicted to cause truncation of the encoded protein, acceptor splice site mutations and non-truncating mutations not identified in control populations. Cancer-causing mutations in kinases are classically activated by mutations. For example, dominantly-inherited disorders such as multiple endocrine neoplasia type 2 (MEN2) and familial papillary renal cell cancer are caused by activating mutations in the tyrosine kinases *RET* and *MET* respectively (see below). Fascinatingly, in PJS, the mutations in *LKB1* are clearly inactivating. From this and other data, *LKB1* is probably acting as a tumour suppressor gene and is the first cancer susceptibility gene that is known to have its effect by loss of kinase activity.

A novel type of mutation causing an increased susceptibility to colorectal cancer (CRC) was recently uncovered in an Ashkenazi Jewish man with eight colorectal adenomas and a family history of CRC. He was found to have a germline missense *APC* mutation (I1307K). However, protein truncation test assays (see Chapter 8) showed that there were several truncated proteins formed in vitro, which were not detected in lymphocytes from the patient, and thus was an in vitro phenomenon. The mechanism for such instability in *APC* appears to be 'slippage' during replication due to the conversion of an AAATAAAA sequence to (A)8, resulting in gains or losses of repeat units during replication. This polymorphism is frequently found in the Ashkenazi Jewish population (6%), but as yet not in other populations, and the detection of the potential pathogenic effects of an apparently 'benign' variant in *APC* raises the question about such an effect in other variants in cancer susceptibility genes (Laken et al., 1997).

Very recently, a new locus underlying autosomal dominant colorectal cancer susceptibility with variable numbers of colorectal adenomas has been identified by linkage analysis supplemented by loss of heterozygosity studies in tumours in a single large family. This putative susceptibility gene has been named *CRAC1*, for colorectal adenoma and carcinoma, and maps to 15q14-q22 (I.P.M. Tomlinson, pers. comm., 1998).

One of the important questions in the expression of hereditary cancer susceptibilty is the genetic influences on gene expression. A study of mice with the inherited Min locus causing the mouse model of familial adenomatous polyposis – FAP (i.e. with germline *apc* mutations) – has shown that mice bred to inherit the *Mom1* gene have significantly reduced numbers of intestinal adenomas compared with those without. In a recent experiment, a plasmid containing the *Pla2g2a* gene was introduced into an Apc^{min}/+ background. Mice overexpressing *Pla2g2a* had a significant reduction in tumour load, which was dose-dependent, and was similar to the effect of introducing a resistance allele of *Mom1* (Cormier et al., 1997). Thus *Mom1* is probably *Pla2g2a*, which encodes a secretory phospholipase A2, involved in the prostaglandin synthesis pathway. However, inhibition of adenoma formation by phospholipases may not be mediated by prostaglandins, as might be expected, as *Pla2g2a* produces a COX-2 lipid substrate (cyclooxygenase 1 and 2 catalyse the conversion of arachidonic acid to prostaglandin H2) and would be expected to have a positive effect on polyp formation. This is so because *apc* null mice also null for COX-2 have fewer and smaller adenomas than mice with *apc* mutations alone (Oshima et al., 1996). COX-2 inhibitors have a similar effect on *apc* null mice, and are exceptionally promising candidates as CRC prevention agents.

Our understanding of colorectal carcinogenesis in HNPCC families has progressed. In a recent study of hMSH2-deficient tumour cell lines, no increased frequency of mutations was detectable in cell lines growing actively with no increase in cell density, but there was an accumulation of mutations in cells growing at increased density. This indicates that the development of mutations in mismatch repair-deficient cell lines only overcomes the normal cellular checkpoints when cells are growing in stressed conditions of impaired nutrition and oxygenation (Richards et al., 1997). Fibroblasts also show a similar phenomenon (Reimair et al., 1997).

How common is HNPCC? This important epidemiological question appears to be approaching resolution. Two papers – from Manchester, in the UK and Orange County, in California, USA – show convincingly that when individuals are ascertained systematically through hospital or population-based registries, families that fit the Amsterdam criteria are rare, comprising certainly not more than 2% of all CRC. Interestingly, in a sample of 10 of the Californian families, only half were RER+ and had mismatch repair gene mutations, further suggesting that some 'Amsterdam positive' families are either due to other genes or are chance accumulations (Evans et al., 1997; Peel et al., 1997). However, some families that do not fit the Amsterdam criteria may contain mutations in mismatch repair genes. In 1995, mutations in another mismatch repair gene, *GTBP/MSH6* were identified in sporadic CRCs (Papadopoulos et al., 1995). These mutations tend to occur in mononucleotide tracts. Germ-line mutations have now been identified in two Japanese patients with CRC (Akiyama et al., 1997; Miyaki et al., 1997), both with a positive family history that did not fit the Amsterdam criteria for HNPCC (the ages of onset of colorectal cancer appeared to be slightly older and there was a predominance of extra-colonic cancers). Undoubtedly, there will be more CRC predisposition genes identified.

It seems possible to live with two germ-like *MLH1* mutations, as a woman has recently been found to be a compound heterozygote for two *MLH1* missense mutations (Hackman et al., 1997). Interestingly, she developed breast cancer at 35 years of age and has no colonic tumours at age 45 and unlike the knockout mice, is fertile and has two children. It is probable that the fact she has two missense, rather than nonsense or frameshift mutations is relevant to the phenotype. It may be of relevance that, as discussed in Chapter 9, individuals with germ-line *MLH1* mutations who develop CRC have a better five-year survival than individuals with apparently sporadic CRC.

Finally, controversy exists as to whether or not the gene for juvenile polyposis coli (JPC) has been identified. Previous linkage information had indicated that the JPC locus mapped to distal chromosome 10q, making *PTEN*, the gene mutated in Cowden disease and Bannayan–Zonana syndrome, an attractive candidate. Lynch et al. (1997) found a nonsense *PTEN* mutation in one family with features of both CD and JPC. The phenotype of JPC families without *PTEN* mutations was not discussed. In addition, a French team has identified one truncating mutation and one missense mutation in *PTEN* in two individuals with apparently sporadic JPC (Olschwang et al., 1998). The difficulty is that the convincing truncating mutation was identified in a male who first presented with symptoms at age 74. Although 15% of JPC cases can present in adulthood, the age at diagnosis is problematic in this case, especially as there is no family history of JPC. The other affected individual was more convincingly diagnosed with JPC at age seven, but again there is no family history and the mutation could possibly represent a rare polymorphism. However, JPC may be genetically heterogenous, as most JPC families appeared to be linked to a locus distal to *PTEN*. A recent study showed that 18 of 23 JPC patients examined clinically and radiologically had significant extracolonic abnormalities. Of these, two had Bannayan–Riley–Ruvalcaba syndrome, two had Gorlin syndrome and one had hereditary haemorrhagic telangiectasia (HHT). A further four patients had some features of these conditions, suggesting that some individuals with JPC may have well-recognized genetic syndromes, and that in these patients germline mutations may be detectable. Currently, no mutations have been identified in *PTEN*, *PTC* or in HHT genes *ENG* and *ANK-1* in these families (Desai et al., 1998).

Chapter 10: Cancers of the breast, ovary and uterus – *BRCA1, 2* and *3*?

There has been an enormous amount of work carried out in the last year on *BRCA1* and *BRCA2*. In addition, the search for a third breast cancer gene has begun. A single issue of the *American Journal of Human Genetics* (May 1997) contained eight full papers, four letters, and an editorial devoted to mutation frequencies of *BRCA1* and *BRCA2* in different populations. Several founder mutations (other than the previously-reported Ashkenazi Jewish mutations) have now been identified. In particular, a large proportion of Swedish and Dutch families can be explained by a single founder mutation in each country, and virtually all hereditary breast cancer in Iceland is due to one mutation, 999del5 in *BRCA2*. By contrast, most of the mutations identified in Italy are unique, reflecting the city-state political structure that existed in Italy for many generations.

An important question for women at risk is, 'How likely am I to carry a *BRCA1* mutation given my personal and family history?' Two papers have addressed this question, both studying high-risk populations. Myriad Genetics tested 798 probands from families with numerous cases of breast and/or ovarian cancer. They identified 102 disease-associated mutations, 24 of which had not been previously reported. In 71 Ashkenazi Jewish women who were tested, only two different mutations were detected (185delAG and 5382insC). A multivariate model was created, which enabled the authors to determine the most important factors in considering whether a woman is likely to carry a *BRCA1* mutation (Shattuck-Eidens et al., 1997). The three most discriminating features were: (1) proband's age at diagnosis of breast or ovarian cancer (the odds of carrying a mutation decrease by 8% for each year added to the year of diagnosis, so for example, a risk of 20% becomes 18.4% if the diagnosis is made a year later); (2) The number of relatives with ovarian cancer but not breast cancer; and (3) Ashkenazi Jewish descent (about three times more likely to carry *BRCA1* mutations). Of note was the relative unimportance of the number of relatives with breast cancer, confirming previous studies carried out in the Ashkenazim. Very similar results were achieved in a smaller, clinic-based study from Philadelphia (Couch et al., 1997).

A study from England suggested that mutations in *BRCA1* in sporadic ovarian cancer were rather uncommon (only 3% of cases had mutations; Stratton et al., 1997). But recent data from Ontario show that mutations are more common, particularly in the serous papillary type, where 14.1% of cases had mutations in *BRCA1* or *BRCA2*. Just over 4% of women with ovarian cancer who had no first-degree relatives with breast or ovarian cancer had mutations (S.A. Narod and colleagues, unpub. data).

For those who have mutations, there are several pressing questions, for example, 'What are my risks of cancer and how do the cancers behave?' Initial data from linkage studies showed that the risks to age 70 for breast cancer for *BRCA1* carriers was about 85% and for ovarian cancer, 45%. Risks from population-based studies are likely to be lower. By studying 5000 Ashkenazi Jewish volunteers, it has been demonstrated that the risks of breast and ovarian cancer may be lower in the absence of a strong family history (Struewing et al., 1997), but it has been pointed out that in fact, the linkage data and population data have overlapping confidence intervals (Easton, 1997). There may be risk modifiers that explain the observed differences. Some of these may be genetic, such as HRAS, but interest has focused on hormonal and reproductive factors that might modify risk. A small study recently suggested that *BRCA1* mutation carriers who were oral contraceptive pill (OCP) users were more likely to develop breast cancer than carriers who were non-users (Ursin et al., 1997). This preliminary observation requires confirmation, because the OCP appears to be strongly protective against ovarian cancer in the very same women! (S.A. Narod, pers. comm., 1997.) Hereditary breast cancers are distinct from their sporadic counterparts. Early work had indicated that *BRCA1*-positive breast cancers were high grade. These findings were confirmed and extended in a large collaborative study from the UK (Lakhani et al., 1997), where it was found that *BRCA1*- and *BRCA2*-associated breast cancers were significantly more likely to be high grade than age-matched controls, although the difference was of borderline significance for *BRCA2* tumours. Medullary carcinomas were significantly more commonly seen in *BRCA1*-mutation carriers than in *BRCA2* mutation carriers or controls. Ductal carcinoma in situ (DCIS) was less commonly seen in *BRCA1* mutation carriers than in controls, and lobular carcinoma in situ was under-represented in familial cancers when *BRCA1* and *BRCA2* cases were combined. It has also been shown that *BRCA1* mutation-positive breast cancers are overwhelmingly oestrogen receptor (ER) negative (Jóhannsson et al., 1997b; Karp et al., 1997; Tirkkonen et al., 1997), but the TP53 status of *BRCA1* mutation-positive tumours is less certain. *BRCA2*-related breast cancers are more likely to be ER+ than *BRCA1*-positive tumours (Jóhannsson et al., 1997b; Karp et al., 1997). Finally, do these poor prognostic factors translate to a poorer survival? Prognostic studies performed using families that were thought to have a high probability of carrying mutations in breast cancer genes (before the genes were identified) indicated a better prognosis for hereditary breast cancer, and recent studies indicate *BRCA1*- related hereditary ovarian cancer has a better prognosis than sporadic ovarian cancer (Rubin et al., 1996), although some data point in the other direction for both ovarian (Brunet et al., 1997; Jóhannsson et al., 1997a) and breast cancer (Foulkes et al., 1997). Cohort studies will be required to definitvely answer the question.

Mice with a disrupted exon 5 and 6 of *Brca1* on one chromosome and a normal *Brca1* allele on the other, were normal, fertile, and lack tumours to age 11 months. However, mice that were homozygous null died before day 7.5 of embryogenesis, showing reduced cellular proliferation with overexpression of the cyclin-dependent kinase inhibitor P21. The authors explained the findings as a failure of proliferative burst (Hakem et al., 1996). Very similar results were seen when *Brca2* was knocked out (albeit resulting in a slightly milder phenotype) and there was partial rescue of the phenotype by crossing the mice with *P53* or *P21* null mice, suggesting some of the effects of BRCA1 may be mediated via the P53/P21 regulation of the cell cycle (Hakem et al., 1997; Ludwig et al., 1997; Sharan et al., 1997; Suzuki et al., 1997). The localization of the BRCA1 protein has been the subject of much debate, but it now appears to have a nuclear/ perinuclear localization, in endoplasmic reticulum/golgi-derived structures (Coene et al., 1997). This is supported by evidence that the protein encoded by *BRCA1* has the properties of a transcription factor, and transactivates expression of P21 independently of P53. In P21-competent human cancer cell lines, BRCA1 inhibits cell-cycle progression into S-phase in human cancer cells (Somasundaram et al., 1997). Both BRCA1 and BRCA2 interact directly or indirectly with RAD51 (Mizuta et al., 1997; Scully et al., 1997; Sharan et al., 1997), a protein implicated in maintaining genome integrity through repair of double-strand DNA breaks. Therefore, these two genes may act as 'caretakers' rather than rate-limiting 'gatekeepers' in the current argot (Kinzler and Vogelstein, 1997).

Chapter 11: Cancers of the kidney and urothelial tract – MET and *TSC1*

One of the most interesting findings during 1997 is the identification of *MET* as the gene for familial papillary renal carcinoma. As might be guessed from its name, *MET* is from the same tyrosine kinase gene family as *RET* (see Chapter 16) and mutations have been identified in codons homologous to those commonly mutated in MEN2 and variants. As the mutations are missense mutations and are not accompanied by loss of heterozygosity, it is likely that *MET* is acting as a dominant oncogene and thus is the second clearly dominant cancer susceptibility gene to be identified (Schmidt et al., 1997).

Our understanding of the genetic aetiology of renal cancer has continued with the identification of the tuberous sclerosis (TS) gene, *TSC1* on chromosome 9q34, completing the molecular characterization of TS that began with the identification of *TSC2* (on chromosome 16p13) in 1993. About half of TS families are due to *TSC1* and half to *TSC2*. The *TSC1* gene encodes hamartin, a novel protein without homologies, and in particular no homology to the *TSC2* product. Loss of heterozygosity (LOH) at the TSC2 locus in the associated hamartomas suggested that *TSC2* is a tumour suppressor gene, but the lack of LOH at 9q34 indicated that this might not be the case for *TSC1*. However, truncation mutations in *TSC1* have now been identified in over 30 individuals with TS and in one patient with a renal cell carcinoma, a somatic mutation in the wild-type allele accompanied a germ-like mutation. This and other data support the notion that *TSC1* is also a tumour suppressor gene (Vanslegtenhorst et al., 1997). The low frequency of LOH at *TSC1* may be accounted for by a high frequency of intragenic somatic mutations.

Chapter 12: Cancers of the prostate and testis – no easy solutions

Linkage analysis has recently confirmed the location of a prostate cancer susceptibility gene on chromosome 1q (Cooney et al., 1997). As in the original study, some of the linked families are of African–American descent, and are particularly large. These positive findings have not been confirmed by the Seattle, Mayo or Canadian/UK groups (McIndoe et al., 1997; Thibodeau et al., 1997; Eeles et al., 1998). There are several possible reasons why this is so, but the most convincing is that the linked families in the first report are large, multigenerational pedigrees, whereas most of the families collected by other groups are small. Secondly, the chromosome 1q-linked families have a mean age of diagnosis of less than 65 years of age (Grönberg et al., 1997), whereas few of the other families fitted this criteria. Because large, early-onset families are rare, it will be difficult to locate *HPC1* further by linkage alone. Fortunately, a new area of research into the causes of prostate cancer has been opened up by the finding that in a nested case-control study, plasma insulin-like growth factor I (IGF-I) levels were highly predictive of the subsequent occurrence of prostate cancer. Men in the highest quartile of IGF-I levels had a significantly elevated relative risk of 4.3 compared with men in the lowest quartile (Chan et al., 1998). It will now be important to study the genetic regulation of IGF-I levels in more detail.

The situation in cancer of the testis is even less clear. It now seems unlikely that there is one gene associated with a high risk of testicular cancer (Bishop et al., 1997). In fact, the International Testis Cancer Linkage Consortium reports that, assuming two genes are interacting multiplicatively, the majority of the genome has now been excluded as the site of these genes. The majority of the 100-plus families studied comprise two affected individuals only, and as with prostate cancer, linkage alone may not be enough to locate the putative genes.

Chapter 14: Malignant melanoma – are there other genes involved?

There have been a number of studies addressing the questions: (1) how common are *CDKN2A* mutations in melanoma families?; and (2) how broad is the phenotype associated with germ-line *CDKN2A* mutations? Firstly, germ-line *CDKN2A* mutations are not very common, even in families with several cases of cutaneous malignant melanoma (CMM). A large, comprehensive study from Australia has shown that the frequency of *CDKN2A* mutations in families with four, three, and two cases of CMM are roughly 15%, 10%, and 5% respectively (Mann et al., 1997). A similar study from Sweden found equivalent results – only 5 of 64 (7.8%) melanoma families with two or more first-degree relatives with CMM and dysplastic naevi (DN) had mutations in *CDKN2A* (Platz et al., 1997). In fact, four of the five mutations were identical and represent a previously-reported founder mutation (113insArg). The data from Australia could possibly be explained by the large number of phenocopies, but this seems an unlikely explanation for the low frequency seen in Swedish families. In keeping with these findings, only 6 out of 28 (21%) highly selected UK melanoma families had mutations in *CDKN2A* (Harland et al., 1997). Other plausible candidate genes such as *CDKN2B* and *CDK4* do not account for the families without mutations in *CDKN2A*. As familial melanoma is not particularly common (Cutler et al., 1996), it is now doubtful that *CDKN2A* has any important role in the prevention or diagnosis of CMM in the general population. The identity of other putative CMM/DN genes is unknown.

The second question, how broad is the phenotype, has not been completely answered. For example, there is debate as to whether pancreatic cancer seen in excess in some pedigrees is truly related to germ-line *CDKN2A* mutations. The balance of opinion is probably in favour of a causal relationship. However, a study of 67 multi-site cancer families without multiple cases of CMM indicated a limited role for *CDKN2A* mutations in families without at least one case of CMM (Sun, S. et al., 1997). So although *CDKN2A* is altered in a wide variety of cancers, there is a much more specific pattern of malignancy associated with germ-line mutations, as has been seen for other tumour suppressor genes, such as *P53*.

Chapter 15: Non-melanoma skin cancers – patched, sonic hedgehog and skin cancer

In this chapter, the story of patched (*Ptc*) and basal cell carcinoma (BCC) was left at the point where a significant proportion of sporadic BCCs were found to have mutations in *Ptc*. It had also been shown that patched is a sonic hedgehog (*Shh*) receptor, and overexpression of Shh can induce BCC in mice. Another gene, *Gli1*, originally identified as an overexpressed gene in glioma (hence *Gli1*) was known to be a target and mediator of Shh signalling. Now it has been shown that ectopic expression of *Gli1* can cause skin tumours in frogs, and *Gli1* is expressed in human BCCs (Dahmane et al., 1997). Since inactivation of Ptc and/or overexpression of Shh are not absolutely essential for BCC formation, *Gli1* expression may be a key event in BCC formation. The occurrence of BCCs in the field of radiotherapy of patients with Gorlin syndrome may be related to induction of *Gli1* and if so, this might have importance for attempts to prevent and treat BCCs occurring in this condition.

Chapter 16: Hereditary endocrine tumours – MEN1, Carney complex and goitre

The cloning of *MEN1* was the major event in this field in 1997. Interestingly, there is a variant of MEN1 in which prolactinomas predominate: a founder mutation, R460X in exon 10 of *MEN1*, has now been identified in families from the Burin Penninsula of Newfoundland (Green et al., 1997). Two other developments of note were the finding that Carney complex appears, surprisingly, to be genetically heterogeneous (Milunsky et al., 1997; Taymans et al., 1997); and the identification of the first locus for familial multinodular thyroid goitre, on chromosome 14q (Bignell et al., 1997).

Chapter 17: Tobacco-related cancers of the respiratory and upper aerodigestive tract – a role for α1-anti trypsin?

Generally, there has been little progress in the genetics of lung and other tobacco-related cancers. One possible avenue has been explored by researchers at the Mayo Clinic, in the US. They found a higher frequency (12.5%) of α1-anti-trypsin carriers (carrying the S or Z alleles) in lung cancer cases than would be expected by comparison with historical control frequencies reported (~ 2–4%) (Yang et al., 1997). However, selection of the correct control group will be crucial.

Chapter 18: Ataxia-telangiectasia – further news on cancer risk

Michael Swift's reports of an excess of breast cancer cases in the relatives of individuals with ataxia-telangiectasia (A-T) has generated an enormous amount of interest over the years. Recent mutation studies of *ATM* in early-onset breast cancer seem to have ruled out a large relative risk for breast cancer associated with a mutation in *ATM* (see Chapter

10), but the possibility of smaller risks, or larger risks in later-onset breast cancer have not been excluded. Recent studies from Malcolm Taylor's group add further weight to the possibility of a relationship – he describes two families with A-T where both heterozygous and homozygous females have developed breast cancer (one homozygous woman developed bilateral breast cancer in her mid-40s). Interestingly, the missense mutation results in an otherwise mild phenotype, and some of the affected women have had children (Stankovic et al., 1997). Perhaps the A-T and breast cancer story will be resolved when germ-line DNA from women diagnosed with breast cancer at a slightly older age (45–65 years) is analysed for *ATM* mutations.

One cancer that homozygous individuals do commonly develop is T cell prolymphocytic leukaemia (T-PLL) which in the general population is a late-onset, aggressive cancer with a median survival of eight months. It has now been shown that both copies of *ATM* are inactivated in some cases of sporadic T-PLL and one woman, diagnosed at the much younger-than-usual age of 45, probably has a germ-line *ATM* mutation, with inactivation of the other copy, suggesting that *ATM* is a tumour suppressor gene (Stoppa-Lyonnet et al., 1997).

Chapter 19: Childhood cancer – Beckwith–Wiedemann nearing resolution

There have been a number of key developments towards the understanding of the rare but fascinating childhood overgrowth and cancer predisposition disorder, Beckwith–Wiedemann syndrome (BWS). At the time of writing of this chapter, it was not clear what were the individual roles of two key genes, *IGF2* and *H19*. The roles of these, and two other genes, *CDKN1C* (also known as p57^{Kip2}) and *INS*, the insulin gene, (all of which are situated close to one another on chromosome 11p15.5) are now clearer. The central observation in BWS is that, in contrast to the usual situation, both alleles of *IGF2* are expressed (biallelic expression, or loss of imprinting). In some cases, both the alleles are derived from one parent. When this happens, it is the paternal allele that is duplicated (paternal uniparental disomy). Hence the maternal allele is normally silenced. Molecular and clinical analysis has confirmed that many, if not all the features of BWS can be explained by genetic alterations affecting one or more of these genes. Mutations in *CDKN1C* have been reported in familial and sporadic BWS (Hatada et al., 1996; O'Keefe et al., 1997) and recently Maher's group has demonstrated that exomphalos is more common in BWS cases with *CDKN1C* mutations than in those without, but interestingly, no BWS children with Wilms' tumour (WT) had *CDKN1C* mutations (Lam et al., 1997), and no *CDKN1C* mutations are reported in sporadic WT (O'Keefe et al., 1997). These findings fit with dramatic results from mouse experiments where *Cdkn1c* null mice develop omphalocele (similar to exomphalos), renal dysplasia, adrenal overgrowth, and bone defects (Yan et al., 1997; Zhang et al., 1997). More pieces have been added to the puzzle by the creation of a chimeric mouse which overexpresses *Igf2*. These mice have overgrowth of tissues normally affected by BWS, and levels of *Igf2* mirrored the size of the organ (Sun, F.-L. et al., 1997). So now it is clear that *IGF2* is indeed the key player in BWS, with biallelic expression being the commonest single cause of BWS. *H19* and *CDKN1C* may act partly or wholly through an IGF2 signalling pathway. An *IGF2*-independent *CDKN1C* effect is possibly limited to exomphalos alone (Reik and Maher, 1997) and dysregulation of *INS* may result in the hypoglycaemia seen in BWS.

Other recent developments of note include data suggesting that the familial WT gene on chromosome 17q may not be acting as a tumour suppressor gene, since the segregating (abnormal) allele was subject to loss of heterozygosity (LOH) in the tumour (Rahman et al., 1997). Most WTs are not hereditary. A recent study of sporadic WT has demonstrated that in some WT, many if not all of the histological components of the tumour (including striated muscle) show LOH at 11p13, the site of the *WT1* gene (Zhuang et al., 1997). Since *WT1* mutations are so uncommon in sporadic WT and are not seen in these tumours, it must be argued that LOH predates any *WT1* mutation. As a *WT1* mutation is not a necessary event for Wilms' tomourigenesis, 'two hits' at 11p13 may not be required for WT formation, but instead, the LOH is a more general, permissive phenomenon occurring in the abnormal tissues within which the tumour arises (S.A. Narod, pers. comm., 1997).

Acknowlegement

We thank Jennifer Ozaki, M.S. and Nora Wong, M.S. for helpful comments on earlier versions of the text.

References

Akiyama, Y., Sato, H., Yamada, T., Nagasaki, H., Tsuchiya, A., Abe, R. and Yusa, Y. (1997). Germ-line mutation of the HMSH6/GTBP gene in an atypical hereditary nonpolyposis colorectal cancer kindred. *Cancer Research* **57**: 3920–3.

Association of British Insurers (1997). *Information Sheet. Life Insurance and Genetics.* London: Association of British Insurers.

Beardsley, T. (1996). Vital data. *Scientific American* **274**: 100–5.

Bignell, G.R., Canzian, F., Shayeghi, M. et al. (1997). A familial non-toxic multinodular thyroid goiter locus maps to chromosome 14q but does not account for familial non-medullary thyroid cancer. *American Journal of Human Genetics* **61**: 1112–30.

Bishop, D.T., Rapley, E., Crockford, G. et al. (1997). Candidate regions for testicular cancer susceptibility genes: the results of two genomic searches. *American Journal of Human Genetics* **61S**: A268–1563.

Brunet, J.S., Narod, S.A., Tonin, P. and Foulkes, W.D. (1997). BRCA1 mutations and survival in women with ovarian cancer. *New England Journal of Medicine* **336**: 1256.

Burke, W., Daly, M., Garber, J. et al. (1997a). Recommendations for follow-up care of individuals with an inherited predisposition to cancer. II. BRCA1 and BRCA2. Cancer Genetics Studies Consortium. *JAMA* **277**: 997–1003.

Burke, W., Petersen, G., Lynch, P. et al. (1997b). Recommendations for follow-up care of individuals with an inherited predisposition to cancer. I. Hereditary nonpolyposis colon cancer. Cancer Genetics Studies Consortium. *JAMA* **277**: 915–19.

Chan, J.M., Stampfer, M.J., Giovannucci, E. et al. (1998). Plasma Insulin-like Growth Factor-I and prostate cancer risk: a prospective study. *Science* **279**: 563–6.

Coene, E., Van Oostveldt, P., Willems, K., van Emmelo, J. and De Potter, C.R. (1997). BRCA1 is localized in cytoplasmic tube-like invaginations in the nucleus. *Nature Genetics* **16**: 122–4.

Cooney, K.A., McCarthy, J.D., Lange, E. et al. (1997). Prostate cancer susceptibility locus on chromosome 1q: a confirmatory study. *Journal of the National Cancer Institute* **89**: 955–9.

Cormier, R.T., Hong, K.H., Halberg, R.B. et al. (1997). Secretory phospholipase Pla2g2a confers resistance to intestinal tumorigenesis. *Nature Genetics* **17**: 88–91.

Couch, F.J., DeShano, M.L., Blackwood, M.A. et al. (1997). BRCA1 mutations in women attending clinics that evaluate the risk of breast cancer. *New England Journal of Medicine* **336**: 1409–15.

Cutler, C., Foulkes, W.D., Brunet, J.S., Flanders, T. Y., Shibata, H. and Narod, S.A. (1996). Cutaneous malignant melanoma in women is uncommonly associated with a family history of melanoma in first-degree relatives: a case-control study. *Melanoma Research* **6**: 435–40.

Dahmane, N., Lee, J., Robins, P., Heller, P. and Altaba, A.R.I. (1997). Activation of the transcription factor GLI1 and the sonic hedgehog signalling pathway in skin tumours. *Nature* **389** 876–81.

Desai, D.C., Murday, V., Phillips, R.K.S., Neale, K.F., Milla, P., and Hodgson, S.V. (1998). A survey of phenotypic features in juvenile polyposis. *Journal of Medical Genetics.* (In press.)

Easton, D.F. (1997). Breast cancer genes – what are the real risks. *Nature Genetics* **16**: 210–11.

Eeles, R.A., Durocher, F., Edwards, S. et al. (1998). Does the hereditary prostate cancer gene, HPC1 contribute to a large proportion of familial prostate cancer? *American Journal of Human Genetics.* (In press.)

Evans, D.G.R., Walsh, S., Jeacock, J., Robinson, C., Hadfield, L., Davies, D.R. and Kingston, R. (1997). Incidence of hereditary non-polyposis colorectal

440   W. Foulkes and S. Hodgson

cancer in a population-based study of 1137 consecutive cases of colorectal cancer. *British Journal of Surgery* **84**: 1281–5.

Foulkes, W.D., Wong, N., Brunet, J-S. et al. (1997). Germ-line *BRCA1* mutation is an adverse prognostic factor in Ashkenazi Jewish women with breast cancer. *Clinical Cancer Research* **3**: 2465–70.

Geller, G., Botkin, J.R., Green, M.J. et al. (1997). Genetic testing for susceptibility to adult-onset cancer. The process and content of informed consent. *JAMA* **277**: 1467–74.

Green, J.S., Joyce, C., Olufemi, S.E. et al. (1997). A common ancestral mutation in four Newfoundland families with the prolactinoma variant of MEN-1 (MEN 1$_{Burin}$). *American Journal of Human Genetics* **61S**: A67–359.

Grönberg, H., Isaacs, S.D., Smith, J.R. et al. (1997). Characteristics of prostate cancer in families potentially linked to the hereditary prostate cancer 1 (HPC1) locus. *Journal of the American Medical Association* **278**: 1251–5.

Hackman, P., Tannergard, P., Oseimensa, S. et al. (1997). A human compound heterozygote for two MLH1 missense mutations. *Nature Genetics* **17**: 135–6.

Hakem, R., de la Pompa, J.L., Sirard, C. et al. (1996). The tumor suppressor gene Brca1 is required for embryonic cellular proliferation in the mouse. *Cell* **85**: 1009–23.

Hakem, R., de la Pompa, J.L., Elia, A., Potter, J. and Mak, T.W. (1997). Partial rescue of Brca1 (5–6) early embryonic lethality by p53 or p21 null mutation. *Nature Genetics* **16**: 298–302.

Harland, M., Melono, R., Gruis, N. et al. (1997). Germline mutations of the CDKN2 gene in UK melanoma families. *Human Molecular Genetics* **6**: 2061–7.

Hatada, I., Ohashi, H., Fukushima, Y. et al. (1996). An imprinted gene p57KIP2 is mutated in Beckwith–Wiedemann syndrome. *Nature Genetics* **14**: 171–3.

Hemminki, A., Markie, D., Tomlinson, I. et al. (1998). A serine/threonine kinase gene defective in Peutz–Jeghers syndrome. *Nature* **391**: 184–7.

Järvinen, H.J., Mecklin, J.P. and Sistonen, P. (1995). Screening reduces colorectal cancer rate in families with hereditary nonpolyposis colorectal cancer. *Gastroenterology* **108**: 1405–11.

Jenne, D.E., Reimann, H., Nezu, J.-I. et al. (1998). Peutz–Jeghers syndrome is caused by mutations in a novel serine threonine kinase. *Nature Genetics* **18**: 38–43.

Jóhannsson, Ó., Ranstam, J., Borg, A. and Olsson, H. (1997a). BRCA1 mutations and survival in women with ovarian cancer. *New England Journal of Medicine* **336**: 1255–6.

Jóhannsson, O.T., Idvall, I., Anderson, C., Borg, A., Barkardottir, R.B., Egilsson, V. and Olsson, H. (1997b). Tumour biological features of BRCA1-induced breast and ovarian cancer. *European Journal of Cancer* **33**: 362–71.

Karp, S.E., Tonin, P.N., Bégin, L.R. et al. (1997). Influence of BRCA1 mutations on nuclear grade and estrogen receptor status of breast carcinoma in Ashkenazi Jewish women. *Cancer* **80**: 435–41.

Kelves, D.J. (1985). *In the Name of Eugenics: Genetics and the Uses of Human Heredity*. Harmondsworth: Penguin.

Kinzler, K.W. and Vogelstein, B. (1997). Cancer-susceptibility genes. Gatekeepers and caretakers. *Nature* **386**: 761.

Laken, S.J., Petersen, G.M., Gruber, S.B. et al. (1997). Familial colorectal cancer in Ashkenazim due to a hypermutable tract in APC. *Nature Genetics* **17**: 79–83.

Lakhani, S.R., Easton, D.F., Stratton, M.R. and the Breast Cancer Linkage Consortium (1997). Pathology of familial breast cancer – differences between breast cancers in carriers of BRCA1 or BRCA2 mutations and sporadic cases. *Lancet* **349**: 1505–10.

Lam, W.W.K., Hatada, I., Ohishi, S. et al. (1997). Germline CDKN1C (p57KIP2) mutations in the human imprinting disorder: Beckwith–Wiedemann syndrome provides a novel genotype–phenotype correlation. *American Journal of Human Genetics* **61S**: A3–3.

Lehrman, S. (1997). Jewish leaders seek genetic guidelines. *Nature* **389**, 322.

Ludwig, T., Chapman, D.L., Papaioannou, V.E. and Efstratiadis, A. (1997). Targeted mutations of breast cancer susceptibility gene homologs in mice: lethal phenotypes of Brca1, Brca2, Brca1/Brca2, Brca1/p53, and Brca2/p53 nullizygous embryos. *Genes and Development* **11**: 1226–41.

Lynch, E.D., Ostermeyer, E.A., Lee, M.K. et al. (1997). Inherited mutations in PTEN that are associated with breast cancer, Cowden disease, and Juvenile Polyposis. *American Journal of Human Genetics* **61**: 1254–60.

Mann, G.J., Holland, E.A., Becker, T.M., Grulet, O.M., Rizos, H. and Kefford, R.F. (1997). Mutation and linkage analysis of CDKN2A and CDK4 in 119 Australian melanoma kindreds. *American Journal of Human Genetics* **61S**: A73–397.

McIndoe, R.A., Stanford, J.L., Gibbs, M. et al. (1997). Linkage analysis of 49 high-risk families does not support a common familial prostate cancer susceptibility gene at 1q24–25. *American Journal of Human Genetics* **61S**: A347–53.

Mckinnon, W.C., Baty, B.J., Bennett, R.L. et al. (1997). Predisposition genetic testing for late-onset disorders in adults – a position paper of the National Society of Genetic Counsellors. *Journal of the American Medical Association* **278**: 1217–20.

Milunksy, J., Huang, X., Baldwin, C., Farah, M.G. and Milunsky, A. (1997). Evidence for genetic heterogeneity of the Carney complex (familial atrial myxoma syndromes). *American Journal of Human Genetics* **61S**: A72–406.

Mijyaki, M., Konishi, M., Tanaka, K. et al. (1997). Germline mutation of *MSH6* as the cause of hereditary nonpolyposis colorectal cancer. *Nature Genetics* **17**: 271–2.

Mizuta, R., Lasalle, J.M., Cheng, H.L. et al. (1997). RAB22 and RAB163/mouse BrCA2 – proteins that specifically interact with the RAD51 protein. *Proceedings of the National Academy of Sciences of the United States of America* **94**: 6927–32.

Muller-Hill, B. (1988). *Murderous Science. Elimination by Scientific Selection of Jews, Gypsies and Others, Germany 1933–1945: Oxford: Oxford University Press.*

Oddoux, C., Struewing, J.P., Clayton, C. M. et al. (1996). The carrier frequency of the BRCA2 6174delT mutation among Ashkenazi Jewish individuals is approximately 1-percent. *Nature Genetics* **14**: 188–90.

O'Keefe, D., Dao, D., Zhao, L. et al. (1997). Coding mutations in P57(KIP2) are present in some cases of Beckwith–Wiedemann syndrome but are rare or absent in Wilms' tumors. *American Journal of Human Genetics* **61**: 295–303.

Olschwang, S., Serova-Sinilnikova, O.M., Lenoir, G.M. and Thomas, G. (1998). *PTEN* germ-like mutations in juvenile polyposis coli. *Nature Genetics* **18**: 12–14.

442   W. Foulkes and S. Hodgson

Oshima, M., Dinchuk, J.E., Kargman, S.L. et al. (1996) Suppression of intestinal polyposis in Apc delta716 knockout mice by inhibition of cyclooxygenase 2 (COX-2). *Cell* **87**: 803–9.

Papadopoulos, N., Nicholaides, N.C., Liu, B. et al. (1995). Mutations of GTBP in genetically unstable cells. *Science* **268**: 1915–17.

Peel, D., Kolodner, R., Li, F. and Anton-Culver, H. (1997). Relationship between replication error (RER) and MSH2/MLH1 gene mutation in population-based HNPCC kindreds. *American Journal of Human Genetics* **61S**: A208–1203.

Platz, A., Hansson, J., Mansson-Brahme, E. et al. (1997). Screening of germline mutations in the CDKN2A and CDKN2B genes in Swedish families with hereditary cutaneous melanoma. *Journal of the National Cancer Institute* **89**: 697–702.

Rahman, N., Arbour, L., Tonin, P., Baruchel, S., Pritchardjones, K., Narod, S.A. and Stratton, M.R. (1997). The familial Wilms' tumour susceptibility gene, FWT1, may not be a tumour suppressor gene. *Oncogene* **14**: 3099–102.

Reik, W. and Maher, E.R. (1997). Imprinting in clusters – lessons from Beckwith–Wiedemann syndrome. *Trends in Genetics* **13**: 330–4.

Reitmair, A.H., Risley, R., Bristow, R.G. et al. (1997). Mutator phenotype in MSH2-deficient murine embryonic fibroblasts. *Cancer Research* **57**: 3765–71.

Richards, B., Zhang, H., Phear, G. and Meuth, M. (1997). Conditional mutator phenotypes in HMSH2-deficient tumor cell lines. *Science* **277**: 1523–6.

Roa, B.B., Boyd, A.A., Volcik, K. and Richards, C.S. (1996). Ashkenazi Jewish population frequencies for common mutations in *BRCA1* and *BRCA2*. *Nature Genetics* **14**: 185–7.

Rosenblatt, D.S., Foulkes, W.D. and Narod, S.A. (1996). Genetic screening for breast cancer. *New England Journal of Medicine* **334**: 1200–1.

Rubin, S.C., Benjamin, I., Behbakht, K. et al. (1996). Clinical and pathological features of ovarian cancer in women with germ-line mutations of BRCA1. *New England Journal of Medicine* **335**: 1413–16.

Schmidt, L., Duh, F.M., Chen, F. et al. (1997). Germline and somatic mutations in the tyrosine kinase domain of the MET proto-oncogene in papillary renal carcinomas. *Nature Genetics* **16**: 68–73.

Scully, R., Chen, J., Plug, A. et al. (1997). Association of BRCA1 with Rad51 in mitotic and meiotic cells. *Cell* **88**: 265–75.

Selby, J.V., Friedman, G.D., Quesenberry, C.P., Jr. and Weiss, N.S. (1992). A case-control study of screening sigmoidoscopy and mortality from colorectal cancer. *New England Journal of Medicine* **326**: 653–7.

Sharan, S.K., Morimatsu, M., Albrecht, U. et al. (1997). Embryonic lethality and radiation hypersensitivity mediated by Rad51 in mice lacking Brca2. *Nature* **386**: 804–10.

Shattuck-Eidens, D., Oliphant, A., McClure, M. et al. (1997). BRCA1 sequence analysis in women at high risk for susceptibility mutations – risk factor analysis and implications for genetic testing. *Journal of the American Medical Association* **278**: 1242–50.

Somasundaram, K., Zhang, H.B., Zeng, Y.X. et al. (1997). Arrest of the cell cycle by the tumour-suppressor BRCA1 requires the CDK-inhibitor P21(WAF1/CIP1). *Nature* **389**: 187–90.

Stankovic, T., Byrd, P.J., Kidd, A.M.J. et al. (1997). ATM mutations and phenotypes in A-T families in the British Isles; expression of mutant ATM and the risk of leukaemia, lymphoma and breast cancer. *American Journal of Human Genetics* **61S**: A83–456.

Late-breaking developments   443

Stoppa-Lyonnet, D., Soulier, J., Lauge, A. Dastot, H., Garand, R., Sigaux, F. and Stern, M.M. (1997). Inactivation of the *ATM* gene in T-cell prolymphocytic leukaemias. *American Journal of Human Genetics* **61S**: A47–247.

Stratton, J.F., Gayther, S.A., Russell, P. et al. (1997). Contribution of BRCA1 mutations to ovarian cancer. *New England Journal of Medicine* **336**: 1125–30.

Struewing, J.P., Abeliovich, D., Peretz, T., Avishai, N., Kaback, M.M., Collins, F.S. and Brody, L.C. (1995). The carrier frequency of the BRCA1 185delAG mutation is approximately 1 percent in Ashkenazi Jewish individuals. *Nature Genetics* **11**: 198–200.

Struewing, J.P., Hartge, P., Wacholder, S. et al. (1997). The risk of cancer associated with specific mutations of BRCA1 and BRCA2 among Ashkenazi Jews. *New England Journal of Medicine* **336**: 1401–8.

Sun, F.L., Dean, W.L., Kelsey, G., Allen, N.D. and Reik, W. (1997). Transactivation of IGF2 in a mouse model of Beckwith–Wiedemann syndrome. *Nature* **389**: 809–15.

Sun, S., Pollock, P., Liu, L. et al. (1997). CDKN2A mutation in a non-FAMMM kindred with cancers at multiple sites results in a functionally abnormal protein. *International Journal of Cancer* **73**: 531–6.

Suzuki, A., de la Pompa, J.L., Hakem, R. et al. (1997). Brca2 is required for embryonic cellular proliferation in the mouse. *Genes and Development* **11**: 1242–52.

Taymans, S., Macrae, C.A., Casey, M. et al. (1997). A refined genetic, radiation hybrid and physical map of the Carney complex (CNC) locus on chromosome 2p16: evidence for genetic heterogeneity in the syndrome. *American Journal of Human Genetics* **61S**: A84–461.

Thibodeau, S.N., Wang, Z., Tester, D.J. et al. (1997). Linkage analysis at the HPC1 locus in hereditary prostate cancer. *American Journal of Human Genetics* **61S**: A297–1733.

Tirkkonen, M., Johannsson, O., Agnarsson, B.A. et al. (1997). Distinct somatic genetic changes associated with tumor progression in carriers of BRCA1 and BRCA2 germ-line mutations. *Cancer Research* **57**: 1222–7.

Ursin, G., Henderson, B.E., Haile, R.W., Pike, M.C., Zhou, N.M., Diep, A. and Bernstein, L. (1997). Does oral contraceptive use increase the risk of breast cancer in women with BRCA1/BRCA2 mutations more than in other women? *Cancer Research* **57**: 3678–81.

Vanslegtenhorst, M., Dehoogt, R., Hermans, C. et al. (1997). Identification of the tuberous sclerosis gene TSC1 on chromosome 9q34. *Science* **277**: 805–8.

Yan, Y., Frisen, J., Lee, M.H., Massague, J. and Barbacid, M. (1997). Ablation of the CDK inhibitor p57Kip2 results in increased apoptosis and delayed differentiation during mouse development. *Genes and Development* **11**: 973–83.

Yang, P., Wentzlaff, K.A., Marks, R. et al. (1997). Higher rate of alpha-1-antitrypsin (α1AT) deficiency carriers found in lung cancer patients. *American Journal of Human Genetics* **61S**: A15–72.

Zhang, P., Liegeois, N.J., Wong, C. et al. (1997). Altered cell differentiation and proliferation in mice lacking p57KIP2 indicates a role in Beckwith–Wiedemann syndrome. *Nature* **387**: 151–8.

Zhuang, Z.P., Merino, M.J., Vortmeyer, A.O. et al. (1997). Identical genetic changes in different histologic components of Wilms' tumors. *Journal of the National Cancer Institute* **89**: 1148–52.

Index

445